FIFTH EDITION

American Diabetes
Association
COMPLETE GUIDE
TO DIABETES

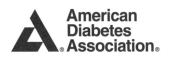

American
Diabetes
Association.

Writer, Kate Ruder; *Director, Book Publishing,* Robert Anthony; *Managing Editor,* Abe Ogden; *Acquisitions Editor,* Victor Van Beuren; *Production Manager,* Melissa Sprott; *Editor,* Greg Guthrie; *Composition,* Naylor Design, Inc.; *Cover Design,* Jody Billert; *Illustrations,* Pam Little, CMI.

Printed in Canada

3 5 7 9 10 8 6 4 2

The suggestions and information contained in this publication are generally consistent with the *Clinical Practice Recommendations* and other policies of the American Diabetes Association, but they do not represent the policy or position of the Association or any of its boards or committees. Reasonable steps have been taken to ensure the accuracy of the information presented. However, the American Diabetes Association cannot ensure the safety or efficacy of any product or service described in this publication. Individuals are advised to consult a physician or other appropriate health care professional before undertaking any diet or exercise program or taking any medication referred to in this publication. Professionals must use and apply their own professional judgment, experience, and training and should not rely solely on the information contained in this publication before prescribing any diet, exercise, or medication. The American Diabetes Association—its officers, directors, employees, volunteers, and members—assumes no responsibility or liability for personal or other injury, loss, or damage that may result from the suggestions or information in this publication.

⊗ The paper in this publication meets the requirements of the ANSI Standard Z39.48-1992 (permanence of paper).

ADA titles may be purchased for business or promotional use or for special sales. To purchase more than 50 copies of this book at a discount, or for custom editions of this book with your logo, contact the American Diabetes Association at the address below, at booksales@diabetes. org, or by calling 703-299-2046.

American Diabetes Association
1701 North Beauregard Street
Alexandria, Virginia 22311

DOI: 10.2337/9781580403306

Library of Congress Cataloging-in-Publication Data

American Diabetes Association complete guide to diabetes / American Diabetes Association. —5th ed.
    p. cm.
  Includes bibliographical references and index.
  ISBN 978-1-58040-330-6 (alk. paper)
 1. Diabetes—Popular works. I. American Diabetes Association. II. Title: Complete guide to diabetes.
  RC660.4.A485 2011
  616.4′62—dc22
                                                                2010041272

Contents

Foreword

I t is with both pride and a great sense of service to the diabetes community that all of us at the American Diabetes Association provide this all-new, fully revised 5th edition of the *Complete Guide to Diabetes*. As recently reported, the diabetes epidemic now reaches both across the country and around the globe. Even more individuals are affected by diabetes and many more can be identified as "at risk" for diabetes—particularly for type 2 diabetes.

The tools available for diabetes care continue to improve, and knowing exactly what tools are available to treat your diabetes is more important than ever. In this 5th edition, we have updated the entire contents and provided even more insight into the use of the many tools available to those affected by diabetes.

This edition emphasizes the important role the diabetes patient plays in his or her own care. In this era of patient-centered care, we trust that this will help you become an ever more important resource for improving your diabetes control. The *Guide* offers insights and advice, reviews all of the new and old tools for management, and gives a personal perspective on how to live well with diabetes. This edition includes updated discussions of:

- The many important components of managing diabetes—including treatment goals, eating healthy, remaining active, and understanding the medications used for treating both type 1 and type 2 diabetes

- Information on new and improved technology for monitoring and controlling diabetes

- Helpful ways to stay on track—and track blood sugar/glucose control, maintaining a healthy weight, and keeping blood pressure and cholesterol under control

- The role of the health care team—and living a happy, healthy life with diabetes

We are grateful for all of the effort the contributors have put into this *Guide* and extend our sincere thanks to the many patients and health professionals who treat, research, and teach about diabetes for their help in making this book possible. The American Diabetes Association is leading the fight to Stop Diabetes and its complications—and we know that you have in your hands an incredibly valuable toolbox that provides you with the information you need to work with your health care team to achieve the best care possible.

David Kendall
Chief Scientific and Medical Officer
American Diabetes Association
January 2011

Introduction

I t's a time of empowerment for people living with diabetes. Patients have never had so many tools and choices at their disposal. Every year, we see new technology for monitoring and treating diabetes. We also see more choices for people to manage diabetes on their own terms—whether it's an application on a mobile phone that tracks readings or a better insulin pump for swimming laps in the pool.

At the same time, scientists and health care providers are finding that tried-and-true methods in diabetes care—such as keeping your blood glucose on target and maintaining a healthy weight—will help you live a long life.

This is all great news for people with diabetes. After all, you are the person most responsible for keeping yourself healthy day to day and into your nineties.

What's New

This newest edition of the *American Diabetes Association Complete Guide to Diabetes* explains the latest advancements in managing and treating diabetes. More importantly, perhaps, the book provides the kind of trusted, in-depth, and essential information that you'd expect from the American Diabetes Association.

Here's what's new: You'll find a new chapter on women's health that describes what to keep on your radar if you're a woman with diabetes. And you'll find a similar chapter for men with diabetes. A more comprehensive discussion of mental health and how it affects people with diabetes is also included.

There are updates on health insurance: how to make it work for you and your diabetes and the impact of health care reform. A few changes to workplace laws and airport security are also tucked inside.

The book provides updates on the latest blood glucose technology, including features to consider when buying a new meter. New to the book also is a section on continuous blood glucose monitors—how they work and who is using them.

How to Read This Book

Of course, how you read this book depends on your goals and time. If you've just been diagnosed with diabetes, you may want to start with chapter 1 to get the most comprehensive picture. However, if you've been living with diabetes for a while, you may want to skip to a topic that interests you, such as medications for type 2 diabetes or carbohydrate counting.

Keep in mind that this book is meant to be a resource for educating yourself as a patient. You should always discuss any changes to your routine or medications with your health care provider. Together, you can come up with the best plan for handling your day-to-day care and emergency situations.

At the beginning of each chapter, you'll find a list of the topics that are covered. Use these lists to quickly determine the content of specific chapters and to prepare yourself for what will be covered.

Definition boxes are strategically placed throughout the text to give you concise descriptions of technical terms so that you won't have to turn to a glossary in the back or look them up in the dictionary. There are more facts and tips on living with diabetes than ever before.

Improved Organization

We've revised and improved the organization of the *ADA Complete Guide to Diabetes*. You'll find shorter chapters that discuss specific topics in diabetes care rather than longer chapters on broad issues. You'll also see the chapters organized into eight distinct parts.

Of course—just like in the last edition—you'll find basic information about diabetes and blood glucose up front. And you'll find the more specific issues of work, school, and travel in the back. Here's a preview.

Part I: Diabetes 101
Chapter 1: Diabetes Facts
Chapter 2: Glucose Facts

Part II: Types of Diabetes
Chapter 3: Type 1 Diabetes
Chapter 4: Type 2 Diabetes
Chapter 5: Gestational Diabetes

Part III: Monitoring Diabetes
Chapter 6: Basics of Blood Glucose Monitoring
Chapter 7: Self-Monitoring Tools
Chapter 8: Blood Glucose Emergencies

Part IV: Managing Your Diabetes
Chapter 9: Setting Blood Glucose Goals
Chapter 10: Healthy Eating
Chapter 11: Physical Activity and Exercise
Chapter 12: Medications for Type 2 Diabetes
Chapter 13: Insulin

Part V: Complications of Diabetes
Chapter 14: Diabetes Complications and Prevention
Chapter 15: Women's Health
Chapter 16: Men's Health

Part VI: Diabetes and Health Care
Chapter 17: Your Health Care Team
Chapter 18: Health Care System

Part VII: Life with Diabetes
Chapter 19: Coping with Diabetes
Chapter 20: Family Life and Children with Diabetes
Chapter 21: Work, School, and Travel

Part VIII: Resources
Sample Forms
Resources
Index

Dive In

Now that you know what's new and how things are laid out, it's time to dive in. Turn to the first chapter, "Diabetes Facts," to find out what diabetes is, who has it, and how it's affecting people worldwide.

Part I
Diabetes 101

CHAPTER 1

CHAPTER 1
Diabetes Facts

When you were first diagnosed with diabetes, your doctor probably sent you home with a lot of information. That's a great place to start. Even if you've been living with diabetes for years, you may still have very basic questions about what diabetes *is*. Or who else has diabetes.

This chapter will work to answer some of your initial questions, helping you brush up on the facts about diabetes. In the following chapters we'll discuss more about how diabetes works and, most importantly, how it affects you.

What Is Diabetes?

In a nutshell, diabetes is a disorder in which the body does not make or correctly use insulin. But what is insulin? Insulin is a hormone. Your body needs insulin to help turn the food you eat into the energy and energy reserves that your body needs to function properly. When your insulin is out of balance, your whole body is out of balance.

Sounds simple enough, right? Well, not everyone with diabetes has the same type of problem using insulin. Some people don't make any insulin at all; other people make too little insulin or don't use that insulin efficiently.

This is why diabetes is broken down into different types, with the most common forms being type 1 and type 2 diabetes. Some women also get diabetes when they become pregnant; this is called gestational diabetes. Most cases of diabetes fall within these three types, which will be explained in more detail in chapters 3, 4, and 5.

There are some other types of diabetes, which can be caused by genetic defects, diseases such as cystic fibrosis, organ transplantation, or AIDS treatment. Still other people don't fit neatly into the categories of type 1 or type 2 diabetes. In fact, there are more than ten different forms of diabetes!

Who Has Diabetes?

Although you may feel like you're the only one dealing with diabetes—you're definitely *not* alone. Millions of Americans and hundreds of millions of people worldwide have diabetes. In the United States, eight out of every 100 people aged 20 years or older have diabetes. That works out to nearly 26 million adults and children with diabetes, according to recent statistics from the Centers for Disease Control and Prevention.

So, it's very likely that you know someone else with diabetes. It could be someone at your school or in your yoga class or in your apartment building. Diabetes affects children and adults, people who are fit or out-of-shape, and people of all races and ethnicities.

However, not everyone with diabetes is wearing a big neon sign screaming: "I have diabetes too!" Each person with diabetes has different symptoms and treatments. The people you know with diabetes are probably managing it in personal and discreet ways.

Famous People with Diabetes

However, some people are quite outspoken about their diabetes—celebrities. There are hundreds of famous people with diabetes, many juggling the demands of entertainment, sports, or politics while keeping on top of a serious disorder.

Famous People with Diabetes

- Halle Berry, actress
- Nicole Johnson, Miss America 1999
- Jay Cutler, NFL quarterback
- Aretha Franklin, singer
- Larry King, talk show host
- Mike Huckabee, former governor of Arkansas
- Nick Jonas, singer
- Gary Hall, Jr., Olympic gold medalist swimmer
- Chris Matthews, news anchor
- Billie Jean King, tennis player
- Anne Rice, author
- Neil Young, singer
- Elizabeth Taylor, actress
- B.B. King, musician
- Bret Michaels, singer

It may sound corny, but this list makes you realize how much you can accomplish with diabetes. It's nice to know that diabetes won't keep you from winning a gold medal in the Olympics like Gary Hall or headlining an '80s glam rock band like Bret Michaels.

Undiagnosed Diabetes

Nearly 26 million people have diabetes in the United States. Yet, there are only 18.8 million diagnosed cases of diabetes. That means that nearly one-quarter of the people with diabetes do not even know they have diabetes. How could all these people go undiagnosed? Unlike many diseases, diabetes doesn't always have obvious symptoms in the beginning.

Over 7 million people have diabetes but don't know it. They are walking around with signs and perhaps mild symptoms of diabetes, but they have not been to a health care provider for the proper tests and diagnosis because few realize that anything is wrong.

Most undiagnosed people have type 2 diabetes. In contrast, few cases of type 1 diabetes go undetected for long. As you'll see in later chapters, the symptoms of type 1 diabetes are so severe that the person goes to a doctor for help.

Diabetes More Common in Elderly People

Older people are still affected most by diabetes. For example, 26.9% of people aged 65 years and older have diabetes, as opposed to 11.3% of people aged 20 years and older.

Rise in Diabetes

You may have heard that more and more people are getting diabetes. Unfortunately, this is absolutely true. The number of people with diabetes in the United States increased by 3 million over two years, according to recent statistics from the Centers for Disease Control and Prevention.

However, children are increasingly getting type 1 and type 2 diabetes. Certain ethnic groups are also seeing an increase in diabetes. Native Americans have the highest rate of diabetes at 16.1%, followed by African Americans at 12.6% and Hispanics at 11.8%. In contrast, 8.4% of Asian Americans and 7.1% of whites have diabetes in the United States.

A Global Epidemic

The rise in diabetes is happening beyond our borders. In 2010, the International Diabetes Federation estimated that 285 million people worldwide have diabetes and more than 430 million people will have diabetes by 2030. Diabetes deaths are likely to double between 2005 and 2030, according to the World Health Organization (WHO). As you may expect, the United States has some of the highest rates of diabetes. But it's still not at the top of the list.

Five Countries with the Highest Rates of Diabetes in 2000

- India
- China
- United States
- Indonesia
- Japan

The WHO and other groups, such as the International Diabetes Federation, are working to raise awareness and help prevent and control diabetes worldwide. For example, the International Diabetes Federation's Life for a Child Program helps supply children with diabetes

with insulin and other equipment throughout the world. The Federation also supplies
grants to fund research on diabetes prevention and treatment.

Early History of Diabetes

As much as diabetes is widespread, it is also
age old. Diabetes is one of the oldest known
diseases in the world. In fact, people wrote down early descriptions of
the disorder before they really understood what it was. References to
diabetes can be found in some of the oldest surviving medical writings
in the world.

World Diabetes Day

The United Nations passed a
Diabetes Resolution in 2006 declaring
November 14th as World Diabetes
Day and encouraging member states
to develop policies to prevent and
treat diabetes.

Early References to Diabetes

- An early Egyptian medical text written around 1550 BCE describes
  a condition of "passing too much urine."

- The Greek physician Aretaeus, who lived in the second century CE,
  gave diabetes its name from a Greek word meaning "siphon" or
  "pass through." Aretaeus observed that his patients' bodies ap-
  peared to "melt down" into urine.

- People observed early on that the urine from people with diabetes
  was very sweet. In fact, one way to diagnose diabetes was to pour
  urine near an anthill. If the ants were attracted to the urine, it meant
  that the urine contained sugar.

- By the 18th century, physicians added the Latin term *mellitus* (honey-
  sweet) to diabetes, which describes its sugary taste.

Up Next

In the next few chapters, you'll find out a lot more about the science of
diabetes. We've come a long way from pouring urine on anthills! One
of the most important scientific discoveries in diabetes was glucose.
Chapter 2 gets down to the basics of glucose and its role in diabetes.

Glucose Facts

It sounds like a technical term, but glucose is just a fancy name for sugar. Your health care provider tested the glucose in your blood when he or she diagnosed you with diabetes. Perhaps it was the first time you heard the term. In any case, you'll probably hear it a lot more.

Glucose is probably the most important term you'll need to understand for managing your diabetes. In this chapter, we'll discuss what it is and how it affects your diabetes. We'll also cover the tests that measure glucose in your blood.

What Is Glucose?

Glucose is a simple sugar in your blood and your body's main source of energy. It is called blood glucose or sometimes blood sugar. It comes primarily from carbohydrates in many of the foods that you eat, including sugary treats like cupcakes, starchy things like vegetables, and grains like breakfast cereal.

How Glucose Works

Glucose: A simple sugar found in the blood that serves as the body's main source of energy.

The purpose of glucose is to provide energy. The key to providing energy is eating food. Yes, food!

When people eat certain foods, their bodies break them down into simple sugars called glucose. Glucose goes into their bloodstream, where it travels to all of the cells in their body. Cells use this glucose for energy to do all the big and small jobs that keep the body humming. To operate at peak performance, your body needs to keep blood glucose levels within a normal range. If you have too little glucose, you run out of energy; too much, and the extra glucose will be stored and cause weight gain. In people with diabetes,

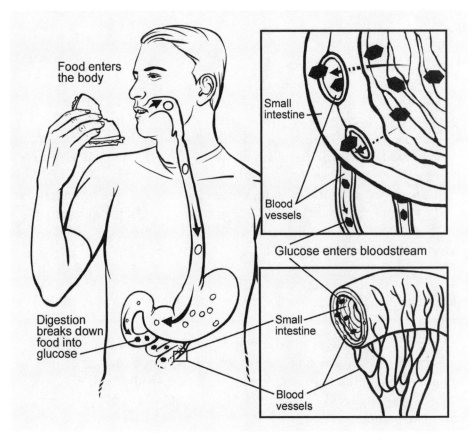

Food enters the body

Small intestine

Blood vessels

Glucose enters bloodstream

Digestion breaks down food into glucose

Small intestine

Blood vessels

excess glucose stays in the blood and may also damage different parts of the body, such as blood vessels and nerves.

The optimal, "normal" range of blood glucose is measured using a plasma glucose test. A normal fasting glucose level is 70–99 milligrams per 1 deciliter of blood, which is abbreviated as 70–99 mg/dl. Fasting means that you haven't eaten for at least eight hours before the test.

But how does the human body regulate glucose levels? This feat requires a delicate balance of hormones and stored glucose.

Pancreas

The pancreas is an organ that does not get much attention—unless it stops doing its job. It is an important player in your digestive system, and it sits right behind your stomach.

The pancreas secretes many hormones, including two very important hormones for regulating glucose: insulin and glucagon. These hormones are made by cells in the pancreas known as the islets of Langerhans. Within the islets of Langerhans, alpha cells produce glucagon and beta cells produce insulin.

Insulin and Glucagon

Insulin and glucagon are two important hormones that help keep your blood glucose on target. Insulin helps move glucose (energy) to your cells and glucagon helps raise blood glucose.

Insulin is the "special key" to make sure glucose effectively gets to cells. Insulin also prevents the liver from making too

Islets of Langerhans

The islets of Langerhans are named for the German physician Paul Langerhans, who first described them in 1869 while still a medical student. He presented a thesis that described these cells as looking different than other cells in the pancreas. However, Langerhans could not determine what these cells did.

Islet Cell: Any of the many types of cells located in the pancreas that make hormones to help the body break down food for energy. Examples include alpha cells that make glucagon and beta cells that make insulin.

Insulin: A hormone that helps the body use glucose for energy. It is produced in the beta cells of the pancreas.

Glucagon: A hormone produced by the alpha cells in the pancreas that raises blood glucose levels. An injectable form of glucagon, available by prescription, may be used to treat severe low blood glucose (hypoglycemia).

much glucose when you are not eating. The pancreas needs to produce the right amount of insulin to move glucose from the bloodstream to cells. It releases insulin in response to rising blood glucose levels during snacks and meals. It also releases a small, steady stream of insulin throughout the day. This keeps your liver from making too much glucose between meals or overnight.

Conversely, the pancreas produces glucagon to raise blood glucose levels between meals or during exercise when your body uses a lot of energy. Glucagon raises blood glucose by stimulating the liver to release stored glucose.

We've only just recently begun to understand the delicate and complicated process of insulin and glucagon secretion. Together, these processes work to maintain a steady level of glucose in the blood all the time. This process is central to understanding how diabetes develops and how to treat it.

People have known about diabetes since antiquity. Unfortunately, for thousands of years, they didn't know how it worked or how to treat it. Beginning in the Enlightenment (17th and 18th centuries), this began to change.

Early Glucose Discoveries

- In 1776, scientists discovered that glucose was in the blood of both people with and people without diabetes. That led them to suspect that people with diabetes pass glucose from blood into urine. But they didn't know how.

- Over one hundred years later, in 1889, two German physiologists, Oskar Minkowski and Joseph von Mering, accidently discovered that the pancreas is involved in diabetes. As part of their experiments on how the body uses fat, they removed the pancreas of a laboratory dog. Much to their astonishment, the dog urinated again and again. Luckily, the scientists tested the dog's urine for glucose. Sure enough, the dog had developed diabetes when its pancreas was removed. This led the scientists to suspect that some substance in the pancreas somehow prevented diabetes.

- It would take another 30 years for scientists to find this magic pancreatic substance—insulin. This discovery, one of the greatest of modern medical history, is discussed in chapter 13.

Too Much Glucose

People with diabetes don't produce enough or don't produce any insulin. Or they don't use insulin effectively. This results in a buildup of too much glucose in their blood.

In all types of diabetes, glucose does not get into the cells that need it and instead builds up in the bloodstream. In addition, cells don't have the energy they need to do their work.

The buildup of glucose in blood can have various effects, depending on its severity. For one thing, the body may try to flush out excess glucose by filtering it through the kidneys and expelling it from the body in urine. Therefore, people with high levels of glucose in their blood may urinate a lot or feel thirsty because of dehydration.

In other cases, the body may try to "grab" energy from muscle and stored fat cells because it can't get energy from glucose in the blood. This can cause muscle deterioration and weight loss.

Symptoms of High Blood Glucose

People with very high blood glucose levels share many similar symptoms. You may have had some of these symptoms before you were diagnosed with diabetes.

Some Early Symptoms of Diabetes

- Extreme thirst
- A frequent need to urinate
- Blurred vision
- A feeling of being tired most of the time for no apparent reason

However, some people do not have any symptoms of high blood glucose. Because the signs of diabetes can be so mild, many people walk around for years with dangerously high glucose levels, which can lead to long-term damage. In fact, many people don't realize they have diabetes until they begin to suffer from complications of the disease.

Of course, only a health care provider can make an accurate diagnosis of diabetes. A trip to the doctor is the next logical step if you or someone you love has symptoms of diabetes or you run a risk of developing diabetes.

Glucose Tests

Although you or your health care provider may suspect that you have diabetes because of your symptoms, the only sure way to tell is with glucose tests.

Diabetes causes your blood glucose levels to be above normal some or all of the time. Your blood glucose levels may be high even though you haven't eaten recently. So, checking the amount of glucose in your blood can determine whether you have diabetes or not. There are four types of tests used to diagnose diabetes: A1C test, fasting plasma glucose test, random plasma glucose test, and two-hour oral glucose tolerance test.

Plasma glucose tests measure the amount of glucose in the plasma of your blood to determine whether the level is higher than normal. Plasma glucose is different from whole-blood glucose, which contains blood cells. In the laboratory, your blood sample is spun in a machine to remove blood cells, platelets, and cell debris. Only the plasma is left. Scientists measure the amount of glucose in the plasma, and these numbers can be 15% higher than whole-blood readings.

A1C Test

- The A1C test can be used to diagnose diabetes.

- Blood is collected from a fingerstick or vein.

- A1C values represent average blood glucose levels over the past 2–3 months.

- The test measures the concentration of hemoglobin molecules that have glucose attached to them. The measure is given as a percentage.

An 8% level means that 8% of your molecules are glycated (sugar coated).

- An A1C of 6.5% or higher is used to diagnose diabetes.

Fasting Plasma Glucose Test

- In diabetes, extra glucose remains in the blood, even after fasting.

- For this test, you will be asked not to eat or drink anything but water for at least 8–10 hours. Then, a sample of your blood is taken and the amount of glucose in the blood is measured.

- For those without diabetes, the amount of glucose after fasting is usually less than 100 mg/dl.

- However, when the amount of fasting plasma glucose is 126 mg/dl or higher, diabetes is suspected. A firm diagnosis of diabetes is made when two fasting plasma glucose tests, done on different days, are at least 126 mg/dl.

Random Plasma Glucose Test

- The simplest way to detect diabetes.

- This test measures the amount of plasma glucose at any given time and is done without fasting.

- You may be diagnosed with diabetes if your plasma glucose is 200 mg/dl or higher and you have obvious symptoms, such as frequent urination, intense thirst, blurred vision, unexplained weight loss, and extreme tiredness.

Oral Glucose Tolerance Test

- This test can also be used to diagnose diabetes.

- For this test, you will be asked not to eat or drink anything overnight. Then, in the morning, a sample of your blood is taken before and two hours after you have a drink that contains glucose.

- If your fasting plasma glucose is 126 mg/dl or higher and/or your post-drink plasma glucose is 200 mg/dl or higher, then you will be diagnosed with diabetes regardless of your symptoms.

Categories of Increased Risk for Diabetes

Sometimes increased risk for diabetes is apparent before diabetes develops. If your fasting plasma glucose test is greater than 100 mg/dl but less than 126 mg/dl, you may have impaired fasting glucose. Some people also have impaired glucose tolerance, a condition in which blood plasma glucose levels are higher than normal (140 mg/dl to 199 mg/dl) 2 hours after the start of an oral glucose tolerance test. If your A1C is 5.7–6.4%, you may be at similar risk.

If you have impaired fasting glucose and/or impaired glucose tolerance, you may be diagnosed with prediabetes. This is not the same as having diabetes, but it sometimes occurs before diabetes develops.

If you have been diagnosed with prediabetes, you will want to have your blood glucose tested routinely and watch for symptoms of diabetes. Also, you need to talk with your health care provider about reducing your risk of heart disease. Keeping your weight in the healthy range and exercising regularly will lower your chances of developing diabetes.

> ### → Prediabetes
>
> Some people with prediabetes never get diabetes, especially if they make lifestyle changes that help improve their health, such as exercising more, making healthier food choices, and losing some unwanted weight. However, some of the same problems that result from having diabetes also occur in people with prediabetes.

Which Type of Diabetes?

If tests reveal that you have diabetes (and you're not pregnant), the next question is whether you have type 1, type 2, or another type of diabetes. Although the symptoms and blood test results can be similar for both type 1 and type 2 diabetes, the causes are very different.

Types of Diabetes

CHAPTER 3

Type 1 Diabetes

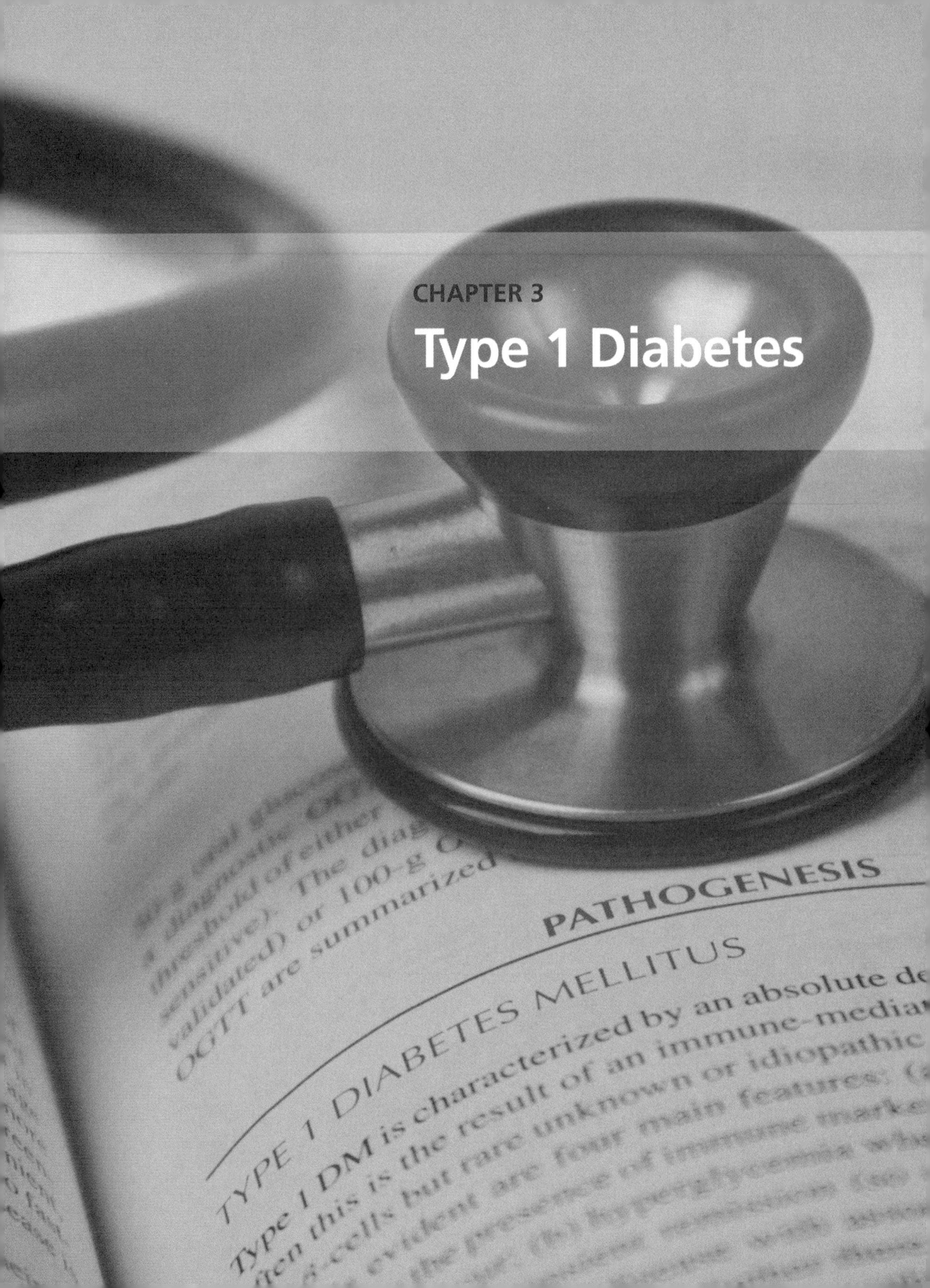

Now, that you've brushed up on some of the basics of diabetes and glucose, you're probably wondering about your specific type of diabetes. In this chapter, you'll find out all about type 1 diabetes.

Type 1 diabetes used to be called juvenile diabetes. Half of all people with type 1 diabetes are diagnosed during childhood or their early teen years.

As you know, being diagnosed with diabetes can be a scary—no matter how old you are when you find out. However, being diagnosed with type 1 diabetes *as a child* can be downright terrifying. For example, it might have come on so fast that you went into a coma before anyone suspected diabetes. After asthma, type 1 diabetes is the second most common chronic disease in children.

Keep in mind, type 1 diabetes can occur at any age. About 5% of adults with diabetes have type 1 diabetes.

Early Symptoms and Tests

People with type 1 diabetes make very little or no insulin, which means that the symptoms of diabetes are often serious and swift. Without insulin, the cells in your body can't do their essential work. Most people with type 1 diabetes will feel quite sick and may even be rushed to the hospital due to high blood glucose.

Common Symptoms of Type 1 Diabetes

- Frequent urination as the body tries to flush out excess glucose in the blood

- Extreme thirst due to dehydration

- Fatigue because the necessary glucose is not getting to your cells

- Blurred vision because of a buildup of fluid in your eyes or elevated glucose levels

- Weight loss, even with increased appetite

- Nausea and vomiting

Tests for Type 1 Diabetes

If your doctor suspects diabetes, he or she will perform a blood test, such as the A1C, fasting plasma glucose test, or the random plasma glucose test. These tests are discussed in more detail in chapter 2. If a fasting plasma glucose test is 126 mg/dl or higher or the random plasma glucose test is 200 mg/dl or higher, you may be diagnosed with diabetes.

Your own description of the way your diabetes symptoms developed will help your health care provider classify your diabetes as type 1.

Your health care provider may also take a urine sample to check for the presence of ketones. Ketones are byproducts produced

A Different Type 1 Diabetes

Some people with type 1 diabetes may have a slow and relentless progression of symptoms. In fact, they may not need to start insulin right away. This condition is called latent autoimmune diabetes of the adult (LADA). As its name suggests, it occurs in adults. Scientists are still trying to clearly define the disorder to improve diagnosis and treatment of people with LADA.

by the body when it breaks down fat for energy. The presence of ketones could be a clue that you have type 1 diabetes. However, keep in mind that ketones are also common in people with type 2 diabetes who are under stress or who have a medical emergency.

In addition, once diabetes has been diagnosed, your health care provider may take a blood sample to test for the presence of autoantibodies in your blood (see more about autoantibodies in the next section). The presence of autoantibodies could mean you have type 1 diabetes. However, some people with type 1 diabetes do not have autoantibodies.

Another measurement, called the "C-peptide" test, measures the amount of insulin produced by the body. It may be ordered if you've just been diagnosed with diabetes and is sometimes ordered in conjunction with a diagnosis of type 1 diabetes.

Causes and Risk Factors

Scientists do not know the exact cause of type 1 diabetes. They suspect that it is a combination of factors due to a person's genetics and environment.

However, scientists *do* know that in people with type 1 diabetes, their immune system mistakenly destroys the insulin-producing cells of their pancreas. The destruction can happen over months and years. The body treats these insulin-producing cells as foreign invaders (not good!). This is called an autoimmune response.

Autoantibodies

In fact, the body creates specific proteins called autoantibodies. When certain autoantibodies are present, they indicate an autoimmune response is helping to kill cells in the pancreas.

Four antibodies are particularly common in people with type 1 diabetes: islet cell autoantibodies, insulin autoantibodies, glutamic acid decarboxylase autoantibodies, and tyrosine phosphatase autoantibodies. Doctors often test for the presence of these autoantibodies to determine whether someone has type 1 diabetes.

Autoantibody: A self-recognizing antibody that targets the cells of the body; indicates a risk that the body's immune system may attack itself.

Celiac Disease

One in 20 people with type 1 diabetes has celiac disease.

Gene: The basic biological unit of heredity composed of a sequence of DNA.

Autoimmune responses can occur in other diseases, such as multiple sclerosis and lupus. In fact, people with other autoimmune disease, such as thyroid disease and celiac disease, are more likely to have type 1 diabetes.

Scientists do not know what causes autoimmune diseases. However, in diabetes, researchers have found a few triggers that may point to why the body starts attacking itself.

Genes and Family History

Scientists have long suspected that family history and genes play a role in type 1 diabetes. For example, if your parent or sibling has diabetes, you are more likely to develop the disease than someone without a family history.

The way in which genes interact to cause diabetes is an extremely complex process that scientists are only just beginning to unravel. Some of the most promising discoveries have been made with a group of genes called HLA that are involved in the body's immune response. Scientists can test a person's DNA for specific mutations in HLA genes that would indicate that that person might get type 1 diabetes.

Race and Ethnicity

In addition to family history, race and ethnicity appear to play a role in who develops type 1 diabetes. White people are much more likely to develop type 1 diabetes than other racial groups. For example, 1 in 100,000 people in Shanghai, China, has type 1 diabetes, but more than 35 in 100,000 people in Finland have type 1 diabetes. Most likely, certain racial groups pass down genes that either trigger or protect against type 1 diabetes.

Viruses

Many scientists suspect that viruses may cause type 1 diabetes. Some people who develop diabetes have often had a recent viral infection. Also, cases of diabetes have frequently occurred after viral epidemics.

Viruses—such as those that cause mumps, German measles, and a virus related to the one that causes polio—may play some role in causing type 1 diabetes. Nonetheless, there is no virus known that specifically triggers type 1 diabetes.

Chemicals and Drugs

Several chemicals, in rare cases, have been shown to trigger diabetes. Pyriminil, a poison used to kill rats, can trigger type 1 diabetes. Two prescription drugs, pentamidine (used to treat pneumonia) and L-asparaginase (an anticancer drug) can also cause type 1 diabetes.

Prevention

There is no way to prevent type 1 diabetes. However, scientists are deeply interested in finding ways to delay or reduce the severity of type 1 diabetes.

People without outward symptoms of type 1 diabetes often produce autoantibodies that can be detected in the blood. The autoantibodies may be present several years before diabetes is diagnosed. Currently, scientists can screen people who may be at high risk because they have a family member with type 1 diabetes or because they carry mutations in certain HLA genes.

For example, if you have a parent or sibling with type 1 diabetes, you are 10% more likely to get diabetes. However, if you also carry certain HLA genes or autoantibodies in your blood, you are even more likely to get type 1 diabetes.

Several studies currently underway are testing whether treating these people early may improve their lives. One study is treating people with insulin in a pill form, and other studies are examining whether certain diets could affect the development of type 1 diabetes. Still other studies are aimed at vaccines to slow the progression of diabetes after diagnosis.

In summary, it is unlikely that either genetics or environment alone causes diabetes. Instead, it is probably a complicated inter-

Early Antibodies

People without symptoms of type 1 diabetes can produce autoantibodies in their blood several years before being diagnosed.

play between the genes you were born with and the world in which you live.

Management and Treatments

How you manage your diabetes depends on your personal goals and needs. No two people with diabetes are exactly alike. Therefore, everyone with diabetes needs an individualized diabetes care plan.

Common Goals for People with Diabetes

• Prevent short-term problems, such as a glucose level that is too low or too high.

• Prevent or delay long-term health problems, such as heart disease and damage to the nerves, kidneys, and eyes.

• Maintain a healthy lifestyle and keep doing enjoyable activities, such as exercising, working, and socializing.

Work with your health care providers to come up with a plan for managing your diabetes and meeting your goals. You'll find more about this topic in chapter 9. For now, though, let's talk about some of the treatments for managing type 1 diabetes.

• People with type 1 diabetes must take insulin. Therefore insulin injections play a big role in your diabetes care plan. How much insulin you need to take depends on your blood glucose level or what you predict the level will be after a meal.

• Naturally, certain food choices also play an important role in your diabetes management plan, because they can add glucose to your blood.

• Usually, exercise can lower your blood glucose level and, in turn, decrease your dose of insulin. So, you'll need to account for exercise and physical activity in your diabetes management.

Insulin

Most people with type 1 diabetes take insulin by injecting it with a needle and syringe or an insulin pen. The goal is to mimic normal insulin release as closely as possible.

People without diabetes have a low level of insulin available in the blood most of the time. This is a background, or basal, level of insulin. After meals, a bolus (extra dose) of insulin is released, just enough to clear the glucose in the blood after eating.

To imitate this sequence, you can develop a regular schedule of insulin injections using different forms of insulin. Read on in chapter 13 for a lot more about insulin and insulin plans. Other people use insulin pumps to dispense insulin at a steady background, or basal, rate and to provide extra insulin to cover meals. More about insulin pumps can be found in chapter 13.

Although today's insulin pumps are worn externally, researchers are developing and testing pumps that are placed inside the body. Ideally, the pump would sense the amount of glucose in the blood and deliver the right amount of insulin, as needed. These pumps are called closed-loop systems.

Your type of insulin therapy should relate directly to your health and your lifestyle choices. Your chosen therapy may aim to keep your blood glucose levels from shooting too high after meals or falling too low between meals. Or your therapy may aim to keep after-meal blood glucose levels as close as possible to those of someone without diabetes.

The food you eat and the exercise you get go hand in hand with your insulin therapy. Of course, healthy eating and regular exercise are a part of everyone's healthy living plan. But for you, knowing how these two daily features move your blood glucose level up and down is essential.

Insulin Pen: A device for injecting insulin; it resembles a fountain pen and holds cartridges of insulin; a dial is often used to set the insulin dose; some pens are disposable and some pens have replaceable cartridges.

Insulin Pump: An insulin-delivering device about the size of a deck of cards that can be worn on a belt, kept in a pocket, or worn on your skin. It carries a reservoir of insulin connected to narrow, flexible plastic tubing (cannula) that is inserted just under the skin. Users set the pump to give a basal amount of insulin continuously throughout the day. Pumps also release bolus insulin to cover meals and at times when blood glucose levels are high, based on programming done by users.

To know how much insulin you'll need to have, it helps to know:

• Your current blood glucose level (you know this by blood glucose testing).

• What you plan to eat (so you can estimate how much your blood glucose will increase).

• What physical activities you plan to do.

There is more information about insulin therapy and different insulin plans in chapter 13, and more about healthy eating in chapter 10. Read about physical activity and exercise for people with type 1 diabetes in chapter 11.

Pancreas Transplants

So far, the only way to treat type 1 diabetes is to give the body another source of insulin. Usually, this is done through insulin injections. However, new experimental approaches also show some promise.

Some patients with type 1 diabetes have experienced positive results from pancreas transplants. Typically, part or all of a new pancreas is surgically implanted. The old pancreas is left alone; it still makes digestive enzymes, even though it doesn't make insulin. Most organs are obtained from someone who has died but decided to be an organ donor.

A transplant of the pancreas is usually reserved for those with serious complications. Pancreas transplants are most often done when a patient also receives a new kidney. The pancreas transplant adds little further risk and offers big benefits. However, transplant surgery is risky. Each person needs to carefully weigh the potential benefits and risks.

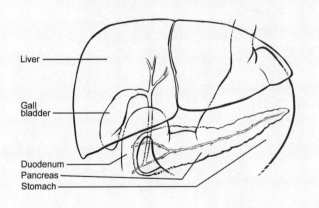

Liver

Gall bladder

Duodenum
Pancreas
Stomach

Benefits of Pancreas Transplants

• You may be able to maintain a normal blood glucose level without taking insulin.

• Many of the diabetes-related side effects are prevented or delayed.

• Most people with nerve damage who receive a pancreas transplant do not get worse and sometimes show improvement.

Downsides to Pancreas Transplants

• The body treats the new pancreas as foreign and the immune system attacks the transplanted pancreas.

• Transplant patients must take powerful immunosuppressant drugs to prevent rejection of the new pancreas. Drugs that suppress the immune system can lower resistance to other diseases, such as cancer, and to bacterial and viral infections.

Islet Transplants

Researchers are testing transplanting only the islet cells of the pancreas. These are the cells in the pancreas that secrete insulin. The islets also sense glucose levels in the blood and dispense the right amount of insulin to the blood.

Islets from a deceased person are taken out, purified, and then transferred to a person with type 1 diabetes. These cells then go on to make insulin.

The procedure has been beneficial for some people—allowing them to take less or sometimes no insulin. However, islet transplantation is still considered experimental.

Organ Donors

One of the biggest problems with both pancreas and islet cell transplantation is the shortage of organ donors. About 7,000 bodies are donated for organ transplants each year in the United States—too few to supply islet cells for everyone with type 1 diabetes.

CHAPTER 4
Type 2 Diabetes

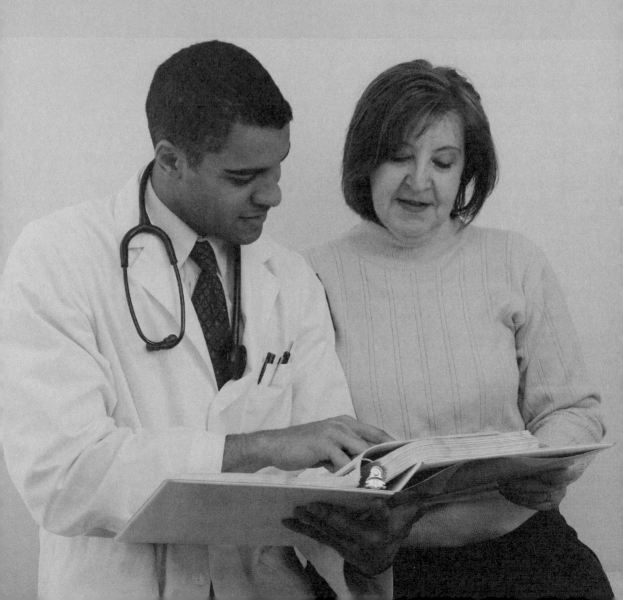

M ost people (about 95%) with diabetes have *type 2* diabetes. Type 2 diabetes tends to develop in people over 40 and used to be called adult-onset diabetes. If you're reading this chapter, you or someone you love has probably been diagnosed with type 2 diabetes.

However, in recent years, more children and teens are developing type 2 diabetes. Much of this has to do with kids becoming obese and inactive.

Early Symptoms and Tests

Usually, type 2 diabetes does not appear suddenly. Instead, you may have no noticeable symptoms or only mild symptoms for years before diabetes is detected, perhaps during a routine exam or blood test.

Common Symptoms of Type 2 Diabetes

- Frequent urination due to the body trying to flush out excess glucose

- Increased thirst due to dehydration

- Fatigue because the necessary glucose is not getting to your cells

- Blurred vision due to a buildup of fluid in your eyes or elevated glucose levels

- More frequent or slower-healing infections

Tests for Type 2 Diabetes

If your doctor suspects diabetes, he or she will perform a blood test, such as the A1C, fasting plasma glucose test, or the random plasma glucose test, as discussed in chapter 2. If your A1C is 6.5% or higher, your fasting plasma glucose test is 126 mg/dl or higher, or your random plasma glucose test is 200 mg/dl or higher, you will be diagnosed with diabetes. Usually, a second test will be done to confirm the diagnosis.

Causes and Risk Factors

Initially, people with type 2 diabetes will usually make insulin for some time, unlike people with type 1 diabetes, who stop making insulin once their diabetes fully develops. However, sometimes people with type 2 diabetes do not respond properly to insulin (this is called insulin resistance), or their body doesn't produce enough insulin, or both. These problems lead to the same outcome: insulin cannot deliver glucose to the cells that need it and glucose builds up in the blood.

Many cells in the body contain special proteins called receptors that bind to insulin. They work like a lock and key. In order for glucose to enter a cell, insulin (the key) must first fit into the insulin receptor (the lock). In addition to working as a key in a lock, insulin performs other important jobs. It inhibits the release of glucose and other substances from the liver and helps make proteins in the body. So, prob-

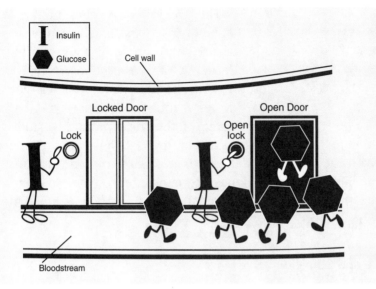

How insulin allows glucose to function in the body.

lems with insulin production or resistance can also make the liver release too much glucose.

Diabetes is a progressive disease. Initially, the pancreas produces
enough insulin to overcome these problems. But over the course of
several years, the pancreas no longer makes enough insulin or releases it too slowly. Without enough insulin to meet the body's needs,
glucose levels rise and diabetes develops.

Scientists do not know why the pancreas stops working in people
with type 2 diabetes. Some believe that the system that tells the pancreas to make more insulin is broken. Others think that the pancreas—after many years of working overtime to overcome insulin resistance—simply burns out.

Genes and Family History

Genes and family history appear to play a strong role in the development of type 2 diabetes—an even stronger role than in type 1 diabetes.
For example, if a person with type 1 diabetes has an identical twin,
there is a 25–50% chance that the twin will develop diabetes. But if a
person with type 2 diabetes has an identical twin, there is a 60–75%
chance that the twin will develop diabetes.

Human Genome: The genetic information of humans, as contained in the DNA of every cell. Each person has his or her own genome.

The way in which genes interact to cause diabetes is an extremely complex process that scientists are only just beginning to understand. There is no known "type 2 diabetes gene." And it is likely that a large number of genes interact to cause type 2 diabetes. Some of the most promising studies have been done since scientists decoded the DNA of the human genome.

With the sequence of the human genome in hand, scientists have been able to link mutations in certain genes to type 2 diabetes. It appears that people pass these mutations down to family members through their DNA.

Race and Ethnicity

More evidence for the role of genes in type 2 diabetes comes from studying certain ethnic groups. African Americans, Asian Americans, Hispanics (except Cuban Americans), and Native Americans all get type 2 diabetes more than whites.

Incidence of Diabetes by Ethnicity

- 7.1% of non-Hispanic whites have diabetes

- 8.4% of Asian Americans have diabetes

- 11.8% of Hispanics have diabetes

- 12.6% of African Americans have diabetes

- 16.1% of Native Americans have diabetes

   According to the "National Diabetes Fact Sheet, 2011," from the Centers for Disease Control and Prevention.

The unusually high rate of diabetes in Native Americans also holds true for their children. Unfortunately, 4.5 out of 1,000 Native American children have diabetes, with rates as high as 50 out of every 1,000 children in the Pima Indian tribe in Arizona.

Obesity

Type 2 diabetes tends to develop in people who have extra body fat. Three-fourths of all people with type 2 diabetes are or have been obese. Body mass index measures your body's amount of fat based on your height and weight. A body mass index of 30 or above is considered obese.

Scientists also think that some people may have genes that put them at a higher risk for obesity—and thus diabetes.

In some way, having too much body fat promotes resistance to insulin. This is why, for so many years, type 2 diabetes has been treated with changes to food and physical activity. Losing weight and increasing muscle while decreasing fat helps your body use insulin better.

Age and Lifestyle

Age is also a risk factor for type 2 diabetes. Half of all new cases of type 2 diabetes occur in people over 55 years of age. People also tend to gain weight as they get older, so perhaps diabetes occurs more often in older people as they put on extra pounds.

Leading an inactive, sedentary lifestyle can also lead to obesity and diabetes. You'll find out more about getting and staying in shape with your diabetes in chapter 11.

Body Shape and Obesity

Your body shape may help determine your risk of developing type 2 diabetes. Extra fat above the hips (central body obesity or having a body shaped like an apple) is riskier than having extra fat in the hips and thighs (having a body shaped like a pear). Central body obesity, as well as overall obesity, is more common in African Americans than whites, which helps explain why diabetes is more common in African Americans.

Sweet Tooth

You can't get diabetes from eating too much sugar. However, eating too much sugar isn't good for anyone. Sweets contain lots of carbohydrates and calories, which can lead to excess pounds. Eating too much of anything (including sweets) can lead to obesity—and diabetes.

Prevention

It may sound like a no-brainer, but the best way to prevent type 2 diabetes is to be fit and to maintain a healthy weight. Okay, that's a lot easier said than done. However, knowing it *can* be done is encouraging!

Studies show that people at high risk for diabetes may be able to prevent diabetes with weight loss, healthy eating, and exercise.

One of the most famous studies that looked at the prevention of type 2 diabetes is called the Diabetes Prevention Program or DPP. Scientists studied whether changing lifestyle habits, such as choosing healthier foods and physical activity, or taking diabetes medication could delay or prevent type 2 diabetes in people at high risk for the disease. The study ended a year early, when scientists discovered some amazing results!

DPP Study Results

- People who lost about 7% of their body weight through eating well and increasing their physical activity (30 minutes a day five times a week) had a 58% lower incidence of diabetes than people who took a placebo (dummy pill).

- People in the study who took the diabetes medication metformin had 31% lower incidence of diabetes than people who took a placebo.

Management and Treatment

With all the talk about the importance of eating well and exercising, you're probably guessing that these two areas play a big role in managing your diabetes. Yes, living a healthy lifestyle is one of the most important things that you can do for yourself and your diabetes. If needed, there are additional options for managing your diabetes, including diabetes pills and insulin. Pancreas or islet transplantation is not usually an option in type 2 diabetes.

Common Goals for Living with Diabetes

- Prevent short-term problems, such as too low or too high glucose.

- Prevent or delay long-term health problems, such as heart disease and damage to nerves, kidneys, and eyes.

- Maintain a healthy lifestyle and keep doing things you enjoy, like exercising, working, and socializing.

How you manage your diabetes depends on your personal goals and needs. There are a number of different options for treating type 2 diabetes. Work with your health care providers to come up with a plan for managing your diabetes and meeting your goals (you'll find more about this topic in chapter 9).

For now, though, let's talk about some of the basics in managing type 2 diabetes.

Tips on Managing Type 2 Diabetes

- Not everyone with type 2 diabetes needs pills or insulin when they are diagnosed.

- Some people who are newly diagnosed can begin with new meal and physical activity plans. For many, eating healthy food portions and exercising regularly keep blood glucose levels near normal.

- Your treatment plan is based on your usual blood glucose levels. Ideally, you will want to keep your blood glucose levels as close to normal as possible.

- For most people, the goal is to keep blood glucose levels between 70 and 130 mg/dl before meals and less than 180 mg/dl after meals. Your doctor may have different goals for you.

Food and Physical Activity

For many, treatment for type 2 diabetes means a balance of healthy eating and exercise. Most people with type 2 diabetes are advised to lose weight and improve their physical fitness, which can decrease weight and resistance to insulin. The severity of type 2 diabetes can be greatly reduced by maintaining a healthy body weight.

Losing a Few Pounds

Even a modest weight loss of 10–15 pounds can have benefits for your health and diabetes.

Benefits of Physical Activity and Healthy Eating

- Physical activity, such as exercise, helps by taking some glucose from the blood and using it for energy during a workout, an effect that lasts well beyond the workout.

- As your physical fitness improves with regular exercise and activity, so does your body's sensitivity to insulin.

- Healthy eating keeps glucose levels lower.

You'll find out more about healthy eating, physical activity, and exercise in chapters 10 and 11.

Medication for Diabetes

In addition to healthy eating and exercise, some people use pills to help manage their diabetes. These pills are called "oral diabetes medications" or "diabetes pills" because you take them by mouth instead of injecting them like insulin. In addition to pills, people with type 2 diabetes now have the option of taking injectable medications to lower their blood glucose.

If needed, you and your health care provider will work together to find the best medication for your goals and lifestyle. Only your health care provider can prescribe these medications. You'll find out more about these medications in chapter 12.

Tips on Medication for Type 2 Diabetes

- Generally, diabetes pills are only prescribed for people with type 2 diabetes.

- At the time of diagnosis, your health care provider may prescribe a diabetes medication, as well as changes to meals and physical activity.

- Not everyone with type 2 diabetes will be helped by diabetes pills. They are more effective in people who have had high blood glucose levels for less than 10 years.

- They are more effective in people who eat healthy and who produce some insulin.

Insulin

Insulin used to be considered the last resort for people with type 2 diabetes. Now, we know that starting insulin early can help keep you healthier longer.

For example, in the beginning (before you were even diagnosed) your body was becoming more and more resistant to insulin as your blood glucose levels remained high. Then, once you were diagnosed, and perhaps treated with diet and exercise or diabetes pills, your body became less resistant to insulin. Your meal plan or exercise, alone, may have been enough to keep your blood glucose levels under control.

However, for many people, the body becomes more resistant to insulin over time. In fact, you are more likely to use insulin the longer you've had diabetes.

Tips for Getting Started

- Find a health care provider who can help you with insulin instructions, injection techniques, and schedules.

- Taking insulin can be intimidating. Find someone you can talk to about getting started. Often people say they wished they'd started taking insulin sooner because it gave them more energy.

You'll find more information about insulin and insulin plans in chapter 13. There are several different ways to begin taking insulin. You'll work with your health care provider to develop an insulin plan that is best for you.

It's Not Failure

It is a big step, but taking insulin does not mean that you have failed to take care of yourself or that your diabetes is worse. It simply means that your body needs more help to keep your blood glucose levels on track.

Insulin Is Common for Type 2 Diabetes

Around 30–40% of people with type 2 diabetes use insulin. If you take insulin, it doesn't mean your diabetes has changed from type 2 to type 1. You don't necessarily have type 1 diabetes just because you need insulin. Instead, you are one of many people with type 2 diabetes who uses insulin because it is a helpful treatment option.

Gestational Diabetes

Pregnancy is a time of possibility and excitement. You try to eat well and rest as much as possible. You may celebrate the baby's anticipated arrival by decorating a nursery or purchasing new baby clothes. You imagine what kind of mother you'll be to your son or daughter. The last thing you've probably been thinking about is getting diabetes. However, finding out you have gestational diabetes raises a lot of important questions. How will it affect you? How will it affect the baby? Will you have diabetes forever?

This chapter will attempt to answer some of these initial questions. Women who manage their diabetes well during pregnancy can have healthy, normal babies. But it takes effort and planning. Work closely with your health care providers to come up with a strategy for managing your diabetes to keep you and the baby healthy during pregnancy.

Gestational diabetes is the technical term for diabetes that develops during pregnancy. It only refers to women who have never had diabetes before and develop high blood glucose during pregnancy. It *does not* refer to women with preexisting type 1 or type 2 diabetes who become pregnant. Roughly 18% of pregnancies are affected by gestational diabetes, which means about 700,000 American women develop gestational diabetes each year.

Early Symptoms and Tests

Gestational diabetes usually appears around the 24th week of pregnancy. This is when the hormones of pregnancy naturally begin to cause changes in how your body uses insulin (see more about hormones below). Women with gestational diabetes usually don't experience any outward symptoms of the disorder. A test is the only way to diagnose gestational diabetes.

Most women, except those at very low risk for gestational diabetes, will be tested between 24 and 28 weeks of pregnancy. Your health care provider will give you an oral glucose tolerance test to diagnose diabetes.

Some women who are at very high risk for gestational diabetes may be tested during their first prenatal visit. This might include women who are severely obese, have a prior history of gestational diabetes, have polycystic ovarian syndrome or glycosuria, have previously delivered a very large infant, or who have a strong family history of type 2 diabetes. In fact, your health care provider may diagnose you with type 2 diabetes, rather than gestational diabetes, at this point.

Causes and Risk Factors

Scientists do not know the exact cause of gestational diabetes. However, they have a few clues about how it happens and who is at risk.

Hormones

You've probably heard a lot about hormones since becoming pregnant. They are a big part of the changes that occur to help your baby grow. Hormones are chemicals that help the body carry out various functions, like building organs and repairing tissues.

During pregnancy, your body produces lots of hormones in an organ called the placenta. The placenta is also the organ that nourishes the growing baby. These extra hormones are important for the baby's growth. However, some of these hormones also block insulin's action in the mother's body, causing resistance to insulin. All pregnant women—with or without gestational diabetes—have some degree of insulin resistance.

To compensate for all this "resistance," pregnant women make up to three times more insulin than normal. In some cases, a woman's body cannot make enough insulin to keep up. Scientists think this occurs in gestational diabetes.

Without enough insulin, your body cannot convert glucose into energy and the excess glucose builds up in the blood. Women with gestational diabetes have elevated blood glucose, much like people with type 2 diabetes.

Genes and Family History

Family history plays a role in gestational diabetes: women with a parent or sibling with diabetes are more likely to have gestational diabetes. Scientists suspect that gestational diabetes is more like type 2 than type 1 diabetes. For this reason, they think that similar genes are involved in both gestational and type 2 diabetes. However, there have been very few studies on the genes specifically involved in gestational diabetes, and there is no genetic test to detect gestational diabetes.

Obesity and Age

Just like type 2 diabetes, obesity and age are risk factors for developing gestational diabetes. Women who are 25 years or older or overweight are more likely to have the disorder. Obesity contributes to insulin resistance and negatively affects the body's ability to use insulin properly. As discussed above, pregnant women already experience some insulin resistance, so any added resistance through excess weight can put you at higher risk for diabetes.

Prevention and Precautions

The best way to prevent gestational diabetes is to eat nutritious foods, be physically active, and maintain a healthy weight. The goal is to get your body in optimum physical shape before you get pregnant. This may include discussions with your doctor about your weight and wellness before you become pregnant.

Race and Ethnicity

Women who are Hispanic, American Indian, Asian, or African American are more likely to have gestational diabetes than non-Hispanic white women.

Risks for Mom and Baby

Most women with gestational diabetes who manage their glucose levels have healthy babies. However, if you do not actively manage your diabetes during pregnancy, there are significant risks to you and the baby.

Babies born to women with gestational diabetes have a higher risk of jaundice and low blood glucose when they are born. In addition, they are at risk for being born larger than normal. This is called macrosomia. During the last half of pregnancy, the baby grows rapidly. A mother's high blood glucose during the latter half of pregnancy can lead to a larger-than-normal baby. In some cases, the baby can become too large to be delivered vaginally.

Because women with gestational diabetes tend to have larger babies, they also tend to have more cesarean deliveries. A cesarean section (where a baby is delivered surgically) can be a safer option than vaginal delivery when the baby is larger than normal. The baby may also need to be delivered earlier than the due date. Cesarean deliveries, though relatively safe and frequent, put women at higher risk for infections, increased bleeding, prolonged recovery, and other issues.

Also, the baby may need to be delivered early if he or she grows too large too fast. An early delivery puts the baby at higher risk for respiratory distress because the lungs may not be fully matured.

Women with gestational diabetes are also at higher risk for preeclampsia, a condition in pregnancy in which blood pressure is too high. Swelling of legs and arms commonly goes along with this condition. Preeclampsia can be dangerous for the mother and baby and can mean bed rest for the mother until delivery.

In addition, gestational diabetes puts women at higher risk for urinary tract infections and ketones in their urine. Ketones are byproducts produced by the body when it breaks down fat for energy. They can be harmful to the mom and baby, and the best way to prevent them is to keep blood glucose levels on target. Your doctor may ask you to monitor your ketones (see more about ketone testing in chapter 7).

Macrosomia: Abnormally large; in diabetes, it refers to abnormally large babies born to women with diabetes.

Management and Treatments

Overall, gestational diabetes is treated much like type 2 diabetes. Most women start with meal planning and regular physical activity to try to lower blood glucose levels. If these strategies do not work, your doctor may prescribe insulin.

Just like in type 2 diabetes, women with gestational diabetes have a buildup of glucose in the blood because they do not produce enough insulin.

Treatment for gestational diabetes is based on the results of your oral glucose tolerance test. In some cases, your doctor may recommend changes in your meal plan or physical activity. In other cases, your doctor may recommend that you start taking insulin right away in addition to changes in your meal plan and physical activity.

Blood glucose goals are narrower for pregnant women than for most people with type 2 diabetes. This is due to the harmful effects that high blood glucose can have on a mother and her growing baby. Work with your health care provider to develop individualized goals for your blood glucose before and after meals.

You will probably need to monitor your blood glucose frequently, perhaps four or more times a day. You can read all about glucose monitoring in chapters 6 and 7.

Food and Exercise

Your meal plan during pregnancy is *not* designed for weight loss. Instead, the goal is to eat the right food at the right time and in the right amount to manage your blood glucose and promote the healthy development of your baby. Food choices play a key role in managing gestational diabetes because of the importance of controlling blood glucose after meals. It's important that you meet with a registered dietitian. You may set a daily calorie goal based on the amount of weight you should gain during the pregnancy. The dietitian may also help you adjust your carbohydrate intake to help manage your blood glucose levels. For many women, this is enough to keep blood glucose levels within the target range.

A registered dietitian is an important part of your health care team. You will work with him or her to design a healthy eating plan as well as to set weight goals.

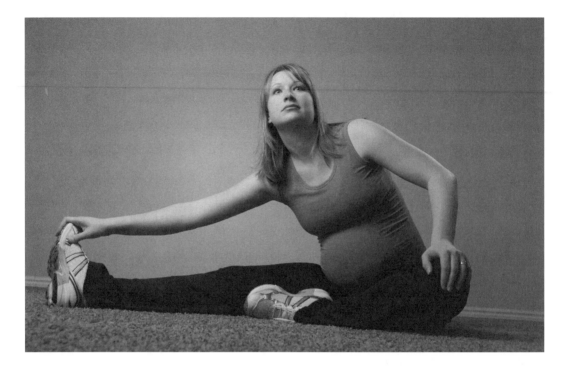

Using moderate exercise to lower blood glucose levels can also help. Most women can swim or walk to keep active. You may also focus on limiting the amount of weight you gain, especially if you were obese before pregnancy. Read more about healthy eating and exercise during pregnancy in chapters 10 and 11, respectively.

Lows in Pregnancy

Luckily, dangerous low blood glucose episodes are relatively rare because insulin resistance is so high late in pregnancy. However, if you seem prone to low blood glucose, remember that the safest time to exercise is after meals, when you are less likely to experience lows.

Insulin

You may need insulin to help you reach your blood glucose goals during pregnancy. It's extremely important to keep glucose levels as close to normal as possible to prevent any complications. Your health care provider will help you decide whether you need to start insulin and, if so, what kind of plan you'll follow.

You'll become more insulin resistant during the third trimester of pregnancy. Therefore, you may need more insulin. This might require a mixture of different types of insulin such as rapid- and intermediate-acting insulin. Look for more information on insulin and insulin plans in chapter 13.

Don't be alarmed if your total insulin dose increases as your pregnancy continues. This does not mean that your diabetes is getting worse, only that your insulin resistance is increasing, which is to be expected. You may need to make changes in your insulin dosage every 10 days or more often.

Future Considerations

After pregnancy, gestational diabetes goes away in most women. Only 5–10% of women have diabetes after giving birth (usually type 2 diabetes). However, your overall risk for developing diabetes in your lifetime goes up dramatically after having gestational diabetes. From 35% to 60% of women with gestational diabetes eventually develop type 2 diabetes.

You should be tested for diabetes 6 weeks after your baby is born. At this visit, you and your health care provider can discuss goals for maintaining a healthy weight and preventing type 2 diabetes. You can prevent diabetes by taking active steps to get in shape and lose weight after pregnancy. You should then be tested for diabetes at least every 3 years thereafter. If you continue to have diabetes after you deliver, you will be referred to a diabetes care provider.

If you had gestational diabetes, your child is also at risk for becoming obese and developing type 2 diabetes. Breast-feeding your baby is one way to protect your child from developing diabetes. Some studies have shown that breast-feeding can reduce the risk of diabetes in children. It will also help you burn extra calories (and perhaps lose weight) and ensure that your baby is getting the proper amount of nutrition.

In the future, remind all of your providers that you had gestational diabetes. Some drugs, such as steroids, can raise your blood glucose levels, just as pregnancy did. Ask to have your glucose levels tested earlier if you become pregnant again.

The message to take home is that both you and your baby have a lifetime risk of developing diabetes. It is important for the whole family to eat well, be active, and maintain healthy weights.

Tips from the National Diabetes Education Program: "It's Never Too Early to Prevent Diabetes"

A Lifetime of Small Steps for a Healthy Family

For You:

- Tell any future health care providers about your gestational diabetes.

- Get tested for diabetes 6–12 weeks after your baby is born, then at least every 3 years.

- Breast-feed your baby. It may lower your child's risk for type 2 diabetes.

- Talk to your doctor if you plan to become pregnant again in the future.

- Try to reach your pre-pregnancy weight 6–12 months after your baby is born. Then, if you still weigh too much, work to lose at least 5–7% (10–14 pounds if you weigh 200 pounds) of your body weight slowly over time and keep it off.

- Choose healthy foods, such as fruits and vegetables, fish, lean meats, dry beans and peas, whole grains, and low-fat or nonfat milk and cheese. Drink water.

- Eat smaller portions of healthy foods to help you reach and stay at a healthy weight.

For the Whole Family:

- Ask your child's doctor for an eating plan to help your child grow properly and stay at a healthy weight. Tell your child's doctor that you had gestational diabetes. Tell your child about his or her risk for diabetes.

- Help your children make healthy food choices and help them be active at least 60 minutes a day.

- Follow a healthy lifestyle together as a family. Help family members stay at a healthy weight by making healthy food choices and moving around more.

- Limit TV, video game, and computer game time to an hour or two a day.

Part III
Monitoring Diabetes

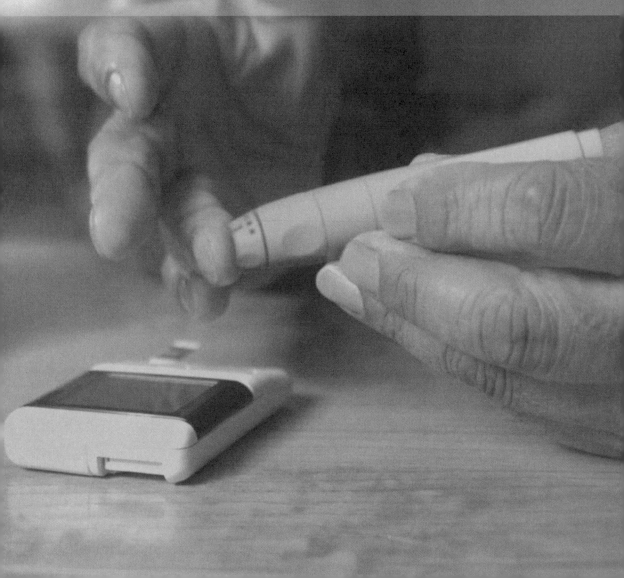

Basics of Blood Glucose Monitoring

Monitoring your blood glucose is an important tool for taking care of yourself and your diabetes. Your health care provider will perform tests to measure your average blood glucose level at most visits, as discussed in more detail in chapter 2. However, the blood glucose monitoring that you do every day—on your own—will form the backbone of your diabetes management plan.

Blood glucose readings help you understand how you respond to different situations: food, exercise, illness, and even stress. Readings also help you make informed choices for treating your blood glucose with insulin or other medications, food choices, and physical activity. Ultimately, these choices help you feel better each day and prevent complications down the road.

This chapter will explain some of the basic guidelines for monitoring blood glucose, such as who should monitor, how often you should monitor, and when to do extra checks. Keep in mind that blood glucose monitoring is up to you. You will be the person most responsible for keeping tabs on your diabetes and making adjustments to fit your lifestyle and health goals.

Who Should Monitor?

The simple answer is . . . you.

People with diabetes who take insulin should always monitor their blood glucose. People with type 2 diabetes who take diabetes pills should check with their health care providers about whether and how often to monitor. Insulin and other diabetes medications are powerful drugs that lower blood glucose. You can tell how well they are doing their job by keeping track of your blood glucose. Also, when you use these medications, you are at risk for low blood glucose (hypoglycemia). Monitoring will tell you if your blood glucose is low, so that you don't have to guess. It can also guide you in deciding how much and which foods to eat at meals.

People with type 2 or gestational diabetes who manage their blood glucose with exercise and meal plans do not need to worry as much about low blood glucose levels. However, monitoring may be helpful. It gives you feedback on how well your diabetes care is working. Positive feedback may be a wonderful source of encouragement for you. You can see the effects of your exercise program or food choices. For pregnant women, it guides the treatment adjustments that will help keep you and your baby healthy.

The best way to lead a healthy life is to take charge of your diabetes. You can do this by managing glucose levels with food, physical

➔ Why Should I Bother?

- If you take insulin or certain diabetes pills and your blood glucose level swings too low over the course of the day, you could develop hypoglycemia. For example, if you take insulin and your blood glucose level drops too low and you don't treat it, you could fall unconscious.

- High blood sugar may not cause an immediate emergency but may lead to severe complications over time. People with a history of chronic high blood glucose can develop debilitating eye disease, kidney disease, circulation problems, or nerve disease. They can also be at risk for dehydration.

activity, and medication. The single most important thing you can do for yourself is to keep track of the amount of glucose in your blood on a regular basis.

Monitoring is the only way to know how your body responds to food, medication, activity, and stress. Without knowing this, you can't make changes in your diabetes care plan. Trial and error—and a little patience—will help you reach your glucose goals.

> → Instead of saying "I feel good" or "I feel terrible," take measurements and keep records. These records will tell you how well your diabetes plan is working.

How Often You Should Monitor

Of course, how often you monitor your blood glucose is highly individual. It depends on: whether you have type 1 or type 2 diabetes, your blood glucose goals, how often you're willing to prick your finger, and what supplies you can afford. How often you monitor also depends on your reasons for checking your blood glucose.

If you have type 1 or type 2 diabetes and you use the results to adjust your next insulin injection or food intake, then you may need to check your blood glucose level each time before you inject or eat a meal (3–4 times a day). You might also monitor after meals to see if you gave the right insulin dose.

If you aim for a blood glucose level close to normal, it's essential to monitor at least four, and sometimes eight, times a day. You would check before and after each meal and before bedtime every day and in the middle of the night (around 3 a.m.) about once a week. Studies in type 1 diabetes have shown a relationship between the number of blood checks a day and blood glucose control. You'll hear more about setting goals for keeping your blood glucose levels as close to normal in chapter 9.

However, you may only be taking one or two insulin shots each day or oral medications, so you may decide to monitor just two times each day. Blood glucose levels in people with type 2 diabetes are often more stable over the course of a day. If you take oral diabetes medications, you may not need to monitor as often because you can't use the results to fine-tune your dose.

People with type 2 diabetes who manage their blood glucose without medications might monitor once or twice a day, three or four times a week, or not at all. However, checking your blood glucose levels regularly will help you keep track of your diabetes and see how all of your efforts are working. One approach is to routinely measure your fasting or pre-breakfast blood glucose levels. It can also help to check your blood glucose at different times of the day: before and after exercise, before and after meals, and at bedtime. This gives you a better idea of what is happening with your blood glucose levels.

Standard Times to Check Blood Glucose

- Before breakfast, lunch, dinner, or an especially big snack
- Before you go to bed
- 1–2 hours after breakfast, lunch, dinner, or an especially big snack
- At 2 or 3 a.m.

Sometimes you may not feel quite right, and you may not know why. Monitoring your blood glucose may help you pinpoint the problem. For example, if you feel sweaty and a little shaky after a three-mile run, you may just be tired from the workout or you could be having a low blood glucose reaction. You simply don't know without monitoring. You may decide to eat because you think your blood glucose is low, but it could actually be high. Only monitoring will give you the information you need to make the right decision about treatment.

Over time, you will gain confidence in your ability to manage your diabetes. You may think it's okay to monitor less often. Beware! It's tempting to think you can tell what your glucose level is by the way you feel, but research shows that most people cannot guess their glucose levels reliably. Guessing is dangerous, especially if your blood glucose level tends to swing with little warning.

→ **Monitoring Goals**

Your goal is to understand the pattern of your blood glucose in response to your daily lifestyle. However, you may also need to capture unusual highs and lows.

When to Do Extra Checks

There are times when you'll need to monitor your blood glucose more often, particularly when you're trying to decipher how new situations affect your blood glucose. In general, changes in medication, food, physical activity, stress, and illness will affect your blood glucose. So, you'll need to perform extra blood glucose checks during these situations. These checks will help you respond to and treat your blood glucose properly. Remember, you should always monitor your blood glucose when you suspect that it is too high or too low.

Extra Checks for Meals

Put most simply, some foods make your blood glucose go up. However, there are quite a few nuances to keep in mind. The amount and type of carbohydrates in certain foods, as well as the amount of food you eat during a meal, will affect your blood glucose level. Sounds complicated, right?

Well, the best way to take charge is to begin to learn how the food you eat affects your blood glucose levels. You'll want to monitor your blood glucose more closely when you eat new foods or eat special meals. You may be surprised at how your glucose level responds to different foods. Measure your blood glucose 1–2 hours after you eat particular foods. Do you find that your blood glucose rises faster after you eat rice or pasta? Does it rise faster after a cookie or a granola bar? By figuring out how your body responds to specific foods, you can have a plan so that your blood glucose will not rise too high, too fast. You can read more about managing your diabetes and food in chapter 10.

Extra Checks for Physical Activity and Exercise

In general, physical activity, including exercise, will lower your glucose and make your body more sensitive to insulin. During exercise, your muscles work harder and use up the glucose they have stored for fuel. Your body uses glucose from the blood when the glucose stored

> ### → High Blood Glucose and Exercise
>
> It sounds strange, but people with type 1 diabetes will also need to check their blood glucose to make sure that it isn't too *high* during exercise. If your blood glucose level is over 250 mg/dl, exercise may cause your blood glucose level to go up rather than down.
>
> Hard exercise with too little insulin can make the liver release stored glucose. Someone with type 1 diabetes whose blood glucose is greater than 250 mg/dl should test for ketones (read about how to test for ketones in chapter 7). Do not exercise if ketones are present. Use caution if your blood glucose is greater than 300 mg/dl, even if no ketones are present.

in muscles becomes low. Exercise can help use up some of the glucose that builds up in the blood.

You need to take special precautions when you exercise. You want to make sure that your blood glucose levels don't drop too low too fast. This can happen in the hours after exercise when your muscles take glucose from the blood to restore their glucose reserves (this is more common in type 1 diabetes). Make sure to check your blood glucose immediately after exercising as well as several hours later.

Doing extra checks before and after physical activity will help you decide if you need to eat a little more or inject a little less insulin. Some people with type 2 diabetes find that they no longer have to take insulin or other diabetes medications once they start a regular exercise program. However, to be safe, talk over your blood glucose readings and exercise program with your health care team before you make changes to your diet, insulin, or other medications. Read more about managing your diabetes and physical activity in chapter 11.

Extra Checks for New Medications or Insulin

If you have type 2 diabetes and take oral medication, finding the best dose can be tricky. You will need to monitor frequently when you are starting a new medication or trying to find the best dose of medication. Check your blood glucose once or twice a day (before breakfast and one other time during the day) to avoid low blood glucose. Occasionally you may want to check 2 hours after meals to see how well the medication works with your meal plan. Your monitoring records will help you and your health care provider decide what changes, if any, are needed.

Starting or changing an insulin plan will also mean more blood glucose monitoring. Read up on the specifics of insulin in chapter 13.

Other Times for Extra Checks

- Before you drive (if you take insulin)

- When you are more physically active than usual

- When you have lost or gained weight

- If you start taking a medication for another condition that affects blood glucose levels or your ability to recognize low blood glucose warning signs

- If you have hypoglycemia at night or wake up with high blood glucose levels

- When your levels have been outside your target range more often than in your range

- If you don't feel well. Checking helps you determine whether your glucose level needs attention

- If you're pregnant

Extra Checks during Stress

Everyone seems a little stressed out these days—and living with diabetes can add even more stress to your life. Stress can produce hormones that raise blood glucose levels. Stress can also be a hidden contributor to unexpected swings in blood glucose levels.

Therefore, you'll want to check your blood glucose more often when you're experiencing stress. The effects of stress on your blood

When you can't figure out why your blood glucose level is so high despite "doing everything right," think about the stresses in your life and how you respond to them. Do you eat when you are under stress? These extra calories, plus stress hormones, could raise your blood glucose.

glucose can't be measured as easily as units of insulin or calories burned during exercise. However, stressful situations could be throwing your blood glucose out of range (for example, if you have a bad day at work), so make sure to check your blood glucose when you feel stressed.

Extra Checks during Illness

Being sick is another kind of stress on your body that can raise blood glucose. Your body releases hormones to fight the illness, but these hormones also counteract the effect of insulin and raise blood glucose. Sickness can cause your diabetes to go out of control. Extremely high blood glucose levels caused by illness can also lead to diabetes emergencies, including coma and death.

Blood glucose monitoring is especially important during any illness. Even if you have type 2 diabetes and only monitor once a day, you may want to check more often during times of illness. In general, you'll want to check your blood glucose every 3–4 hours. Read more about handling sickness under the "Illness" section in chapter 8.

Tips on Using Results of Self-Monitoring

Throughout the book, you'll find more advice about using the results of self-monitoring. Your results will help you develop your diabetes management plan, including your goals for meals, physical activity, and treatment.

Sometimes, you'll need to take immediate action based on a blood glucose reading, while many other times you'll use the information to interpret a pattern and make future adjustments. This is particularly true for people who are not taking multiple, daily injections of insulin.

Self-monitoring is also important for identifying blood glucose emergencies. Chapter 8 will describe some common blood glucose emergencies and how to handle them.

Self-Monitoring Tools

N ow that you've read about the importance of monitoring your blood glucose, you probably want to know exactly how to measure your blood glucose. There are a handful of tools that will help you accurately and easily measure your blood glucose every day. These tools are now smaller and more sophisticated than anyone would have dreamt of 30 years ago.

New products are always being developed, so keep in mind that this chapter just covers the most essential tools. Every year the American Diabetes Association's magazine *Diabetes Forecast* publishes a Consumer Guide for patients that describes the latest devices, as well as most devices currently on the market. The Consumer Guide is published in print and online, and it is a patient's best resource for researching blood glucose monitoring tools (http://forecast.diabetes.org/consumerguide).

Essential Tools

Lancet: A device that pricks the skin with a small needle to obtain a blood sample.

Test Strip: A strip (with a blood sample) that is inserted into a blood glucose meter.

Blood Glucose Meter: A small, portable machine used to display blood glucose readings on a digital display.

Blood Glucose Log: A record of your blood glucose readings over time. Some people prefer a paper log, whereas others prefer a digital log.

→ Lancets are sterile the first time only, so don't share lancets or lancing devices. Lancets can become dull after multiple uses, making future fingersticks more painful, so change them when needed to fit your comfort level.

Not all lancets fit all devices, so do your homework. Make sure that you can easily get replacement lancets to fit your device. Check the prices for replacement lancets as you compare devices.

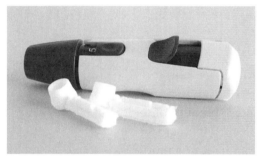

A lancing device with lancets.

Lancets

Lancets allow you to take a sample of blood with minimal discomfort and optimal discretion. The spring-loaded device contains a needle or lancet, a way to select how deep the needle goes, and a release button. You'll want to use the shallowest poke possible to draw blood. This hurts less and causes less scarring on your fingers.

Many blood glucose meters come with lancing devices. However, there are quite a few lancets on the market, so shop around if you don't like the one that came with your meter or if you want more than one. Some allow you to prick sites other than your fingers. Others are designed for people who have trouble drawing blood or who have sensitive or calloused skin. Still others have retractable needles or easy disposal systems. Different lancets produce different sizes of blood drops. Make sure the device you are considering will help you get a drop of blood that is large enough for your meter.

Test Strips

Test strips are disposable strips that take a sample of blood. You insert a test strip into a meter to get a digital reading of your blood glucose level. Test strips are made to work with specific meters, so you'll need to buy the appropriate brand and type.

Here are some things to consider when purchasing a meter and test strips. Some test strips are designed with a curve to help patients guide their fingers more easily to the application site. Other test strips are extra large to make them easier to handle. The packaging of the test strips may also be an important consideration for you. Some come packaged in a vial, whereas others are individually wrapped in foil. The foil wrappings can be more portable, but also more difficult to open. Some meters take a testing "disc" (containing enough room for multiple blood samples) or a drum with preloaded strips.

You'll want to research the price of test strips as you consider which blood glucose meter to purchase (see more on this topic below). Test strips usually come in boxes of 50 or 100, and you can buy them online or in stores. The box of test strips will have an expiration date, and individually packaged strips usually last about 2 years. In the past, the U.S. Food and Drug Administration uncovered schemes to distribute counterfeit test strips. Always buy your strips from a reputable retailer, and check the FDA website (www.fda.gov) for updates on test strips or call the manufacturer if you have any concerns.

Sometimes, in rare cases, people who take certain medications containing sugars that aren't glucose or who are undergoing medical procedures may receive false high readings with certain strips. Be sure to discuss your strips with your health care provider if you are put on a new medication or if there is a change in your health status.

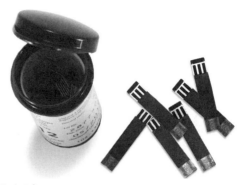

Test strips.

> ### → Generic Test Strips
>
> You can also buy generic brands of test strips that are manufactured to work with specific meters. Make sure that the generic brand lists your meter on the packaging or in the product information.

> ### → Test Strip Storage
>
> Test strips should be stored in their covered container and kept in a dry area. Not keeping your strips safe and dry could affect their accuracy. For example, keeping strips in the bathroom with the container uncovered may result in false blood glucose readings.

Blood Glucose Meters

If your doctor has told you that you need to frequently self-check your blood glucose, then a blood glucose meter is an essential tool for taking

→ Plasma Versus Whole Blood

Meters measure the amount of glucose in *whole blood,* which is the complete composition of the blood flowing through the body. More simply, whole blood is the blood that is directly drawn from the body without further treatment. Several blood-glucose testing methods, however, measure the glucose contained in *blood plasma.* Plasma is a yellow liquid component of whole blood that has to be separated from blood using laboratory methods. The issue is that tests yield different blood glucose results when performed on whole blood versus blood plasma. Plasma test results tend to be 10–15% higher than results from whole blood.

Even though they measure the glucose levels in *whole blood,* today's meters are adjusted to provide results in the plasma glucose equivalent, so blood glucose test results are consistent among all testing measures.

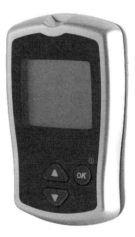

A blood glucose meter.

care of your diabetes. Only by keeping close tabs on your blood glucose levels and recognizing when they are out of range can you take steps to remedy the situation.

The meter measures an electric current in the blood that depends on the amount of glucose present. A sample of blood is placed on a small area of a test strip or disk. A special enzyme transfers electrons from glucose to a chemical in the strip, and the meter measures this flow of electrons as current. The amount of current depends on how much glucose is in the blood. This weak current flows through the strip and is measured in the meter. The meter produces an electronic reading of blood glucose levels in milligrams per deciliter (mg/dl).

There are also several meters that check more than blood glucose. One meter measures blood glucose and ketones (a byproduct that can indicate a serious medication problem). Another meter measures blood glucose, ketones, and lipids (including HDL and LDL cholesterol and triglycerides).

The sheer number of blood glucose meters on the market can be overwhelming. But the good news is that consumers now have more choices than ever in finding a device that fits their budget and lifestyle. Considerations for a blood glucose meter break down into roughly three categories: cost, performance, and your lifestyle. The following section will explore each category in detail.

Considerations for Buying a Blood Glucose Meter

- *Cost:* Insurance coverage, price of test strips

- *Performance:* Accuracy, batteries, and meter replacement

- *Lifestyle:* Meter size, your vision and language, test site, user-friendliness, meter memory, and data management system

Cost Considerations

The cost of your blood glucose meter should be a consideration as you research different brands. Your health insurance may cover the cost of a meter and maybe the test strips. Meters are usually deeply discounted by the manufacturer through rebates and coupons, but you'll want to analyze the long-term costs of any meter and the strips before you purchase it.

Insurance Coverage
Check with your insurance plan or company health program before you invest in a meter. For example, Medicare covers the cost of meters, strips, and lancets. Your insurance may pay for only specific meters or have a cost allowance. Also find out if you are covered for the test strips and how many you are allowed per year. Your insurance may cover more of the cost of meters and strips through a mail-order program. However, you will need to get a prescription to be reimbursed.

Price of Test Strips
In the long run, your meter's test strips will cost you much more than the meter itself. You may be surprised by the cost when you go to buy replacement strips for your meter. The meter that seemed like a bargain at the time of purchase may turn into a major expense when it comes time to pay for strips (especially if you don't get reimbursed for

them by your insurance). Make sure you check the cost of the strips your meter uses before you buy it. Check *Diabetes Forecast's* Consumer Guide and ads for lists of companies that sell discounted strips.

Performance Considerations

The U.S. Food and Drug Administration (FDA) regulates all meters made and distributed in the United States. Manufacturers are required to list devices with the FDA, as well as follow guidelines for marketing, labeling, safety, and efficacy. However, you—as the primary user—will be responsible for checking the performance of your meter over time.

Accuracy
Some machines require that you code each new batch of test strips with your meter in order to maintain accuracy (some do not). Test strips can vary from batch to batch. There may be differences in the amount of chemical on the strips in each batch. So you must standardize (or code) your meter to make up for these small differences when you open a new batch of strips. If you don't code, all your results with the new strips may read higher or lower than they really are. Instructions for coding are included in every new package of strips. Some meters automatically code themselves—you don't have to do anything when you open a new batch of strips or the disk.

You'll also want to check the accuracy of your meter from time to time. You can do this one of three ways: perform an electronic check, use a "control" solution or strip, or compare your meter with a laboratory meter.

Your meter should perform an electronic check every time you turn it on. It will give you an error code if something is wrong. You can check the owner's manual for instructions for correcting errors.

Meters often provide a standard solution, known as a "control" solution. This solution contains a known amount of glucose to help check for accuracy. Other meters use a control strip to check for accuracy. If you measure the amount of glucose in this standard solution or strip in your meter and your meter shows a reading that is too high or too low, your machine may be giving you a faulty reading. The manufacturer's instructions will tell you how often to check with the control solution or strip for the best accuracy.

If you are having a problem with accuracy, first check to see if your problems are being caused by old or damaged test strips. Then call the manufacturer of your meter. There may be something wrong with your meter. You can usually order a vial of standard glucose solution by calling your meter's manufacturer.

In some cases, your health care provider can help you check the accuracy of your meter by using a laboratory meter in his or her office. Your health care provider might ask you to perform a blood glucose test just as you would on your own. Then, he or she might check your blood glucose using the laboratory machine. If the two results match, your meter is probably accurate.

> Write the date on your control solution when you open it and remember that it is usually good for one to three months, depending on the manufacturer.

> Other factors can affect the accuracy of your meter. Altitude, temperature, and humidity can have unpredictable effects on glucose results.

In some cases, *you,* not the meter, may be giving inaccurate results. Researchers have found that practice, at least in the area of blood glucose monitoring, does not make perfect. Fresh from training by a diabetes educator, people start off getting accurate results. But as time goes by, people begin to get sloppy. Accuracy usually decreases over time.

Take your meter with you for checkups, and ask your health care provider to observe your technique from time to time. Or measure your blood glucose level with your own meter when your blood is drawn for laboratory glucose tests. Record your results. The two readings are best compared when you are fasting. When your lab-tested blood results are available, compare the numbers.

Comparing Home and Lab Results

- Make sure that you are comparing plasma blood readings (not whole blood) from your meter to your lab results.

- If your result was off by more than 5–10%, go over your technique with your diabetes educator or provider. If he or she can't find any problems with your technique, it's time to consider whether something may be wrong with your meter.

Monitoring: Problem Areas to Watch

- **Your blood.** Are you getting enough blood on the test strip? To increase blood flow, wash your hands in warm water, hang your hand down, and massage your hand from your palm out to your fingertip before pricking. You may find it less painful to prick the side of your finger rather than the fleshy pad. For some strips, once the drop is on the strip, you can't add more blood. Washing your hands will also help prevent any perfumes or food residue from affecting your test results.

- **Test strips.** Are your strips fresh? Be aware of the expiration date. Avoid exposing the strips to light and moisture. Are you coding your meter to each new batch of test strips? Variations occur from one batch to another, even when made by the same manufacturer.

- **Your meter.** Check your meter regularly with the control solution specified by the meter's manufacturer. Look in the instructions that came with the meter if you've forgotten the technique. If your meter can be cleaned, do it periodically. You may find a buildup of blood, dust, and lint that can affect the readings.

Batteries and Meter Replacement

Meters run on batteries, but each model handles batteries differently. Find out what kind of battery your meter takes before purchasing it. Consider the cost and ease of replacing the batteries.

Some models allow you to buy the battery and insert it into the meter yourself. These batteries might be specific to the meter and therefore could be more expensive and difficult to find. Or these batteries might be standard batteries (such as AA or AAA) that run in devices like flashlights or remote controls and therefore are cheaper and easier to find. Still other meters have no replacement batteries.

> With daily use, batteries generally have to be replaced every 1,000 readings.

Most manufacturers will tell you how long the meter's batteries will last. Some meters tell you when the battery needs replacing. Some companies will replace batteries for you, and others simply replace the whole meter.

Lifestyle Considerations

Your lifestyle is one of the most important considerations for choosing a blood glucose meter. With so many meters on the market today, you are bound to find a meter with at least a few of your preferred features.

Size
Some glucose meters are so small that they fit on a vial of strips, while others are larger, so people with big hands can handle them easily. Small meters are easy to slip into your pocket or purse. However, if you have trouble with small hand and finger movements, you may want to consider a larger meter. Larger meters may be heavier and clumsy to carry around. Some meters have rubber grips that make them easy to hold.

Your Vision and Language
Whether you have severe visual impairment or just have a hard time focusing on small print, you may want to consider this when choosing a meter. Some meters completely talk users through monitoring with both voice set-up commands and readings. The meter may also have buttons with raised imprints. Others have a large screen to make reading the numbers easy. If you have any degree of color-blindness, test a few different models. Make sure that you have no trouble reading the digital display.

Some meters display or speak in different languages, such as Spanish. Others use symbols instead of words to display information.

Test Site
Alternative blood glucose monitoring, such as the upper arm, thigh, calf, and palm, is available with some meters. Make sure to check your meter for the availability of this feature before using alternate sites. Alternate sites will give you more options, but these sites may not be as consistently accurate as your fingertips. For example, readings from alternate sites may vary after eating, after taking insulin, or during low blood glucose periods.

User-Friendliness
Make sure your meter or monitoring system is easy to handle, especially if you have arthritis. Several features can make meters easier to

> ### → Blood Contamination
>
> Contamination can be a serious concern if you have an illness such as hepatitis or HIV infection. So, choose a system that will keep handling of blood samples to a minimum. Don't share lancet devices or meters in which blood can contaminate the device. Always dispose of sharps properly.

use. Some models require a smaller-sized drop of blood. Ask how much blood is required for each model you might be considering. With some models, too little blood may give a faulty reading, and you may need to repeat the test. This can be inconvenient at best, but it could be a problem for people with poor circulation in their hands or those who must check their blood glucose in cold environments.

Other models may require more hands-on time than others. For example, stay away from devices that require too much time if you're always in a hurry. Some meters can measure blood glucose just seconds after a drop of blood lands on the strip. These devices can be very useful when you test often or in work and social situations, where a few seconds here and there really make a difference. If you are always on the move, you may want to consider a meter and insulin pen combination.

Support System

If you are using a meter for the first time, consider one that offers a video that teaches you how to do the reading. A picture or visual image can make a seemingly complicated procedure crystal clear. Also make sure that the company has a 24-hour toll-free number to call for any questions about the meter. Sometimes a quick phone call clears up a simple problem. Also check that your health care team is familiar with the model you purchase and that supplies are easily available in your area or by mail order.

Meter Memory and Data Management System

Your meter can do much more than give you a blood glucose reading. It can also store and manage these readings and sometimes even make recommendations for food or insulin doses based on this information.

Some meters can store up to 3,000 glucose readings. A big memory can be helpful for people who carry their meters around with them during the day. Some models have one-button memory recall to review recent results.

Your meter's data management system is also important to consider. Some models will help you upload the information to a web portal that only you and your health care provider can access. Some models come with software programs that you download to your computer to help you track and visualize your results.

> → Don't buy a high-end blood glucose data management system unless you can afford the extra cost. Many people find that they can get along with a good logbook. This is especially true if you have type 2 diabetes and monitor less often.

These programs can provide trend analysis, averages, graphs, printouts, and more. This can make it easier for you and your health care team to pinpoint any problem areas that might arise. You'll read more about keeping records of your readings in the logbook section below.

Surprisingly, data management systems don't cost too much more than regular meters. Before you buy a system, check to see if your health care team uses or recommends one system over another. Also call the manufacturer's toll-free number, and ask them what you will be getting. They should answer any questions you may have.

How to Use a Blood Glucose Meter

Follow your meter manufacturer's instructions for calibrating, setting date and time, and using control solutions. Check to make sure your strips are not outdated, and store them within the proper temperature limits. Strips can be ruined if they are kept outside the range of acceptable temperatures. If you have problems, there is a toll-free number on the back of the meter that you can call for help. Read the instructions for possible test sites.

Equipment
- Lancet
- Test strip
- Cotton ball or tissue
- Blood glucose meter
- Logbook

Instructions
1. Make sure your hands and skin are clean and dry. Soap or lotion on your skin can cause incorrect test results.

2. Puncture the skin where testing is to be done with the lancing device. If there is a problem with potential hypoglycemia, use your finger for testing.

3. Squeeze or milk out the amount of blood needed by the individual meter. With alternative sites, follow manufacturer's instructions.

4. Follow instructions to see if blood needs to be dropped on the test strip or if the finger or other site should be held so the strip can absorb the blood.

5. Apply firm pressure with a cotton ball or tissue to the lanced site until bleeding stops.

6. Dispose of the lancet and test strip according to local waste disposal laws.

7. Record your test results in your logbook. See more about logbooks in this chapter.

Continuous Glucose Monitors

A continuous glucose monitor (CGM) is a small sensor inserted under the skin that measures the fluid between cells called interstitial fluid. This measure correlates to blood glucose. The monitor communicates wirelessly with a handheld device that displays your interstitial fluid level. The sensor must be changed every few days or so. The system can display real-time glucose levels at 1- and 5-minute intervals, and alarms can be set to alert patients of high or low glucose levels. Rapid rate of change can also be displayed. In addition, these systems come with data management software to help patients see readings in trend charts and graphs.

CGMs are more expensive than traditional meters. However, some insurance is beginning to cover these devices.

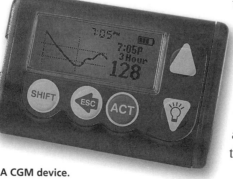
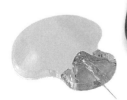

A CGM device.

Although CGMs have not been widely studied, some initial studies have shown that they may beneficial for patients who wear the devices all the time and are highly motivated. For example, continuous glucose monitoring along with tight blood glucose management can lower A1C in adults with type 1 diabetes. Children, teens, and younger adults may benefit, too.

> Currently, the FDA requires users to confirm CGM readings with readings from a traditional blood glucose meter before making treatment decisions because CGM devices are so new.

Logbooks

One of the most important tools in your diabetes toolbox is also the most overlooked. A logbook may not look like much, but it will help you and your health care providers understand your blood glucose levels. It will alert you to any red flags that could signal a serious problem and help you determine whether your treatments are working—and how to fine-tune them.

Your health care provider can provide you with a logbook or your meter may come with one. Call the toll-free number for your meter manufacturer to request more. Some manufacturers have logbooks that you can download to your computer and print.

If you like the idea of keeping a paper logbook, you can photocopy blank pages and compile them in a loose-leaf notebook or create your own custom logbook. You may want a lot of room to write in your logbook. Consider buying a spiral-bound notebook or using a loose-leaf notebook, where you can add pages as needed, to jot down extra notes. You may find it useful to have extra space to record different symptoms and situations that could be relevant to your health. Your logbook is an important tool that can help you spot patterns in your blood glucose control, so be sure that it is easy to use.

Some meters come with an electronic logbook that records your readings and allows you to enter comments about your meals or other situations. Some people may prefer the convenience of using an electronic logbook rather than paper. However, you

> **Logbook:** A book in which readings are kept; for people with diabetes, it can contain blood glucose levels, blood pressure, eating data, and physical activity data.

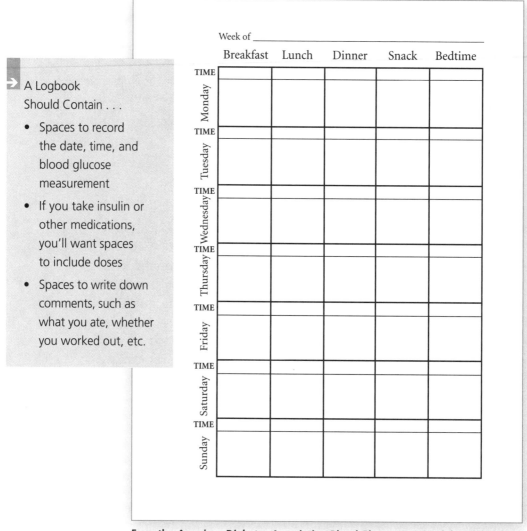

A Logbook Should Contain . . .

- Spaces to record the date, time, and blood glucose measurement

- If you take insulin or other medications, you'll want spaces to include doses

- Spaces to write down comments, such as what you ate, whether you worked out, etc.

From the *American Diabetes Association Blood Glucose Log Book* (available from www.shopdiabetes.org).

should always keep some type of logbook rather then just storing readings in your meter's memory.

Ask your health care provider which readings you should write down in your logbook. You should also bring your logbook with you during doctor's appointments so that you can look over your readings together.

Ketone Tests

People with type 1 diabetes, and occasionally people with type 2 diabetes, can experience a dangerous condition called ketoacidosis. Ketoacidosis is a buildup of ketones in your urine. It can lead to a diabetic coma and death if left untreated. It can happen at any time, but may be more likely during illness, stress, or pregnancy. You can read more about ketoacidosis in chapter 8 about blood glucose emergencies.

Diabetic Ketoacidosis: An emergency condition in which extreme hyperglycemia (high blood glucose), along with a severe lack of insulin, results in accumulation of ketones in the blood and urine. Signs are nausea, vomiting, stomach pain, fruity odor on the breath, and rapid breathing. If left untreated, it can lead to coma and death.

Luckily, you can test the ketones in your urine with a urine test strip to make sure you don't develop ketoacidosis. It's important to detect ketones before they grow to large levels. Checking for urine ketones is especially important for people with type 1 diabetes who do not make any insulin. People with type 2 diabetes usually produce some insulin, so they are less likely to develop ketoacidosis. However, everyone with diabetes needs to know how and when to check for ketones. Read more about when and how to check for ketones in chapter 8.

Urine Ketone Test Strips

You put a test strip in your stream of urine or in a cup to test for ketones. Urine strips vary in how quickly they show a result, so read and follow the directions so you know how long to wait. A change in color will indicate the presence of ketones. Some strips will indicate ketone levels as 0, trace, moderate, or large, whereas others will give a specific reading. Some urine strips also measure glucose and have two test pads on each strip.

Where to Buy Supplies

People with diabetes now have more choices than ever about where to buy their diabetes supplies and devices. You can shop online, in a local

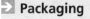

Packaging

Individually foil-wrapped ketone strips are the most expensive up front, but they last longer. They may save you money because you are unlikely to need to test ketones very often. Ketone strips that come in a vial all spoil at the same time, probably 6 months after you open them.

or chain pharmacy, and through the mail. It's up to you to decide which is the most convenient and cost-effective place to shop. Be wary of online marketplaces where people sell and auction personal items. It is not possible to know if testing supplies have been stored properly or have been altered in any way. Only buy from a reputable source.

Pharmacies

Some pharmacies offer a smaller selection of equipment, so check the aisles to see how your pharmacy stacks up. If you have a good relationship with your pharmacist, you may be able to ask him or her to order what you want. Although small pharmacies can be more expensive, establishing a good working relationship with your pharmacist can save you a lot of running around. Pharmacists can often give you information about the ins and outs of different products and models. Local pharmacists will know the products they sell and will be able to spend time training you to use the purchase. This is often a real, convenient advantage.

Diabetes Supply Stores

Another shopping option is to visit a diabetes specialty store. To find one near you, call your local American Diabetes Association office or check in the phonebook under "Diabetes" or "Medical Supplies." If you are lucky enough to have one nearby, you may be able to get many nonprescription items along with diabetes information and support in one easy stop. You may also find a selection of healthy foods, books, and information on local diabetes events and organizations. Many diabetes shops have knowledgeable staff who can help you compare models, answer questions, and provide training on new tools.

Most grocery store and chain pharmacies carry diabetes supplies, which might be convenient if you are shopping for other items.

Mail Order

Purchasing your diabetes supplies, such as test strips, through a mail-order supplier can save you money. However, you'll also have to calculate the extra time it will cost to ship supplies and perhaps the extra time to deal with insurance coverage.

> ### Buying Supplies Online
>
> When purchasing supplies online, make sure to look for an Internet site that is secure and reputable. The FDA recommends purchasing from websites that are located in the United States and provide clear ways to contact the company with questions or concerns.

Making Mail Order Work for You

- Pay extra attention to timing. Some orders will ship automatically, whereas others will take up to 2 weeks. Order your supplies far enough in advance that your current supply won't run out before the new ones arrive.

- The mail-order company should confirm your insurance coverage before filling out your first order. If you use Medicare to help pay for supplies, note that the prices shown in advertisements or quoted over the phone may differ from the amount that Medicare will reimburse for that item.

- If you live in a warm climate or order during the summer, ask how perishable items will be shipped. Strips can spoil in excessive heat, so overnight shipping is best for these items.

- Compare prices by shopping around. Most mail-order firms have toll-free numbers and websites.

- Always keep copies of any orders you send through the mail. If you call in an order, be sure to write down when you placed the order and what you ordered.

- Check the expiration date on each item that arrives. If you'll need the item in 6 months, make sure it doesn't expire in 2 months. Send back all items with expiration dates that are just around the corner.

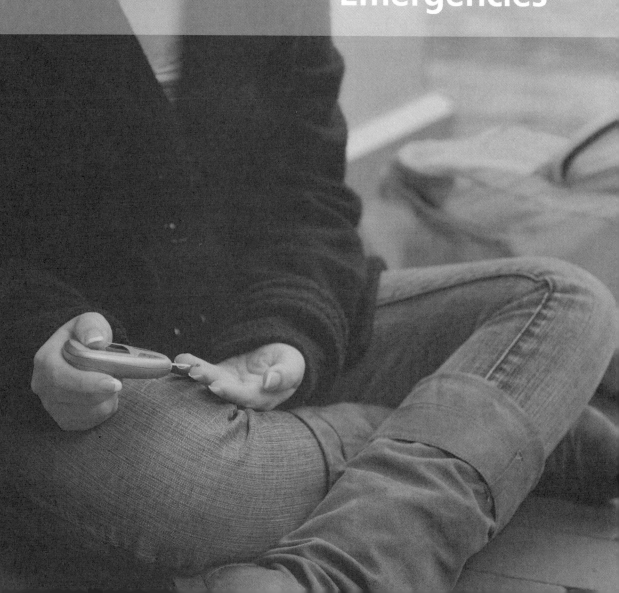

Blood Glucose Emergencies

Dealing with high and low blood glucose levels is a fact of life with diabetes, so you should be aware of possible emergencies that can occur. Emergencies include blood glucose levels that are too high or too low.

It is important that you learn to recognize the warning signs and have a plan for dealing with them. Discuss with your health care team what you should be on the lookout for and what you should do if you suspect an emergency situation may be developing. Also, talk to your family, friends, and coworkers about what to do in an emergency. If you are in danger, you may not always be able to handle the situation yourself.

Hypoglycemia

The most common emergency is low blood sugar, which is called hypoglycemia. It can be a problem for people who take insulin or certain diabetes pills, including chlorpropamide, glipizide, glyburide, glimepiride, repaglinide, and nateglinide.

Being prepared is your best bet, and frequent monitoring of blood glucose will alert you in time to prevent most emergencies.

Hypoglycemia: A condition characterized by abnormally low blood glucose levels, usually less than 70 mg/dl; signs include hunger, nervousness, shakiness, perspiration, dizziness, lightheadedness, sleepiness, and confusion. If left untreated, hypoglycemia may lead to unconsciousness. Sometimes this is called an insulin reaction.

Hypoglycemia occurs when blood glucose levels get too low. At the beginning of a hypoglycemic reaction, you might feel dizzy, sweaty, shaky, or faint. If untreated, you could lose consciousness or have seizures.

Hypoglycemia is usually caused by insulin doing its job too well. In people without diabetes, the body stops releasing insulin before glucose levels fall too low. But if you inject insulin, your body has no way to shut it off. Another interesting, if frustrating, fact about diabetes is that the body uses insulin inconsistently. Even if you always give yourself the same dose of insulin or other diabetes medication, you could end up with more than enough insulin to handle the glucose in your blood. This can happen even when you are doing everything (including eating) the same as usual.

It's impossible to control everything you do to manage your diabetes, no matter how hard you try. Insulin will do its job of clearing glucose from the blood even if it means that blood glucose levels fall too low. Hypoglycemia usually occurs just before meals, during or after strenuous exercise, or when you have too much insulin in your body. Sometimes you may even get hypoglycemia during the night when you are sleeping.

Causes of Hypoglycemia

- Too much insulin
- Too little food
- Too much exercise
- A delayed meal
- Alcohol on an empty stomach

Symptoms of Low Blood Glucose

It's important that you learn your own signs of hypoglycemia. Different people may have different feelings, so it's important to know what signals your body gives during a low glucose reaction. Hypoglycemia can occur at any time. The only sure way to know whether you have hypoglycemia is to check your blood glucose.

Symptoms of Hypoglycemia

- Shakiness
- Nervousness or anxiety
- Sweating
- Irritability or impatience
- Chills and clamminess
- Rapid heartbeat
- Lightheadedness
- Hunger
- Sleepiness
- Anger, stubbornness, or sadness
- Lack of coordination
- Blurred vision
- Nausea
- Tingling or numbness in the lips or tongue
- Nightmares or crying out during sleep
- Headaches
- Strange behavior, including delirium, confusion, or personality change
- Seizures
- Unconsciousness

> Each person's reaction to low blood glucose can cause a different set of symptoms. It is unlikely that you will have them all or that you will have the same ones each time.

Hypoglycemic symptoms can serve as important clues to whether you are having a low glucose reaction, but they are not always the full story. Sometimes the symptoms could be due to something else. Unless you check your blood glucose level, you could overtreat or overreact, causing glucose levels to soar.

Very often, hypoglycemia occurs when blood glucose levels fall below 70 mg/dl. However, many people have glucose readings below this level and feel no symptoms. Others may start to have symptoms of hypoglycemia when their blood glucose is higher than 70 mg/dl. All of this can be very confusing. To start, ask your provider or educator what glucose levels to look out for when you suspect hypoglycemia.

Make note of the symptoms you are experiencing. You will soon learn what level is too low for you.

Hypoglycemia at Night

While it may seem difficult to figure out whether you've had hypoglycemia in your sleep, there are some clues.

- Pajamas or sheets are damp with sweat in the morning

- Restless sleep or nightmares

- A headache or feeling of tiredness when you wake up in the morning

- Ketones in your urine in the morning without a high blood glucose reading

You may want to check your blood glucose around 2 or 3 a.m. a few times to try to match your results with your food intake, physical activity, and medication doses from the previous day and evening. This will help you pinpoint what is really going on.

Hypoglycemia Unawareness

Some people have a hard time knowing when their blood glucose level has fallen to a dangerous level. People who tend to miss these early symptoms are said to have hypoglycemia unawareness. For them, the first symptom of low blood glucose can be impaired thinking.

Hypoglycemia unawareness seems to occur more frequently in people who have had a lot of low blood glucose episodes or who have had diabetes for a long time. In addition to unawareness, a person's body may not respond properly. Someone with hypoglycemia unawareness may not respond immediately to treatment, and the hypoglycemia may last longer.

Hypoglycemia Unawareness:
A state in which a person does not feel or recognize the symptoms of hypoglycemia.

People with hypoglycemia unawareness are less likely to be awakened from sleep when hypoglycemia occurs at night, and they have less strong defenses against hypoglycemia during exercise. It is common in pregnant women and people who intensively manage their diabetes. There is some evidence that frequent episodes of low blood glucose can make someone have hypoglycemia unawareness.

This is a dangerous condition, and if you think you have hypoglycemia unawareness, you should consult with your health care team. Sometimes, just avoiding mild hypoglycemia can help restore a person's awareness of the symptoms of hypoglycemia. Other times, the solution will be to increase blood glucose goals to higher numbers.

Some Safety Nets for Hypoglycemia Unawareness

- Increase the number of times you check every day or check at different times

- Always check before driving. If levels are under 100 mg/dl, eat and test again. If glucose levels are higher than that but falling, eat and test again before driving

- Discuss your hypoglycemic episodes with your health care team so you can look for patterns to use as warning cues

- Educate the people you're with every day about hypoglycemia and how to help you

- Wear an ID bracelet that identifies you as a person with diabetes

- Ask for prescription glucagon, and be sure those around you know how to use it. (Find out more about glucagon later in this chapter.)

- Attend a class on blood glucose awareness training offered at a specialty diabetes clinic

Treatment of Hypoglycemia

Check your blood glucose level if you think you have hypoglycemia. Talk to your health care team about the blood glucose level at which you should begin treating for hypoglycemia. Although it's best to check before treating, this may not always be possible. What if you don't have your monitor with you? Should you wait until you get home? No! Eat or drink something immediately. Never wait until you get home, especially if you have to drive.

After an episode of severe low blood glucose, readings may run high for some hours afterward, as a result of your body fighting back against the low blood glucose. High blood glucose readings immediately following a low reading can lead to a misinterpretation of the pattern. Talk to your health care provider about these patterns, because if you treat for the high readings, you may begin a dangerous cycle of fluctuating blood glucose levels.

Glucose Tablet: A chewable tablet made of pure glucose used to treat hypoglycemia.

You need to eat or drink something that contains carbohydrate that can be rapidly absorbed from your digestive tract and into your blood. However, you shouldn't go overboard. You'll feel worse later on if you send your blood glucose levels soaring. There are many choices of fast-acting carbohydrates.

You're best prepared for low blood glucose if you carry around a measured amount (15 grams) of "pocket carbohydrate." The easiest and most convenient fast-acting carbohydrate is found in glucose tablets or gel, which come in a variety of flavors. Check the annual *Diabetes Forecast* Consumer Guide for a list of current over-the-counter products for treating low blood glucose. Usually, two to five glucose tablets or one package of glucose gel will bring quick relief, but check the instructions and dosing on the package to make sure.

Recheck your blood glucose 15 minutes after you've treated your low blood glucose. If you still have low blood glucose, you may need to take another dose of 10–15 grams. Check again in another hour. If blood glucose is low, you may need another 15 grams of carbohydrate.

Fast-Acting Carbohydrates for Hypoglycemia

Each has about 15 grams:
- 2–5 glucose tablets
- 1 gel tube
- 2 tablespoons raisins
- ½ cup regular soda (not diet)
- 4 ounces orange juice
- 5–7 Lifesavers
- 6 jellybeans
- 10 gumdrops
- 3 teaspoons sugar, honey, or corn syrup
- 6–8 ounces nonfat or 1% milk

Special Considerations for Hypoglycemia

Physical Activity

Exercise and other physical activity lowers blood glucose levels, so you have to be extra careful to avoid hypoglycemia during and sometimes after exercise (if you take insulin). When you first begin an exercise program, you will need to monitor your blood glucose levels after exercise to find out how your body responds. If you feel as though you are becoming hypoglycemic while you are working out, stop at once. Don't say, "I'll just do one more lap" or "Just 5 minutes won't hurt." Stop.

Treating Hypoglycemia during Physical Activity

- Check your blood glucose right away and treat hypoglycemia if you need to.

- If you want to continue your workout, eat a snack, take a 15-minute break, and check to make sure your blood glucose has come back up above 100 mg/dl before starting back. If you start too soon, your blood glucose may drop again, quickly.

- Studies show that hypoglycemia is even more likely to occur 4–10 hours after you exercise than during the activity or shortly after.

Sexual Activity

If you are prone to hypoglycemia when you work out or at night, you may also have a low blood glucose reaction following sexual activity. This can be especially true if you have sex at night. This is when your blood glucose levels typically dip, so you may need to adjust your insulin or have a snack before or after sexual activity. Be especially careful if you are combining sexual activity with alcohol.

Avoiding Lows During and After Sex

- If you use insulin, you need to be watchful for low blood glucose during or after sex.

- Check your blood glucose first. This may slow you down a bit, but it's better than having to deal with low blood glucose at an inopportune moment.

- Eat just before or right after active sex, just as you would if you were exercising.

- Consider having a snack before going to sleep for the night.

- If you use an insulin pump, you may want to set a temporary basal or disconnect it during sex to avoid going low. See more about insulin pumps and plans in chapter 13. The length of time you can safely keep the pump off without an injection depends on how active you are. Ask your health care team for advice about this.

Heart Disease

Hypoglycemia can cause your heart to beat faster than normal. If you have heart disease, talk to your doctor about how hypoglycemia might affect you. You may need to keep your blood glucose levels a little higher to reduce the risk of developing hypoglycemia.

Alcohol

Alcohol lowers blood glucose levels. Normally, when your blood glucose levels begin to drop too low, your liver will convert stored glycogen to glucose. This helps protect you from a severe reaction temporarily and gives you time to recognize and treat hypoglycemia. But alcohol interferes with this process. If you drink alcohol, you may have a severe hypoglycemic reaction with little warning. Read more about alcohol and your meal plan in chapter 10.

Dawn Phenomenon

Your body has a normal mechanism that wakes you up and gives you energy to start the day. Your body responds to this wake-up call of hormones. These hormones depress the activity of insulin, allowing blood glucose to rise between around 4 and 8 a.m. This is called the dawn phenomenon. The dawn phenomenon can be one reason for blood glucose readings and ketone levels that are high when you wake up.

If high morning blood glucose levels seem to occur mysteriously, discuss the problem with your health care team and talk about the best way to treat it.

Severe Hypoglycemia

You could develop severe hypoglycemia if your symptoms of low blood glucose go unnoticed or are ignored. People who are elderly or who take diabetes pills, such as sulfonylureas, are more likely to develop severe hypoglycemia. You may lose consciousness if your brain has been deprived of blood glucose for too long. This is a real emergency. The best way to deal with severe hypoglycemia is to take precautions so that it doesn't happen in the first place. Be alert to your symptoms and treat yourself right away. Don't wait to see if it gets worse or put off treatment until a more convenient time.

You may become so confused and irritable that you refuse help during a hypoglycemic reaction. Those around you may have to be persistent to get you the help you need. They can save you from a coma and a trip to the hospital by insisting that you take some form of glucose quickly. Your life will be easier and safer if those with whom you spend the most time can spot a low glucose reaction and know what to do about it.

Someone else must take over if you become unconscious. You will not be able to eat or drink anything, but your blood glucose levels need to go up immediately. The safest remedy is to get a glucagon injection. Your helper should call for emergency help at once if he or she does not know how to inject glucagon. Glucagon will not work on people with type 2 diabetes or someone who has no glucose stored in the liver, which can occur in cases of starvation, chronic hypoglycemia, or in people who struggle with alcoholism.

If you are prone to hypoglycemia, you'll need to train someone you trust to inject glucagon. Talk to your provider about whether you should buy a glucagon kit, which is available by prescription. Ask your family members or friends to learn how to use glucagon, so they know what to do.

> **Severe Hypoglycemia and Sleep**
>
> If you live alone, you may be concerned about having a severe hypoglycemic reaction while you are sleeping. Your best bet is to monitor your blood glucose levels before you go to sleep and occasionally during the night. If your blood glucose level is dropping, eat a small snack before going to sleep. Try mixing uncooked cornstarch into the snack or eat a product that contains slow-digesting carbohydrates. Many people who take insulin are able to reduce their risk of nighttime lows by switching to an insulin pump.

> **Tell a Friend**
>
> Either you or a member of your health care team should instruct family, friends, or coworkers about the signs of severe hypoglycemia—and what to do if it develops.

How to Inject Glucagon

1. Typically, glucagon kits are brightly colored and include step-by-step instructions.

2. A glucagon kit has a syringe filled with diluting fluid and a bottle of powdered glucagon. You must mix the diluting fluid with the powder immediately before it is injected. The instructions for mixing and injecting glucagon are included in the kit.

3. Inject glucagon into the buttock, arm, or thigh.

4. Turn the person on his or her side so if there is vomiting, he or she will not choke.

5. Feed the person with appropriate carbohydrate immediately when he or she wakes up and is able to swallow. Start with nondiet soda, juice, glucose tablets or gels, and then additional carbohydrate.

6. Check blood glucose. If the person does not wake up within 15 minutes, call for an ambulance. The dose may be repeated after 20 minutes.

7. Always call your provider and emergency personnel when a severe reaction occurs in order for help to arrive and appropriate care to be administered. Ask for instructions on emergency procedures when you get the prescription. Read the instructions that come with the glucagon and share them with friends, family, and coworkers.

8. Kits usually last a year before expiring (check the date on the box). However, premixing the glucagon and diluting solution will make the mixture last only 48 hours in the refrigerator.

Glucagon: A hormone produced by the alpha cells in the pancreas that raises blood glucose levels. An injectable form of glucagon, available by prescription, may be used to treat severe hypoglycemia.

Always let your health care providers know if you have taken glucagon and had a severe hypoglycemia episode. Also, tell them if you are having frequent bouts of even mild hypoglycemia. By working together, you might find a pattern in your insulin, meals, or activity routine that may be causing the hypoglycemia. With clues, you and your health care team can do some problem solving and decide on changes to prevent severe hypoglycemia.

Pregnancy and Severe Hypoglycemia
Many pregnant women, who have intensive blood glucose goals, may experience hypoglycemia unawareness. Thus, they are more likely to have mild and moderate bouts of hypoglycemia. Pregnant women should keep up a consistent blood glucose monitoring routine and check their blood glucose when hypoglycemia is most likely (between meals and in the middle of the night). You need to treat any blood glucose level below 70 mg/dl. You'll have to take special precautions if you are pregnant and become unconscious.

Treating Severe Hypoglycemia during Pregnancy

- You may need only half the normal dose of glucagon at the beginning of a severe episode of hypoglycemia.

- After 15 minutes, if you do not regain consciousness or your blood glucose levels do not rise, you need another shot and someone should call 911 for emergency help.

- Make sure that those with whom you spend time know that you are pregnant and know what to do if you have a low blood glucose episode.

- Ask your health care provider about the dose of glucagon you need.

Hyperglycemia

High levels of glucose in your blood over time may lead to long-term complications. But blood glucose levels can also become dangerously high in the short term and cause a life-threatening situation that could result in coma or death. It is important to know the warning signs and treatments for hyperglycemia, which are different for people with type 1 and type 2 diabetes.

Type 1 Diabetes and Diabetic Ketoacidosis

Too little insulin in your body leads to too much glucose in your blood. A rare and serious—but often preventable—emergency can arise when blood glucose levels rise. Diabetic ketoacidosis, also called DKA, occurs when you don't have enough insulin. It is mostly a problem for people with type 1 diabetes. A person with diabetes may have such low levels of insulin that his or her liver may produce unchecked levels of glucose and ketones, especially during illness or stress. It can occur in people with type 1 diabetes who have not yet been diagnosed.

Diabetic ketoacidosis can start innocently enough; you miss a dose of insulin, the insulin you've been using has gone bad, or your insulin pump tubing gets blocked. The lack of insulin leads to an undetected high blood glucose level, which can progress to a coma, shock, pneumonia, difficulty breathing, and even death.

Diabetic ketoacidosis can occur during periods of stress or illness, when the body releases hormones that promote the release of stored glucose and block the effects of insulin. Sometimes when you are sick and can't eat, you may think, "I shouldn't take insulin today." But your body still needs insulin to cover its 24-hour insulin needs, even if you aren't eating. Plus, you are likely producing extra glucose. So, in addition to your usual dose of insulin, you may actually need extra insulin. Drinking plenty of fluids will also help. Talk with your health care providers ahead of time about a plan of action for dealing with ketoacidosis and how to prevent it when you are stressed or ill.

Signs of DKA

- High blood glucose above 240 mg/dl and not falling
- Classic signs of hyperglycemia: intense thirst, dry mouth, need to urinate frequently
- Lack of appetite or pains in your stomach
- Vomiting or nausea
- Blurry vision
- Fever or warm, dry, or flushed skin
- Difficulty breathing
- Feeling of weakness
- Sleepiness
- A fruity odor on your breath

Testing for Diabetic Ketoacidosis
You can use a test strip to measure the amount of ketones in your urine. Urine test strips are available over the counter, and you can find out more about using them in chapter 7. Some blood glucose meters also check for ketones.

You'll want to test your urine for ketones whenever your blood glucose is over 240 mg/dl or you feel ill. If your urine shows trace or small amounts of ketones, it's a sign that you need more insulin or carbohydrate.

When to Test for Ketones

- If your blood glucose is over 240 mg/dl and not falling

- When you are ill, especially if you have a high fever, bouts of vomiting, or diarrhea

- When you have severe fatigue, fruity breath, breathing difficulties, or a hard time concentrating

- During pregnancy, if your blood glucose is over 200 mg/dl or as your health care provider recommends

How to Check for Ketones in Urine

Equipment

- Ketone test strip

- Cup or a clean container to contain the urine, if desired

- Watch or other timing device

Instructions

1. Dip a ketone test strip in a urine sample or pass it through the stream of urine.
2. Time test according to the directions on the package.
3. The strip will change colors if ketones are present. Compare test strip to package color chart.
4. Record the results.
5. Contact your provider as recommended based on your results.

If Your Urine Shows Moderate or Large Amounts of Ketones

- Call your health care team immediately or use the plan that you and your health care team have already put in place.

- You probably need to take extra rapid- or short-acting insulin right away.

- Drink plenty of sugar-free fluids to prevent dehydration.

- Seek emergency help at once if your ketones do not promptly go down or if you are vomiting and can't stop.

- Make sure those who spend time with you know what to look for and what to do if you have signs of diabetic ketoacidosis.

Illness calls for more frequent blood glucose monitoring and urine testing for ketones. Do both at least every 4 hours until you're feeling better. Check your urine for ketones any time you feel queasy or are vomiting (even if your blood glucose isn't high). A buildup of ketones can cause nausea.

Pregnant women should also test for ketones frequently. Daily urine ketone testing can help detect elevated levels and prevent diabetic ketoacidosis, which can be very dangerous for the developing baby.

Blood Ketone Testing

Your doctor may prefer that you check for ketones in your blood rather than in your urine. Testing ketone levels in the blood actually yields more accurate results than checking ketones in urine. Usually, blood ketone levels are checked by drawing blood and testing the sample in a lab—obviously, this is something done at a clinic or hospital. However, some newer blood glucose meters can check blood ketone levels in addition to blood glucose levels, making this test easy to perform at home.

Type 2 Diabetes and Hyperosmolar Hyperglycemic Syndrome

People with type 2 diabetes have less dramatic swings in blood glucose levels compared with people with type 1 diabetes, in general. However, people with type 2 diabetes can sustain high blood glucose levels over prolonged periods without even knowing it. This can wear on the body and may cause diabetes complications. You can guard against chronic hyperglycemia by monitoring your blood glucose levels regularly.

Acute hyperglycemia can occur in people with type 2 diabetes and is life threatening. Hyperglycemia in people with type 2 diabetes does not usually produce ketones. But blood glucose levels can soar to over 600 mg/dl and even as high as 1,000 mg/dl. This sometimes happens before diabetes is diagnosed. Extreme hyperglycemia can cause a coma.

Hyperosmolar hyperglycemic syndrome (HHS) occurs almost exclusively in people with type 2 diabetes. It can happen to people who manage their diabetes with food and exercise only and those who take diabetes medications.

> **Hyperosmolar Hyperglycemic Syndrome:** An emergency condition in which one's blood glucose level is every high, but ketones are not present in the blood or urine. If left untreated, it can lead to coma or death.

One-third of all cases of HHS are caused by undiagnosed diabetes. HHS results from stress, infections, heart attacks, strokes, corticosteroid medications, and even diuretics. Sometimes something as simple as not being able to get a drink of water can contribute to developing HHS. It occurs more often in people who have restricted mobility, such as the elderly, or in people who cannot take good care of their bodies. Also, as you age, your sense of thirst diminishes, and it's harder to sense the need to drink enough fluids.

HHS occurs because rising blood glucose levels cause you to urinate more and become dehydrated. This process may go on for days and weeks. Extreme dehydration eventually leads to confusion and inability to get a drink or make it to the toilet. The blood gets thicker with more glucose and less fluid. Eventually, the severe dehydration leads to seizures, coma, and death.

Signs of HHS

- Dry, parched mouth

- Extreme thirst, although this may gradually disappear

- Sleepiness or confusion

- Warm, dry skin with no sweating

- High blood glucose. If it's over 300 mg/dl on two readings, call your health care team; if it's over 500 mg/dl and not falling, have someone take you to the hospital immediately.

If you experience any of the above signs of HHS, check your blood glucose levels at once and call your provider. Be sure those around you know what to do because you may not be able to react.

You'll be alerted to high blood glucose levels well before HHS sets in if you check your blood glucose even once a day. To be sure, test your blood glucose levels three or four times a day when you are sick. It's also very important to drink plenty of alcohol-free, sugar-free fluids. You may need to take insulin, even if you don't ordinarily use it.

Special Precautions for HHS

- Ask your doctor or pharmacist if certain medications may increase your risk for HHS, such as glucocorticoids (steroids), diuretics, phenytoin (Dilantin), cimetidine (Tagamet), and beta-blockers (especially Inderal).

- HHS can occur in people having peritoneal dialysis or intravenous feedings, so you'll need to check blood glucose frequently.

- About one-third of cases of HHS occur in people living in nursing homes. This can happen when residents are confused or have to wait for staff to offer them something to drink, leading to dehydration. Family members may have to educate staff of the patient's needs and ask for regular blood glucose monitoring.

Illness

When you're sick, your body releases hormones to fight the illness. These hormones also counteract insulin and raise your blood glucose levels. Extremely high blood glucose can lead to diabetic ketoacidosis and HHS.

So, when you're sick, you'll want to check your blood glucose more frequently than ever. Also, be sure to talk to your health care team before you get ill about what you should do in the event of illness. You and your health care team can work together to come up with a plan to help you handle common illnesses, such as colds or the flu.

Sick-Day Action Plan

You and your doctor may want to answer these questions when developing a plan for your next illness.

- How often should I monitor my blood glucose?

- When should I call the doctor?

- Should I test for ketones?

- What medication changes should I anticipate? How should I manage doses of my insulin or other medication?

- Which over-the-counter medications are safe to take?

- How should I choose appropriate foods and fluids while I'm sick?

Tips during Illness

- **Monitor.** Check your blood glucose and ketone levels about every 3–4 hours. If the levels are too high or you are pregnant, you may need to monitor more often.

- **Food.** Make substitutions for your usual food if nausea and vomiting make it difficult to eat. Try to eat or drink your usual amount of carbohydrates. Talk to your dietitian about ways to cover your basic eating plan. Prepare a sick-day plan before you even become sick. Try to keep some comforting foods, like soup, on hand, especially during the cold and flu season.

- **Liquids.** Drink plenty of caffeine-free liquids. You may need regular soft drinks or sports drinks with sugar or carbohydrate if you are losing fluids by vomiting, fever, or diarrhea. These drinks may help prevent the hypoglycemia caused by not eating or taking extra insulin. Try sipping 3–6 ounces an hour to keep your blood glucose even.

- **On Hand.** Keep a thermometer on hand and a small supply of common sick-day medications that are safe to take. Be sure to read the labels. Be sure to consult with your health care team to find out which medications are safe to use.

- **Insulin.** If you have type 1 diabetes, continue to take your insulin—even if you can't eat. You may even need extra insulin to take care of the excess glucose your body releases when you are sick. Ask your provider about what blood glucose levels call for a change in your insulin dose.

Cold Medicines

Some cold medicines sold over-the-counter to treat colds and flu can affect your blood glucose level. Many cough and cold remedies labeled "decongestant" contain ingredients, such as pseudoephedrine, that raise blood glucose levels and blood pressure. Talk to the pharmacist or your provider before you take any over-the-counter medication.

In addition, some cough and cold remedies contain sugar and alcohol. Make sure you read the label and find out exactly what "active ingredients" as well as "inactive ingredients" any medication contains. A small amount of sugar or alcohol is probably fine, as long as you're aware of it.

Pain medications are usually safe in small doses. You don't have to worry about taking an occasional aspirin for a headache or fever. Many people with diabetes take a daily, coated "baby" aspirin to protect against cardiovascular disease. This is safe for people with diabetes, if it is recommend by their health care team. Check with your doctor to see if you can safely take ibuprofen.

Call the Doctor

You'll want to call your health care provider if you experience any of the following:

- You have been sick for 1 or 2 days without improvement.

- You have experienced vomiting or diarrhea for more than 6 hours.

- You have moderate to large amounts of ketones in your urine or blood ketones are 0.6–1.5 mmol/l or higher.

- You are taking insulin and your blood glucose levels continue to be over 240 mg/dl or the level determined by you and your provider.

- You have type 2 diabetes, you are taking oral diabetes medication, and your pre-meal blood glucose levels are 250 mg/dl or higher for more than 24 hours.

- You have signs of extreme hyperglycemia (very dry mouth or fruity odor on the breath), dehydration, or confusion and disorientation.

- You are sleepier than normal.

- You have stomach or chest pain or any difficulty breathing.

- You have doubts or questions about what you need to do for your illness.

Keep records of your condition during your illness so that you'll have the information ready when you call your doctor. These records will make it easier for your doctor to determine how sick you are and to keep track of your progress in getting well.

Things to Tell Your Health Care Provider

- Blood glucose levels and your urine ketone results—starting when you first realized you were ill

- Insulin doses and diabetes pills you have taken and when you took them, as well as any other medications you've taken

- The amount of time you've been sick

- Symptoms such as your temperature, your appetite and fluid intake, any weight loss, or any other problems

- Your pharmacist's phone number

Part IV

Managing Your Diabetes

CHAPTER 9

Setting Blood Glucose Goals

Covered in This Chapter

- ADA Guidelines
- Intensive Diabetes Management

etting your blood glucose goals is one of the first steps you'll make in order to manage your diabetes. Your goals include the blood glucose levels that you want to aim for on a daily basis.

No matter what kind of diabetes you have, your goal will be to keep blood glucose as close as possible to the level of someone without diabetes. This will help prevent long-term diabetes complications, such as heart and nerve disease and foot and eye problems.

However, keep in mind that blood glucose goals are entirely personal, so you'll want to talk with your health care provider about creating reasonable goals and the strategies to achieve these goals. Some people with diabetes find that keeping blood glucose levels close to normal is not realistic or even desirable. For example, elderly people or people who live alone may be more concerned about preventing severe low blood glucose episodes than avoiding long-term complications.

ADA Blood Glucose Goals

Before meals: 70–130 mg/dl

Two hours after the first bite of a meal: less than 180 mg/dl

ADA Guidelines

Choosing blood glucose goals can be easy. You can simply use the guidelines supported by the American Diabetes Association (ADA). These recommendations are based on the findings from research about preventing complications.

However, the ADA's goals may not be easy for you to reach. Or they may not be right for you. Why not see what your blood glucose levels are before and after meals and compare them to the goals in the box on the left? Then choose a realistic goal for the short term. Perhaps you can make a few small changes to slowly lower your blood glucose levels.

Things to Change to Lower Blood Glucose

- How much food you eat
- Kinds of food you eat
- Your activity level
- How much insulin or other medication you take

Write down an acceptable blood glucose range for you at this time. The range could be something like 70–200 mg/dl. This means that any reading below 70 mg/dl is too low. Anything over 200 mg/dl is higher than you want. This range includes lower blood glucose levels before meals and somewhat higher glucose levels 1–2 hours after meals. You should see the high end of the range come down as you work toward reaching your goals.

Children's Blood Glucose Goals

Blood glucose goals for children are broader. For example, the target range may be 100–200 mg/dl. Most children under the age of 6 or 7 are not yet able to be aware of and respond to oncoming low blood glucose. So it's important to limit episodes of low blood glucose. Tailor goals to the age and abilities of the child and be flexible with goals as the child grows.

Intensive Diabetes Management

Some people may want a more rigorous approach to setting goals and managing blood glucose. Intensive diabetes management, also referred to as IDM, can help prevent long-term complications and make you feel better every day. However, it is hard work, and it is *not* for everyone.

You'll find out more about the treatments required for intensive diabetes management in chapter 13 on insulin and chapter 10 on healthy eating. For now, let's discuss why you may or may not want to pursue intensive diabetes management.

Research behind Intensive Diabetes Management

It always seemed obvious that keeping blood glucose levels as close to normal as possible would prevent diabetes complications. Yet, researchers needed to prove it for sure. For example, what if something else related to diabetes caused the complications? What if lowering blood glucose had no effect on complications?

In recent years, two major research studies confirmed what many diabetes health professionals and people with diabetes had long suspected. The two studies are called the Diabetes Control and Complications Trial (DCCT) and the United Kingdom Prospective Diabetes Study (UKPDS).

The DCCT followed 1,441 people with type 1 diabetes for 10 years. Some people received a conventional treatment therapy of 1–2 shots of insulin a day, whereas other people received intensive diabetes therapy, which included either an insulin pump or multiple daily injections of insulin.

DCCT Results

Among those receiving intensive diabetes therapy, the following findings were made:

- Reduced the risk of developing diabetic eye disease, called retinopathy, by 76%.

- Slowed the progression of retinopathy by 54% in people who already had early signs of eye disease.

➔ **DCCT**

The Diabetes Control and Complications Trial showed that people with type 1 diabetes could delay or even prevent many of the complications of diabetes by tightly managing blood glucose levels.

DCCT Results

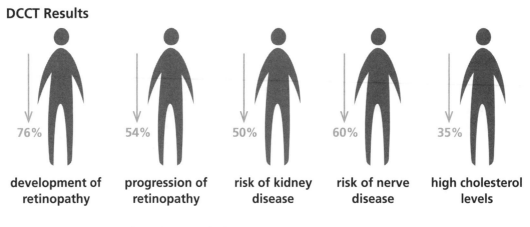

76%	54%	50%	60%	35%
development of retinopathy	progression of retinopathy	risk of kidney disease	risk of nerve disease	high cholesterol levels

- Reduced risk of kidney disease by 50%.

- Reduced risk of nerve disease by 60%.

- Reduced risk of high cholesterol levels by 35% (a major contributor to heart disease).

Before the DCCT, many people with diabetes thought that complications would progress no matter what they did. After the DCCT, we know that way of thinking is wrong. Keeping blood glucose levels close to normal matters.

The other study—the UKPDS—followed 5,102 people with newly diagnosed type 2 diabetes for 20 years. People were treated with conventional therapy of mainly diet alone or intensive therapy of insulin or diabetes pills.

UKPDS Results

- People who on intensive therapy reduced their risk of microvascular complications, such as eye and nerve disease, by 25%.

> **→ UKPDS**
>
> The United Kingdom Prospective Diabetes Study showed that tight blood glucose control and blood pressure management could help people with type 2 diabetes delay or prevent diabetes complications.

- People who lowered their blood pressure reduced their risk of stroke by 44% and their risk of heart failure by 56%.

- Improved blood glucose control also reduced the risk of heart attacks and diabetes-related deaths.

UKPDS Results

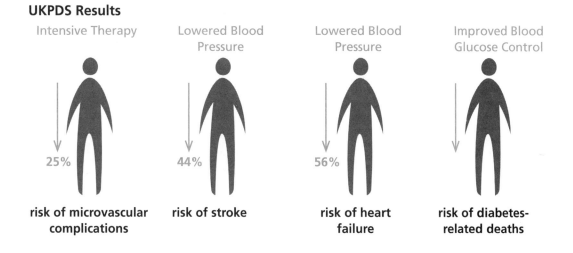

| Intensive Therapy | Lowered Blood Pressure | Lowered Blood Pressure | Improved Blood Glucose Control |

25% — risk of microvascular complications

44% — risk of stroke

56% — risk of heart failure

risk of diabetes-related deaths

- The long-term benefits of glucose control were seen even 10 years after the study ended.

What do all these numbers mean? Intensive management of blood glucose and blood pressure can significantly reduce your risk of diabetes complications. However, intensive diabetes management has some negatives.

Drawbacks to Intensive Diabetes Management

- It is more expensive.

- It takes more time and effort.

- You'll have more hypoglycemia episodes. People in the DCCT using intensive diabetes management had three times as many severe low blood glucose episodes than those on the conventional treatment program. This happened because their overall blood glucose levels were much lower.

- You may gain weight. People in DCCT following intensive management tended to gain more weight than those using a conventional treatment program because they were no longer losing calories in the form of glucose in their urine. Taking more insulin also made their bodies more efficient at capturing and storing calories.

Is Intensive Management Right for You?

Are you already reaching your blood glucose and blood pressure goals? Do you firmly believe that you are doing fine without intensifying your diabetes management? Do you dislike the idea of having your life dictated by your diabetes care or schedule? If you answered yes to any of these questions, then intensive management may *not* be right for you.

However, if you want to reduce the long-term risk of complications, you may decide that intensive diabetes management is worth the extra effort, time, and side effects. In the end, intensive management may offer you more flexibility in your day-to-day living. You monitor your blood glucose more frequently so that you can make adjustments in your insulin dose to accommodate variety in your eating and activity patterns.

Intensive diabetes management can benefit almost anyone with diabetes. For years, women with type 1 or type 2 diabetes who were planning a pregnancy and women who developed gestational diabetes have been advised to take an intensive approach to their diabetes. It is particularly important during pregnancy to keep glucose levels close to normal to avoid problems in the development and growth of the baby.

Keep in mind, intensive diabetes management is not safe for some groups of people: children, elderly people, and people experiencing severe complications of diabetes, such as life-limiting illnesses or trouble with cognition or function.

Intensive Diabetes Management May Not Be Right for You If...

• You have a history of severe hypoglycemic episodes or hypoglycemia unawareness.

• You are younger than 10, unless you have motivated parents and/ or caregivers.

• You are elderly, with other health problems or impairments.

• You have cardiovascular disease, angina, or other medical conditions complicated by hypoglycemia or you take certain medications like beta-blockers.

- You have severe complications of diabetes. Although intensive therapy can slow down the development of complications, there is no evidence that it can reverse the process.

- You have conditions, such as debilitating arthritis or severe visual impairment, that would make it difficult to carry out tasks.

- You have drug or alcohol abuse problems or are unable to make reasonable decisions about your everyday diabetes management.

- You are unable or unwilling to carry out the tasks associated with intensive management.

Intensive diabetes management in children can be risky because it raises the risk of hypoglycemia. Severe hypoglycemia can interfere with normal brain development, particularly in very young children. Intensive diabetes management in children also requires close supervision, usually from a diabetes specialist.

The increased risk of hypoglycemia can also be an issue with the elderly. Hypoglycemia may make it harder to live alone or be independent. Some older people may find the potential benefits are not worth the risk, particularly if they have other health problems or impairments. However, if you are in good health, believe the benefits are worth the wait (they may take 10 years), and are willing to take on the responsibility, then let your health care team know.

Intensive Diabetes Management Education

The idea of embarking on an intensive diabetes management plan may seem overwhelming. There is a lot to remember, but keep in mind that it is an ongoing process. You can't learn it overnight, and no one expects that of you. Your health care team is there to help you.

You'll have many questions as you begin. How many units of insulin should you take if you blood glucose is a little high? How should you change what you eat for your next meal? It will require trial and error and coordination and advice from your health care team as you learn to make adjustments. Over a short period of time, you will gain the confidence to make these adjustments on your own.

Talk to your health care team about the best way to approach intensive management. Maybe your local community hospital or health

For people without diabetes, blood glucose levels rarely go over 120 mg/dl, even after eating a meal.

care team offers classes in intensive management. Maybe your diabetes educator wants to arrange several one-on-one sessions with you.

Intensive Diabetes Management Classes

Look for these topics when considering an intensive diabetes management class.

- Nutritional guidelines and carbohydrate counting to determine the effect of food on blood glucose levels.

- Insulin action and dosage adjustment or dosing of other injectable medications.

- How to measure the effect of exercise.

- Blood glucose and urine ketone monitoring and interpretation of the results.

- Strategies to help you make changes in your lifestyle and cope more effectively with diabetes.

Choosing Intensive Diabetes Management Goals

The goal of intensive diabetes management is to keep blood glucose levels as close to normal as possible. You may want to tailor this approach to goals that are reasonable and safe for you. It is a group decision that you, your family, and your health care team need to make together.

People with diabetes need to take action to lower their blood glucose either by injecting insulin or compensating with food or insulin at the next mealtime. You may hear that keeping your blood glucose below 130 mg/dl is the magic number. In fact, your target range may be a little higher or lower depending on several factors such as your age, capabilities, and life situation.

Factors to Consider When Setting Goals

- Your age
- How long you've had diabetes
- Type of diabetes

- Frequency and severity of hypoglycemia
- Lifestyle and occupation
- Other medical conditions
- How much support you get from family and friends
- Your personal motivation for diabetes self-management

The American Diabetes Association has established recommended targets for glucose levels. The ADA recommends that patients keep blood glucose between 70 and 130 mg/dl before meals and less than 180 mg/dl after meals. You may choose these or different goals. But remember, the DCCT showed that any improvement in lowering blood glucose levels provides real benefits.

Another way to measure blood glucose control is with an A1C test. An A1C test is a test that measures a patient's blood glucose levels over 3 months. It can be used to diagnose diabetes (as mentioned in chapter 2) and to monitor your blood glucose control over time. Usually, your health care provider will give you an A1C test at your appointments. A reasonable goal for most people with diabetes is an A1C of less than 7%, as the risk for kidney disease, eye disease, and other complications increases as A1C goes up.

Type 1 Diabetes and Intensive Diabetes Management

If you have type 1 diabetes, you'll be using insulin and other injectable medication to intensively manage your diabetes. You'll probably be

It Can Be Hard to Reach Goals

Even though your goals may seem reasonable at first, they may be hard to reach on a day-to-day basis. It is difficult to keep blood glucose levels close to those found in people without diabetes, no matter how hard you work at it.

For example, people in the DCCT study had a hard time reaching their goals (near-normal blood glucose levels before and after meals and at bedtimes). Most people just could not consistently reach these goals.

A1C Test: A test that shows a person's average blood glucose level over the past 2–3 months, usually shown as a percentage. The A1C test measures the amount of glycosylated hemoglobin in the blood (also called hemoglobin A1C, glycated hemoglobin, or HbA1C). It can also be used to diagnose diabetes.

Estimated Average Glucose (eAG)

In addition to A1C, patients may also hear the term estimated average glucose (eAG). Estimated average glucose is a new way to report A1C results using the same units as your blood glucose meter (mg/dl).

A1C (%)	eAG (mg/dl)
5	97
5.5	111
6	126
6.5	140
7	154
7.5	169
8	183
8.5	197
9	212
9.5	226
10	240
10.5	255
11	269
11.5	283
12	298

A1C in the DCCT

Researchers took patients' A1C measurements in the DCCT to see how well they were doing with overall control. The study subjects on intensive management lowered their A1C values dramatically—even though they did not often reach their daily blood glucose goals. This improvement was seen after about 3–6 months of intensive management.

taking more and different types of insulin in intensive diabetes management. You'll find more information using insulin plans, insulin pumps, and other injectables in chapter 13.

Keep in mind that you'll also need to monitor your blood glucose much more frequently with intensive diabetes management.

Type 1 Monitoring and Intensive Diabetes Management

- You'll probably want to check your blood glucose often, at least as often as you inject insulin or other injectables and sometimes more.

- You could be monitoring seven times a day depending on how often you eat: before your three meals, after each meal, and before bedtime.

- Bedtime monitoring. You may even check at 3 a.m. once or twice a week. For instance, you will not want your blood glucose level to become too low during the night. So if you've experienced several severe hypoglycemic episodes, you may want to aim for a higher overnight blood glucose level.

- Every bit of checking gives you more knowledge of how your body reacts to food, exercise, insulin, stress, and illness. Once you've settled into a comfortable routine, you may be able to do fewer checks. Remember that monitoring gives you the information you need to make wise decisions in managing your diabetes.

- You may want to wear a continuous glucose monitor that records your glucose level throughout the day and night.

Type 2 Diabetes and Intensive Diabetes Management

If you have type 2 diabetes, your blood glucose targets are not that different from those of people with type 1. However, the way you reach those targets may be different. Talk to your health care provider about strategies you may need to pursue.

Special Considerations for Type 2 Diabetes and Intensive Diabetes Management

- If you manage your blood glucose with food and physical activity, you may need to add an oral diabetes medication.

- If you already take medication, you may need to add another pill, once-a-day insulin, or other injectable medication.

- If you already take insulin, you may need to take a more aggressive approach such as three or four shots a day. Your therapy might even be similar to a person with type 1 diabetes.

- You may choose to wear an insulin pump if you begin taking more frequent insulin shots.

- Watch out for weight gain that accompanies lowered blood glucose levels. You may need to add an extra workout a week to counteract the fact that you're not losing as much glucose in your urine anymore.

Pregnancy, Gestational Diabetes, and Intensive Diabetes Management

Getting and keeping tight blood glucose control is especially important during pregnancy to prevent complications for the mother and baby. Intensive diabetes management is recommended for mothers-to-be with diabetes.

If you have type 1 or type 2 diabetes, it's important to plan your pregnancy. Your blood glucose should be as close to normal as possible before you become pregnant. You increase the baby's risk of birth defects if your blood glucose is too high in the first 2 months of pregnancy. It also increases your risk of miscarriage. It's important to take care of your general health, too. Pregnant women with diabetes who do not closely manage blood glucose are more likely to develop hypoglycemia and a temporary worsening of complications, such as eye disease.

Talk to your health care provider about your individualized goals for blood glucose management and targets. Striving for tight blood glucose control requires extra effort and diligence. Although it is hard work, you are doing all that you can to ensure good health for yourself and your baby. Read more about specific treatments for pregnant women in chapter 13 on insulin and chapters 10 and 11 on food and exercise.

Support for Intensive Diabetes Management

As you embark on an intensive approach to diabetes management, you may find that you need more support and encouragement while adjusting to the new routines. Sometimes you might just need someone to talk to, to discuss common problems, to air your concerns, or to just ask questions. Sometimes it will help to know that someone cares and understands what you are going through.

In Conclusion

Whatever blood glucose goals you choose, remember that your goals will probably change over time. Use this chapter as a resource for

→ Sources of Support for Intensive Diabetes Management

- Family and friends may provide you with the encouragement you need to affirm your commitment to intensive management.

- Your health care team can provide you with technical support, answering questions as they arise and reassuring you that you're doing the right thing and making wise decisions.

- Your health care team can also help you locate financial resources and brainstorm ways to ease financial concerns.

- Support groups may introduce you to other people with whom you can share stories and commiserate. They may also give you the opportunity to help others, which can be therapeutic.

setting and then redefining your goals when necessary. Looking ahead, you will find out more about specific strategies for managing your blood glucose such as healthy eating, exercise, medications, and insulin.

CHAPTER 10

Healthy Eating

Covered in This Chapter

- Food Groups
- Choosing a Meal Plan
- Carbohydrate Counting
- Food Labels
- Eating In and Eating Out
- Special Considerations

Healthy eating is a challenge for everyone. And it's no surprise. It can be difficult to change how and what we eat, as these choices are interwoven with our family and work lives, and even our upbringing.

The truth is that healthy eating for a person with diabetes is no different from healthy eating for a person without diabetes. It's a matter of eating a variety of foods and a balanced amount of carbohydrates, proteins, and fat. It doesn't mean you have to give up all sugars or special treats. You just have to make sure you account for them in your total meal plan for the day.

However, people with diabetes need to work harder to balance the foods they eat with their blood glucose levels. You'll need to make sure that your calorie and carbohydrate intake is balanced with your medication and physical activity. A dietitian or diabetes educator can help you come up with a meal plan that fits your goals and includes foods you like. Dietitians and diabetes educators are discussed in more detail in chapter 17 on your health care team.

Registered Dietitian (RD): A health care professional who advises people about meal planning, nutrition, and weight control. A dietitian who is also a Certified Diabetes Educator (CDE) has additional training in diabetes management and can assist you with your overall diabetes care.

Diabetes Educator: A health care professional who teaches people with diabetes how to manage their disease. A diabetes educator can also be a Certified Diabetes Educator (CDE). This means he or she has additional expertise in all areas of diabetes care and has successfully passed a national exam.

First, let's discuss the different types of foods and their effects on your body. Once you know the food groups and some general guidelines, you'll find out more about developing a meal plan.

Food Groups

The best approach to healthy eating is to eat a wide variety of foods. Your body requires nutrients to repair and replace proteins, tissues, and cells throughout your body and to keep you rolling along. Your body needs three important nutrients to do this: protein, carbohydrate, and fat, as well as vitamins and minerals.

Various combinations of these nutrients are found in different foods. So, by eating a variety of foods, you are sure to get all the nutrients you need. Eating a variety of foods is much better than taking vitamin supplements because nature combines the needed nutrients in food in a way that your body can best use them.

Calories 101

- A calorie is a measurement of the amount of energy in a food.

- Carbohydrates and proteins provide about the same amount of energy—4 calories per gram.

- Fats provide more than twice that amount—9 calories per gram.

Any food that your body doesn't use as energy is stored as fat. So, the trick is to balance the total number of calories you take in with the total number you burn up. Proteins and carbohydrates give you fewer calories per bite than high-fat foods. So, if you're trying to lose weight, cut down on fats. A diet high in saturated fat can also put you at greater risk for developing heart disease and certain cancers.

Carbohydrates

Carbohydrates supply most of the glucose your body uses for energy. Your blood glucose goes up as carbohydrates are broken down into glucose and absorbed. Blood glucose rises within 15 minutes of eating carbohydrates. Several factors affect the way in which carbohydrates work.

Types of Carbohydrates
Carbohydrates include vegetables, fruits, cereals, grains, pastas, breads, and milk. These foods are loaded with nutrition. They provide easily used energy, fiber, vitamins, and minerals. They also tend to be lower in calories than foods in other groups.

Sugar is also a carbohydrate. It has long had a bad reputation, especially among people with diabetes. People used to think that eating sugar would cause blood glucose levels to rise much more rapidly than other types of carbohydrates, such as bread or potatoes. So although bread and potatoes were okay to eat, pure sugar or sugar-laden treats were considered taboo. Well, it turns out that the total amount of car-

Food Groups Preview

Carbohydrates. These include vegetables, fruits, beans, and whole-grain cereals, grains, pastas, and breads.

Proteins. These include beans, meat, eggs, and dairy products. Choose lower-fat versions.

Fats. These include oils, margarines, butter, cream, and chocolate.

More about Carbohydrates

Digestibility. How easily the carbohydrate is digested will affect how quickly glucose is freed and gets into blood. Cooked food digests faster than raw food. Food that stays in bigger pieces, like corn on the cob, breaks down more slowly than smaller pieces, like the bits in creamed corn.

Quantity and quality of carbohydrates. Your blood glucose increases with the amount of carbohydrates you eat. You can get a feel for how the quantity of carbohydrates affects your blood glucose by measuring it 1–2 hours after the first bite of a meal. You may be more concerned about the quality versus the quantity of carbohydrates you eat.

Combination with other nutrients. Fat slows down the absorption of food. Therefore, adding fat to carbohydrate food during preparation or at the table will slow digestion of the carbohydrate and delay the effect on glucose levels.

> **Sugar**
>
> Your dietitian can help you learn how to count sugar as part of your carbohydrate allotment in your meal plan. For example, if you plan on having a small piece of cake for dessert, you might want to skip the rolls you normally have at dinner. Your dietitian or health care provider can also help you decide whether you need to adjust your medication dose to deal with the extra carbohydrates.

bohydrates and its combination with other nutrients, such as fat, are much more important.

Foods that contain sugar can be part of your diabetes plan. You'll just need to account for the calories and carbohydrates. Keep in mind, sugar has little nutritional value, so filling up on sugars won't allow you to eat as much of the nutrient-rich carbohydrates.

Artificial Sweeteners

- Artificial sweeteners give you the sweet taste of sugar without its calories and without raising your blood glucose levels. Depending on the brand used, one packet will usually give the same sweetness as two teaspoons of table sugar.

- There are two classes of artificial sweeteners: noncaloric (non-nutritive) and caloric (nutritive).

- Noncaloric sweeteners, such as aspartame, acesulfame-K, sucralose, and saccharin, do not raise blood glucose.

- Caloric sweeteners, such as sorbitol, mannitol, and xylitol, are sugar alcohols. They have calories and are absorbed into the blood, although more slowly.

- Artificial sweeteners are okay for everyone, except that pregnant or breast-feeding women should not use saccharin and people with phenylketonuria should not use aspartame.

Some carbohydrates are harder to spot in foods. Products such as low-fat and nonfat foods have added carbohydrates that can affect blood glucose. You'll want to keep in mind that even if a product is labeled as low calorie, low sugar, or sugar free, it may contain other substances that raise blood glucose.

Often, these substances are modified forms of carbohydrate that are used as emulsifiers or bulking agents. For example, maltodextrin and polydextrose can be found in products such as sugar-free, nonfat yogurt or low-fat pudding and ice cream. Maltodextrin is digested like a carbohydrate and provides 4 calories per gram. Polydextrose mostly passes through the body and provides just 1 calorie per gram so it does not have much effect on blood glucose.

Protein

Protein is an essential nutrient in any healthy diet. Proteins are used to repair the body. They are not used for energy unless there are not enough carbohydrates and fats present. However, many Americans eat more protein than they need. People who have kidney problems may be advised to limit the amount of protein they eat.

Meat, poultry, milk products, and eggs are all good sources of high-quality protein, but they also come with bad things such as cholesterol and saturated fat (see next section). Select low-fat milk products, lean cuts of meat and poultry, and seafood.

Vegetables, grains, and legumes have protein. They are also low in fat, have no cholesterol, and have other nutrients as well. Nuts are another source of protein. They have fat, but most do not contain saturated fat. See more about types of fat in the next section.

> ### Seafood
>
> Seafood is a good source of protein, and most kinds of seafood are lower in saturated fat and cholesterol than meat. Seafood also contains heart-healthy omega-3 fats.

Fats and Cholesterol

Everyone needs some fat in their diet to make sure their bodies function properly. Fat is used to rebuild the membranes that protect the cells in your body and to help the cells in your body send signals. Fats are also stored and used as energy reserves.

However, too much saturated fat and trans fats can clog up blood vessels and increase your chance of developing heart disease and stroke. Many Americans eat too much fat. You are better off trying to limit the amount of fat you eat, especially unhealthy fats.

Keep in mind that your body also makes its own cholesterol, which is separate from the cholesterol that you eat in food. Your body's cholesterol is used to make and repair cell membranes and to make many of the essential steroid hormones, such as estrogen and testosterone. You'll need to limit the amount of dietary cholesterol and harmful fats you take in from foods in order to keep your cholesterol in check (see more about cholesterol in chapter 14 on heart disease).

Healthy Fats
Healthy fats are better for your heart and blood vessels. They are mostly found in plant foods, such as nuts and oil. They include unsaturated fats—monounsaturated and polyunsaturated—and omega-3 and omega-6 fatty acids. Omega-3 fatty acids, which are found in fish, walnuts, and flaxseed oil, are thought to reduce the risk of heart disease. For this reason, three servings of fish a week are recommended.

Types of Healthy Fats

- Monounsaturated fat is in olive and canola oil, avocados, nuts, and all-natural peanut butter.

- Polyunsaturated fat is in corn, cottonseed, sunflower, safflower, and soybean oils, as well as in margarine and mayonnaise.

- Omega-3 fats are in walnuts, flaxseed oil, and fish such as tuna, bluefish, lake trout, salmon, and sardines. Omega-3 and omega-6 fats are found in fish oil and flaxseed and soybean oils.

Unhealthy Fats
Unhealthy fats can lead to clogged arteries, heart disease, and stroke. They include saturated fats, trans fats, and cholesterol. Saturated fats are mostly found in animal fats, such as red meat and bacon.

Some vegetable products are also high in harmful trans fats. These products are often found in cookies, crackers, cakes, snack chips, and pancake mixes. Be careful when you find cookies marked as "sugar-free" or marketed toward people with diabetes because they may provide more than 60% of their calories from fat.

Types of Unhealthy Fats

• Saturated fats are in bacon, butter, cocoa butter (chocolate), coconut oil, full-fat (regular) cream cheese, lard, meat fat, palm oil, solid shortening, and full-fat (regular) sour cream.

• Trans fats are in margarine sticks; shortening; fast-food French fries; some chips and crackers; some muffins, cookies, and cakes; and any product containing hydrogenated or partially hydrogenated oil.

• Dietary cholesterol is in meat, poultry, egg yolks, and dairy products.

Tips for Reducing Meat Fat in Your Diet

• Choose lean cuts of meat. Look for key words, such as "loin," "round," "lean," "choice," and "select."

• Cut off all visible fat before or after cooking, and remove skin from chicken and turkey.

• Broil, roast, grill, steam, or poach instead of frying.

• Try quick-cooking methods, such as stir-frying, that use marinades or dressings with lots of seasonings to enhance juiciness and flavor.

• Limit your portions of lean meat, fish, or poultry to 3–5 ounces per meal—about the size of a deck of cards. Half of a skinless, boneless chicken breast is about 3 ounces of meat.

• Chill meat broth and drippings so the fat rises and solidifies. Then it can be skimmed off the top before serving or making gravy. You can also use this method to reduce the fat in canned or homemade broths and soups.

Tips for Reducing Other Fat in Your Diet

• Avoid fried foods.

• Limit the number of egg yolks you eat to four per week.

> ### → Margarine
>
> Choose a "light" or reduced-fat tub margarine that includes liquid oil, such as olive oil or soybean oil, as its first ingredient rather than one that includes partially hydrogenated oil or trans fat.

- Use a nonfat cooking spray on pans and cooking utensils to prevent sticking.

- Select reduced-fat or fat-free dairy products, such as salad dressings, baked goods, luncheon meats, soups, and dairy products.

Vitamins and Minerals

People with diabetes have the same requirements for vitamins and minerals as people without diabetes. You are most likely getting all the vitamins and minerals you need if you are eating a diverse diet rich in vegetables, fruits, cereals, and grains. The one exception to this may be calcium (to prevent osteoporosis) or vitamin D (if you live in the north or have a darker complexion), which you may need to get from a supplement, if directed by your health care provider.

If you are thinking about becoming pregnant or you are pregnant, you have slightly different nutritional needs. You may need a prenatal vitamin or multivitamin. Folic acid is generally recommended during pregnancy, so check with your doctor.

> **→ Should You Take a Vitamin?**
>
> Large doses of vitamins or minerals have not been shown to help diabetes or blood glucose levels. In fact, large doses of some vitamins can be harmful. Check with your dietitian before you take any vitamin or herbal supplement. A few changes in your food choices may correct the nutritional deficiency.

Reducing Salt

Too much dietary salt or sodium can increase blood pressure. People with diabetes, especially type 2 diabetes, may already have high blood pressure, so they may need to reduce their sodium intake.

- Put the saltshaker away, and use less or no salt when cooking.

- Read food labels to assess the sodium content (80% of your sodium intake comes from processed foods).

- If you are using canned vegetables, rinse them to remove the salt or choose no-salt-added or reduced-sodium options.

- Avoid fast foods.

- Use flavorings such as herbs and spices to make your food tastier.

- Cook using fresh foods whenever possible.

Choosing a Meal Plan

You are the most important person to consider when choosing a healthy meal plan. Your plan should reflect your goals, needs, tastes, and lifestyle. Your provider and dietitian may recommend certain goals, but you will be the one who chooses a meaningful and realistic plan.

Keep in mind that a healthy meal plan for you is a healthy meal plan for anyone—with or without diabetes. You don't have to worry about following some strange diet involving weird foods that no one else in your family will want to touch. You can choose foods that will benefit everyone in your family. Often, family members will not even realize that they are eating a "diabetes meal plan."

Defining Goals for a Meal Plan

- Do you want to lose or maintain weight?

- What are your blood glucose goals? If you have type 2 diabetes, which foods should you choose to help you manage your blood glucose level? If you have type 1 diabetes, which foods are best to eat when taking insulin or other medication?

- How can you use meal planning to fit in with intensive diabetes management?

After first consulting with your diabetes care provider, you will most likely set up a visit with your dietitian to develop a meal plan. You may feel that you don't really need a dietitian. Maybe you've seen sample meal plans recommended for people with diabetes that look easy enough to use. But remember, your meal plan is not a short-term diet that you can follow for a few weeks. You are developing a new way of eating that will stay with you throughout your life.

Your dietitian can help tailor a meal plan to suit your tastes and schedule. As you reach goals or your lifestyle changes, you can remodel your plan to suit these changes. Products change, your life and health needs change, and you change. As these events occur, your dietary goals will change, and you will probably need a new plan.

Designing a Meal Plan

Your meal plan should make it easier—not harder—to manage your blood glucose.

- Include foods you like and that are important to you.

- Take into account your daily activities and schedule.

- Be flexible.

- A plan should help you keep your blood glucose levels within your target range.

- A plan should help you reach and maintain a healthy weight.

- Choose foods that will help prevent diseases and conditions, such as heart disease, high blood pressure, and cancer.

A dietitian with experience in diabetes care can help you develop new ways to look at food. You might want to get a better sense of matching your carbohydrate intake to your insulin or other medication doses to keep your glucose in balance. Or maybe you'd like to know how to manage your blood glucose using a vegetarian diet. Or perhaps you would like to lose weight.

Topics to Discuss with a Dietitian

- What types of foods and how much you need to eat every day.

- How many grams of carbohydrates to eat each day to keep your blood glucose within your target range—and how to count carbohydrates (see more on carbohydrate counting in the next section).

- How many grams of fat to eat if you want to keep your fat intake low. Generally, this means that the fat in your diet provides no more than 30% of the calories you take in per day. You may also want to discuss how to count fat grams.

- How to adjust your meals for exercise.

- Which foods to have on hand to treat hypoglycemia and sick days.

- New ideas for breakfast, lunch, dinner, and snacks.

- How to reduce your sodium intake—and how to count sodium in milligrams.

- How to read food labels.

- How to meet your nutritional needs when following a specific meal plan such as a vegetarian diet.

Meal Planning and Pregnancy

You will want to pay special attention to the food you eat when you're pregnant. Eating healthy during pregnancy really isn't all that different from a healthy meal plan for anyone. However, you will find that you and your growing baby require more nutrients than you did before pregnancy. For example, you will need more protein, calcium, iron, and vitamins while you are pregnant. Your appetite may increase, especially in the last months of pregnancy.

It is important to talk to your provider and dietitian before you decide to become pregnant, because good nutrition starts even before conception. For instance, your provider or dietitian will advise you to take folic acid. Having near-normal blood glucose levels before conceiving is another safeguard against birth defects. If you are overweight, a calorie-restricted diet may be recommended before you conceive.

Once you are pregnant, your dietitian, your diabetes care provider, and your obstetrician can assess your dietary needs and work with you to develop a meal plan that you can use throughout your pregnancy. You will need to take into account your overall health and nutritional status.

Topics to Discuss for Pregnancy and Meals

- How many calories you need to eat each day

- Whether you will need a prenatal vitamin supplement

> **Small Breakfast**
>
> You may be advised to eat a small breakfast because blood glucose is more likely to be high first thing in the morning.

• How to divide your daily calories and carbohydrates between meals and snacks

• Your goals for your blood glucose readings throughout the day

Your dietitian and other members of your health care team can also help you ease into making lower-fat food choices if controlling weight gain is one of your goals. If you are suffering from nausea, your dietitian can teach you how to incorporate snacks at certain times of the day.

If you are taking insulin, you will also need to learn how to adjust your insulin doses to match the changes in your diet. As your pregnancy proceeds, insulin resistance increases, and you'll need more insulin.

Ask your dietitian and doctor about the use of caffeine, alcohol, and artificial sweeteners during pregnancy. Unless you have special needs, it is safe to use the artificial sweeteners aspartame and acesulfame-K during pregnancy. You need to avoid saccharin during pregnancy and when breast-feeding. Alcohol is generally not recommended for anyone during pregnancy and can increase the risk of hypoglycemia among women with diabetes.

Carbohydrate Counting

Carbohydrate counting, or carb counting, is a specific tool to help you manage your blood glucose. It is based on counting the number of grams of carbohydrates in a meal and the total carbohydrates you eat in a day to balance your blood glucose levels.

> **Carbohydrate Counting:** A method of meal planning for people with diabetes based on counting the number of grams of carbohydrate in food.

Your dietitian should recommend the number of carbohydrates to eat at meals and snacks. As a general guideline, most women need about 45–60 grams of carbohydrate at each meal and 15 grams per snack. Most men need 60–75 grams of carbohydrate at each meal and 15–30 grams for one or two snacks.

So how do you figure out how many carbohydrates are in foods? The easiest way is to examine the food label. Food labels should contain a line that lists the total carbohydrate grams and percent of daily value. You'll also want to take into account the serving size. Reading food labels will be discussed in more detail below.

However, many foods like fresh vegetables and fruit don't have labels. You'll need to keep in mind some guidelines for these foods when planning your meals. Find out the carbohydrate count of your favorite foods and keep the list with you while you're learning.

People with type 1 diabetes and people with type 2 diabetes who take insulin can work with their dietitian or diabetes educator to come up with a plan for how much insulin to inject per gram of carbohydrate. You'll read more about managing your insulin and meals in chapter 13.

You may have heard about the glycemic index of foods. The glycemic index is a tool that may help you fine-tune your blood glucose control while following your current meal planning strategy.

The glycemic index is a tool that may help your current meal plan work a bit better for you. Foods with a high glycemic index raise blood glucose more than foods with a medium or low glycemic index. The total amount of carbohydrate, food composition, and cooking method can affect the glycemic index of foods.

When you eat a carbohydrate food, choose one with a moderate or low glycemic index or eat a small portion of food with a high glycemic index. Your food choice may make it easier for you to meet your

→ Greater Flexibility

Carb counting can provide a lot of flexibility in your meal planning because the most important thing is the total number of carbohydrates in meals.

Foods with 15 Grams of Carbohydrate

Small piece of fresh fruit

½ cup starchy vegetable or black beans

¼ large baked potato

⅓ cup pasta or rice

One slice of bread

One-half banana

4 ounces or ½ cup juice

→ Carbohydrate Choices

Some people prefer to think about their carbohydrates as "choices" rather than grams. This method is based on the concept that a carbohydrate choice contains 15 grams per serving. Your dietitian will recommend how many carbohydrate choices you should eat per meal.

Glycemic Index (GI): A ranking of carbohydrate-containing foods, based on the food's effect on blood glucose when compared with a standard reference food.

→ **Sports Drinks and Juice**

Don't forget to consider the calories and carbohydrates in sports drinks and juices as part of your daily intake. Sometimes people forget that beverages can have significant calories too.

→ **How Foods Measure Up Against Each Other**

Nutrient amounts are shown in grams (g) or in milligrams (mg). A gram is a very small amount, and a milligram is one-thousandth of that. For example, a nickel weighs about 5 grams. So does a teaspoonful of margarine. Use the label to compare labels of similar foods. For example, choose the product with a smaller amount of saturated fat, cholesterol, and sodium and try to select foods with more fiber.

post-meal glucose goal. For reliable sources of glycemic index information, visit the official website of the glycemic index, based at the University of Sydney in Australia (www. glycemicindex.com).

Food Labels

The U.S. Department of Agriculture and the Food and Drug Administration regulate food labels. Most manufacturers are required to display food labels, except distributors of fresh vegetables, fruits, and seafood. You're probably quite familiar with the black and white "Nutrition Facts" labels on foods. The Nutrition Facts label is an essential tool for eating healthfully. Here is the valuable information contained on a food label.

Nutrition Facts Labels

• Serving Size.

• Servings per Container. Keep in mind that there may be many servings per container in a frozen pizza or bag of chips.

• Amount per Serving: Calories and Calories from Fat.

• Daily Values: Total Fat (Saturated and Trans Fat), Cholesterol, Sodium, Total Carbohydrate (Dietary Fiber and Sugars), and Protein.

• Ingredients are listed in descending order by weight. Look for foods with healthier ingredients, such as whole-wheat flour, listed first.

→ Percent Daily Values

The percent daily value tells you how much of the total daily intake you use up when you eat one serving of a food. These numbers assume that you are eating 2,000 calories each day. For many people, the true percentages may be higher or lower depending on how many calories you need, which you can learn from a registered dietitian.

Health Claims

Sometimes you'll see a food label with a health claim such as "calcium helps prevent osteoporosis." Food manufacturers can only make health claims that are supported by scientific research. These claims can suggest a relationship between a potentially helpful or harmful ingredient and a disease.

Examples of Health Claims

Here are a few of the ingredients and linked conditions or diseases that are allowed on food packaging in the United States.

- Calcium and osteoporosis
- Fiber-containing grain products and cancer
- Fruits and vegetables and cancer
- Fruits, vegetables, and grain products that contain fiber—particularly soluble fiber—and the risk of coronary heart disease
- Fat and cancer
- Saturated fat and cholesterol and coronary artery disease
- Sodium and hypertension
- Folic acid and neural tube defects
- Olive oil and coronary heart disease

Nutrition Facts

Serving Size 1 cup (228g)
Servings Per Container 2

Amount Per Serving

Calories 260   **Calories from Fat** 120

	% Daily Value*
Total Fat 13g	**20%**
Saturated Fat 5g	**25%**
Trans Fat 2g	
Cholesterol 30mg	**10%**
Sodium 660mg	**28%**
Total Carbohydrate 31g	**10%**
Dietary Fiber 0g	**0%**
Sugars 5g	
Protein 5g	

Vitamin A 4%	•	Vitamin C 2%
Calcium 15%	•	Iron 4%

*Percent Daily Values are based on a 2,000 calorie diet. Your Daily Values may be higher or lower depending on your calorie needs.

	Calories:	2,000	2,500
Total Fat	Less than	65g	80g
Sat Fat	Less than	20g	25g
Cholesterol	Less than	300mg	300mg
Sodium	Less than	2,400mg	2,400mg
Total Carbohydrate		300g	375g
Dietary Fiber		25g	30g

Calories per gram:
Fat 9   •   Carbohydrate 4   •   Protein 4

Nutrient Content Claims

Manufacturers also make claims about the nutritional value of their products. Sometimes these claims can be a little confusing. What's the difference between low-calorie or "lite"? What is "natural"? Below are some details on what these claims mean.

Calories
- *Calorie free* means that the product has fewer than 5 calories per serving or another designated amount (make sure to note the size of the serving).

- *Low calorie* means 40 calories or less per serving.

- *Light* or *lite* means that the food has one-third less calories, 50% less fat, or 50% less sodium than the food with which it is being compared, usually the full-calorie version of the same food.

- *Less* and *reduced* (as in fat or sugar) mean that the food is at least 25% lower in calories or other ingredients compared with the full-calorie or regular version. When these words are used on a label, the actual percentages must also be included, for example, "50% less salt" or "fat reduced by 25%."

Cholesterol
- *Cholesterol free* means that the food must contain fewer than 2 milligrams of cholesterol and 2 grams or less of saturated fat per serving. For example, although vegetable oils contain no cholesterol, they are 100% fat. Vegetable oils are still preferable to butter or lard because they have less saturated fat. But a tablespoon of vegetable oil still has about 14 grams of fat and the same 126 calories found in a tablespoon of butter or cream.

- *Low cholesterol* indicates that a given serving contains 20 milligrams or less of cholesterol and 2 grams or less of saturated fat per serving.

Fat
- *Low fat* means that a food must have 3 grams or less of fat per serving.

- *Fat free* means that a food has less than 0.5 grams of fat per serving.

- *Low saturated fat* means that a food has 1 gram or less of saturated fat per serving and not more than 15% of its calories come from saturated fat.

Sodium

- *Low-sodium* foods contain 140 milligrams or less of sodium per serving and per 100 grams of food. Ordinary table salt (sodium chloride) is not the only source of sodium. It is also found in monosodium glutamate (MSG), sodium bicarbonate (baking soda), and sodium nitrate and occurs naturally in some foods.

- *Very low sodium* means that a food contains 35 milligrams or less of sodium per serving and per 100 grams of food.

- *Sodium free* or *salt free* items have less than 5 milligrams of sodium per serving.

- *Light in salt* means that the food has 50% less sodium than the regular version.

Other

- *Sugar free* means that the item has less than 0.5 grams of sugar per serving.

- *Dietetic* has no standard meaning. It indicates only that something has been changed or replaced. It could contain less sugar, less salt, less fat, or less cholesterol than the regular version of the same product. For example, if you look at a package of "dietetic" cookies, you might find that they are low in sodium but are not as low in calories or sugar as you might be led to believe.

- *Natural* has no specific meaning except for meat and poultry products. For meat and poultry products, it means that no chemical preservatives, hormones, or similar substances have been added. On other food labels, natural is not restricted to any particular meaning by government regulation.

- *Fresh* can only be used to describe raw food that has not been frozen, heat processed, or preserved in some other way.

Eating In and Eating Out

Once you have a new meal plan in hand, you'll want to start using it whenever you eat in or eat out. Your meal plan is personal, so you will do a fair amount of troubleshooting on your own to figure out how to shop, cook, and dine out. However, there are some guidelines to shoot for as you think about making healthy choices.

Shopping

Cooking and eating at home can be one of life's great pleasures. Dinner is a wonderful opportunity to sit around the table with your family or friends.

Eating in with your meal plan may take some planning and improvisation as you learn to shop for and cook with new foods. It may all seem new and overwhelming. Keep in mind—a meal plan is a chance to discover new foods and rediscover cooking. If you aren't comfortable in the kitchen, your dietitian can adjust your plan to fit your skill level and eating preferences.

Tips for Shopping

Vegetables and Fruits
- **Vegetables.** Fresh and frozen vegetables are the most nutritious per bite. Drain and rinse canned vegetables to reduce sodium content.

- **Fruit and fruit juice.** Choose fresh, frozen, or dried fruit, preferably without sugar added. Look for 100% pure fruit juice. Check labels of brands that say "made with 100% fruit juice." These drinks may list other ingredients first. Look for "no sugar added," but know that the natural sugar in juice will still raise your blood glucose. Check the Nutrition Facts label.

Grains
- **Bread.** Look for products that contain whole grains. Look at the ingredient list for items such as whole wheat, whole grain, or whole corn.

- **Cereal.** Choose brands that list whole grains first on the label and contain (per serving) 3 or more grams of dietary fiber, 1 gram or less of fat, 5 grams or less of sugar.

- **Whole grains, rice, and pasta.** Choose brown or wild rice of any type. Look for fresh or dried pasta made with whole-grain flours. Try to avoid pastas that contain eggs and fat.

- **Crackers and snack foods.** Look for whole grains listed first on the label and 2 grams or less of fat per serving. Consider pretzels or plain popcorn (air popped, with no cheese or butter, 2 grams of fat or less per serving) as low-fat snacks. Check sodium content and try to stay under 400 milligrams per serving.

Dairy
- **Milk.** Choose fat-free or 1% milk, buttermilk made from low-fat milk, and low-fat or fat-free yogurt (artificially sweetened or un-sweetened).

- **Cheese.** Look for fat-free and reduced-fat cheeses with 6 grams of fat per ounce or less.

- **Sour cream and cream cheese.** Try fat-free or light sour cream or cream cheese. As an alternative to sour cream, consider using fat-free or low-fat yogurt, either plain or flavored with chives, herbs, and spices.

Meat and Seafood
- **Red meat.** Meat is graded based on its fat content. Choose lower-fat cuts such as Choice or Select rather than higher-fat Prime. Ask the butcher to cut 4-ounce servings of raw meat (on cooking, they will shrink to a 3-ounce serving).

- *Luncheon meat.* Look for lean or 95% fat-free meats (by weight) with 30–55 calories per ounce and 3 grams of fat or less per ounce.

- **Poultry.** Breast meat is the leanest of all. Removing the skin before cooking lowers the fat content by 50–75% and cholesterol by 12%. Look for ground turkey that is less than 7–8% fat by weight (often the fatty skin is ground in, giving it a higher fat content). When turkey or chicken is used to make salami, bologna, hot dogs, and bacon, these products can be high in fat. Look for ones that are 30% fat or less.

- **Seafood.** Supermarkets offer a wide variety of seafood. Buy fresh fish or shellfish. Look for clear eyes, red gills, shiny skin, and no "fishy" smell. Shrimp is usually shipped frozen to preserve freshness. Choose canned fish packed in water or with the oil rinsed off. Look for low-sodium products.

Other Foods
- **Frozen desserts.** Choose varieties that contain 3 grams or less of fat per 4-ounce serving (1/2 cup). Look for low-fat frozen yogurt or low- or fat-free ice cream. Try frozen fruit juice bars with fewer than 70 calories per bar. Avoid desserts made with cream of coconut, coconut milk, or coconut or palm oil, which are high in saturated fat or contain trans fats.

- **Margarine and oil.** Choose olive, canola, soybean, safflower, sesame, sunflower, or corn oils. Choose brands with liquid oil listed first on the label and that contain no trans fats. Try using nonstick vegetable cooking spray for cooking and cut back on oil.

- **Salad dressings.** Try reduced-calorie and fat-free types. Include the carbohydrates in your meal plan.

- **Soup.** Choose low-sodium, reduced-fat varieties. In preparing soup, use fat-free or low-fat milk or water.

- **Cookies and cakes.** Choose brands that contain 3 grams or less of fat per 100 calories. Angel food cake is made without fat and has no cholesterol. Other cakes can be made without cholesterol (by using egg substitutes) but usually not without fat. Some versions substitute applesauce or nonfat yogurt for oil. Some cake mixes include directions for low-fat and low-cholesterol variations. Some fat-free cookies have more calories than the original recipe because of added sugar. Avoid palm, coconut, and hydrogenated oils.

Restaurants

Eating out is a big part of today's lifestyle—and there is no reason why you should avoid restaurants because you have diabetes. However, it is important to know what you're eating and to make healthy choices from the menu.

Tips for Eating Out

- Don't be afraid to ask about ingredients or the serving size of dishes.

- Try to eat the same portion size you would eat at home. Don't feel you need to clean your plate just to get your money's worth.

- Ask your server if you can order a smaller portion at a reduced price, share a plate with your companion, or put extra food in a "doggy bag" to take home.

- Ask if no or less butter can be used in preparing your meal.

- Ask that sauces, gravy, salad dressings, sour cream, and butter be served on the side or left off altogether.

- Choose broiled, baked, poached, or grilled meats and fish rather than fried.

- Try asking for substitutions, such as low-fat cottage cheese, baked potato, or even extra vegetables, instead of French fries.

- If you take insulin, ask your health care team for guidelines on adjusting your dose when you eat out.

Special Considerations

Without a doubt, special considerations are likely to come up from time to time. Disruptions in your schedule, holidays, and parties are inevitable. Here are some tips to deal with these situations.

Alcohol

A common myth is that people with diabetes can't drink alcohol. This is just not true. If your blood glucose levels are on target, it is unlikely that an occasional alcoholic drink at mealtime will harm you. In fact, some studies have shown that light to moderate alcohol intake is associated with reduced risk of death from coronary heart disease for people with type 2 diabetes.

The key is to drink moderately. Moderate drinking is defined as no more than one drink a day for women and two drinks a day for men. One drink is 12 ounces of regular beer, 5 ounces of wine, or 1.5 ounces of 80-proof distilled spirits (liquor). If you do not tolerate alcohol well or have had problems with it in the past, however, you should avoid drinking.

Tips for Drinking Alcohol

- Alcohol contains calories, almost as many per gram as fat. If weight loss is one of your goals, then you need to think about the extra calories from alcohol. Generally, alcohol is substituted for fat calories, with one drink equal to 2 fat exchanges (about 90 calories).

- Alcohol can affect your blood glucose, most often causing very low blood glucose when consumed on an empty stomach. If you use certain medications or insulin, drink alcohol with food to prevent hypoglycemia.

- The signs of hypoglycemia (no matter what the cause) are very similar to the signs of inebriation. There is the risk that people will think you are intoxicated if they see your behavior suddenly change. They may not consider the possibility that you have low blood glucose and need help quickly.

- Some people have hypoglycemia unawareness, a lack of symptoms of low blood glucose. Drinking alcohol increases their risk for hypoglycemia.

- Some medications, including some diabetes medications, require limits on alcohol use.

- If you have health problems, such as pancreatitis, high triglyceride levels, gastric problems, neuropathy (nerve damage), kidney disease, or certain types of heart disease, you may be advised to abstain from alcohol.

- Not drinking and driving is sound advice for everyone. But because of the added risk for hypoglycemia from alcohol, it is especially true for people with diabetes.

- Alcohol can affect your thought processes and inhibitions. It's easy to overeat when you are drinking. In addition, you need to be able to think clearly enough to monitor your blood glucose levels and to know what to do should they drop too low. If you are drinking, make sure to tell a friend what to do in the event of low blood glucose. Your friend should be prepared to take action, even if you are not able to cooperate.

Eating Later than Usual

You may need a snack if your meal is later than usual. Just make sure to account for it in your overall daily nutrition. Always carry snacks with you. You never know when you might get stuck in traffic or delayed at work and start to go low.

If you plan to go out for brunch, eat an early-morning snack. Then, use your lunchtime meal plan and what is left of your usual breakfast plan. If dinner is going to be very late, have your bedtime snack at your normal dinnertime.

If you take insulin and can't change the timing of your insulin dose, eat a piece of fruit or a starchy low-fat snack. You may need to adjust your insulin later to account for these changes, so ask your health care team how to do this.

Eating More Often than Usual

At holidays, it may seem like you're around food all day long. Try dividing your total food for the day into snack-size meals. Then you can spread the food out a little more than usual without going over your usual amounts.

Eating More Food than Usual

Sometimes going to parties, having friends visit, or just dining out may tempt you to overeat. You are bound to eat a little more than you

> **Eating Until You Are No Longer Hungry**
>
> Instead of eating until you are full, eat until you are no longer hungry.

planned on occasion. Don't let an occasional moment of overeating make you feel guilty or like you are "cheating." Remember, eating healthy is all about making choices. Maybe you can plan some more activity to help with extra food intake if you are working toward losing weight. For people on insulin, covering the extra food with more insulin is a choice too.

Plan ahead what you want to do. If you decide to eat more than usual, think about using your other blood glucose management tools. Do a little more exercise either before or after the event. Regardless of what you decide, think afterward about how your plan worked. Would you try something different the next time?

Eating Disorders

Eating disorders occur among people with diabetes just as they do in the general population. Some researchers believe that individuals with diabetes may have an increased risk for eating disorders because they have to pay more attention to what they eat. Unfortunately, in our society, the self-worth of many people comes from having a "perfect" body. Some people resort to extreme measures to get or stay thin.

> **Anorexia:** An eating disorder in which people refrain from eating in order to stay thin. Their perception of their body is often out of tune with reality. Even very thin women and men sometimes perceive themselves as being overweight.
>
> **Bulimia:** An eating disorder in which people will often eat normal or even excessive amounts of food and then purge the food by inducing vomiting or taking laxatives. Over time, bulimia can cause problems with the esophagus, as well as many dental problems.

There are two main eating disorders: anorexia nervosa and bulimia. Each has a distinct set of warning signs. Both disorders stress the body and deny it the necessary nutrients.

People with diabetes and eating disorders are likely to have more episodes of diabetic ketoacidosis (type 1 diabetes) and hypoglycemia, and their A1C levels tend to be higher. They are also at higher risk for diabetes complications because their blood glucose is high.

If you have an eating disorder or are omitting insulin for weight control, professional help is available. Eating disorders are serious and can lead to serious complications and even death. Please talk to someone with whom you feel comfortable discussing your feelings.

Ask your provider to recommend a mental health counselor who can work with the other members of your health care team. Your entire team will work with you and your family to help you understand your disorder and how to treat it. It may help you to join a support group. Talking to others who have similar problems can help you feel understood.

> ### Diabulemia
>
> An eating disorder called diabulemia has been found in people with diabetes who use insulin. They intentionally reduce or omit insulin doses in an attempt to lose glucose and calories in the urine. As in other eating disorders, people who omit insulin for weight loss have more episodes of diabetic ketoacidosis and have problems managing their glucose levels.

Weight Loss

The best approach to weight management is a combination of physical activity and healthy eating. No one plan works for everyone. Some people find it easier to take in fewer calories. Some find it easier to work out more. Whatever your approach, a cornerstone will be to develop a lifetime plan of healthy eating and regular exercise.

If you are beginning to use a healthy eating plan, you are probably already on your way to losing weight. Talk to your dietitian about your weight loss goals and set up a realistic plan for achieving those goals. But don't try to lose too much weight too quickly. A steady loss of 1–2 pounds per week is a safe and effective means to reach your goal.

Strategies for Losing Weight

- Follow a nutritionally sound, calorie-restricted meal plan designed to achieve gradual weight loss over several months.

- Decrease portion sizes or eliminate certain foods.

- Set behavioral goals.

- The most important thing you can do to lose weight is to choose weekly or monthly goals and short-term strategies to reach those

→ **Are You Obese?**

You definitely need to lose weight if you are obese. More than 75% of all people with type 2 diabetes either are or were obese at one time or another. But what is obesity? In medical terms, obesity refers to people with a body mass index (BMI) of 30 or above. Your doctor can help you determine your body mass index and a healthy weight for you. Or you can use the chart on p. 147 to figure out what your BMI is.

goals. You will be more likely to succeed if you take it one day at a time.

If you use medications to manage your diabetes, you need to monitor your blood glucose levels as you lose weight. You may be able to reduce the dose of your medication as weight loss lowers your glucose levels.

If you have episodes of hypoglycemia, you will need to treat them with food, and this adds calories and can slow down your weight loss. Call a member of your health care team if you start to have more frequent low blood glucose reactions, so they can advise you on decreasing your medication dose.

A Healthy Weight-Loss Plan

Creating a healthy weight-loss plan is not much different than creating a healthy eating plan for someone who doesn't need to lose weight. You will need to eat fewer calories than you are used to. You will still want to eat a variety of foods that includes fruits, vegetables, and grains.

Portion Control: Another Step toward Weight Loss

- Invest in a set of measuring cups and spoons and a food scale that weighs food in ounces or grams.

- Serve yourself your usual portion. Now measure it. Is it more or less than you expected?

- Weigh a piece of bread or a bagel. One serving of bread is 1 ounce. How does yours compare?

- Try dividing and weighing portions of different meats and seafood before cooking. One serving of meat is 4 ounces raw (3 ounces after cooking).

To use the table, find your height in the left-hand column labeled Height. Move across to your weight. The number at the top of the column is the BMI at that height and weight. Pounds have been rounded off.

BMI	19	20	21	22	23	24	25	26	27	28	29	30	31	32	33	34	35
Height (inches)								Body Weight (pounds)									
58	91	96	100	105	110	115	119	124	129	134	138	143	148	153	158	162	167
59	94	99	104	109	114	119	124	128	133	138	143	148	153	158	163	168	173
60	97	102	107	112	118	123	128	133	138	143	148	153	158	163	168	174	179
61	100	106	111	116	122	127	132	137	143	148	153	158	164	169	174	180	185
62	104	109	115	120	126	131	136	142	147	153	158	164	169	175	180	186	191
63	107	113	118	124	130	135	141	146	152	158	163	169	175	180	186	191	197
64	110	116	122	128	134	140	145	151	157	163	169	174	180	186	192	197	204
65	114	120	126	132	138	144	150	156	162	168	174	180	186	192	198	204	210
66	118	124	130	136	142	148	155	161	167	173	179	186	192	198	204	210	216
67	121	127	134	140	146	153	159	166	172	178	185	191	198	204	211	217	223
68	125	131	138	144	151	158	164	171	177	184	190	197	203	210	216	223	230
69	128	135	142	149	155	162	169	176	182	189	196	203	209	216	223	230	236
70	132	139	146	153	160	167	174	181	188	195	202	209	216	222	229	236	243
71	136	143	150	157	165	172	179	186	193	200	208	215	222	229	236	243	250
72	140	147	154	162	169	177	184	191	199	206	213	221	228	235	242	250	258
73	144	151	159	166	174	182	189	197	204	212	219	227	235	242	250	257	265
74	148	155	163	171	179	186	194	202	210	218	225	233	241	249	256	264	272
75	152	160	168	176	184	192	200	208	216	224	232	240	248	256	264	272	279
76	156	164	172	180	189	197	205	213	221	230	238	246	254	263	271	279	287

- Practicing portion control at home will help you estimate how much of your meal to set aside for a doggy bag when eating out.

As you plan your weight loss program, think ahead about how to maintain your new weight. Many people are successful in losing weight but have a hard time keeping it off. What are the strategies used by people who get it off and keep it off?

Weight Loss and Physical Activity Together

Remember that weight loss and physical activity go hand in hand. Studies show that exercise is an important part of both taking the pounds off and keeping them off. People who keep lost weight off say that daily exercise is an essential part of their lifestyle. They also report eating more fruits and vegetables than before, a healthy habit they hung on to even after they went off their "diet." In the next chapter, you'll learn about how to safely pursue physical activity with diabetes—and have fun, too.

Physical Activity and Exercise

The benefits of regular exercise are undeniable. Physical activity improves overall health, helps protect against heart disease, and fights depression. It can increase your energy level and help you lose or maintain weight.

You'll hear the terms "physical activity" and "exercise" throughout this chapter. You may wonder about the difference between these two expressions.

"Physical activity" refers to any activity that gets you moving and helps you burn energy. It could include the time you spend walking from your car to the office, climbing a flight of stairs, or raking leaves in the yard. "Exercise" generally refers to a specific, planned physical activity such as swimming, biking, or running. Both physical activity and exercise are wonderful ways to get in shape and stay healthy.

Aerobic exercise—the kind that makes you breathe harder—gives your heart and lungs a good workout. It makes your heart pump harder and gets the blood flowing through even your smallest blood vessels. This is important for anyone, especially for people with diabetes, who are at greater risk for heart disease. Physical activity can decrease bad cholesterol and increase good HDL cholesterol.

Aerobic Exercise: Rapid physical activity that stresses the heart, lungs, arms, legs, and the rest of the body; typically causes harder breathing and faster heart rate; examples include dancing, jogging, running, swimming, walking, or bicycling.

Physical activity also clears glucose from your blood, which is a real benefit for people with diabetes. It seems to make muscles and other tissues more sensitive to insulin, so less insulin is needed to move glucose out of the blood and into muscle cells. People with diabetes who use insulin may need to use less insulin or eat more on the days they work out. People with type 2 diabetes who exercise regularly may be able to manage their blood glucose without insulin or diabetes pills or they may just take less medication.

Benefits of Physical Activity and Exercise

- It improves blood flow, muscle tone, and flexibility
- It can help prevent heart disease and other health problems
- Decreases bad LDL cholesterol and increases good HDL cholesterol
- Improves mild to moderate high blood pressure
- It can help you look and feel better
- Physical activity can help you handle stress
- It can help improve your quality of sleep

Getting Started

One of the first things you'll need to do is meet with your health care team. You should have a complete medical history done and a physical examination, if you haven't done so recently. You will want to talk to your team about adjusting your eating plan and your insulin or oral diabetes medication to keep your blood glucose levels on target. Also, you may want to discuss the types of physical activity you're considering.

Make sure that you don't have any health problems that could keep you from exercising safely. If you are going to begin a regular exercise program, you need to be tested for evidence of retinopathy and cardiac disease and any problems with kidney or nerve function. If you have any of these problems, it doesn't necessarily mean you can't exercise, but you may need to treat these problems before you start working out regularly.

Physical Activity Topics to Discuss with Your Doctor

- How can I safely be more active?

- What times of the day are best for me? How long should my session last?

- How hard can I safely exercise?

- Is it more effective to stick to the same routine each time, or can I vary the length and intensity of my workouts?

- How can I monitor how hard I exercise? Should I count my heart rate? What's my target heart rate? How often should I monitor?

- Are there types of physical activity I should avoid?

- Are there symptoms of hypoglycemia or heart disease that I should look out for?

- Any special precautions I should take?

- Do I need to take less insulin or other medications or change my injection site before I work out?

- Do I need to modify my meal plan?

- Will diabetes pills or other medications affect me differently if I work out?

In some cases, your doctor may refer you to an exercise physiologist to do a more thorough examination of your health. An exercise physiologist will do a variety of tests to determine your fitness level, including measuring your strength, flexibility, endurance, and body fat. The physiologist may also give you a treadmill stress test, in which you walk on a treadmill while your blood pressure and heart function are monitored. The test detects how a workout affects your heart activity and blood pressure.

Exercise Physiologist:
A specialist trained in the science of exercise and body conditioning who can help patients plan a safe, effective exercise program.

When You Might Need a Treadmill Stress Test

- If you are about to begin a moderate- or high-intensity exercise program.

- If you are over 35 and have heart disease, cardiovascular risk factors, vascular complications, or nerve disease.

You'll need a referral to see an exercise physiologist if your doctor does not perform the test. Many hospitals and universities have wellness programs for people with diabetes or rehabilitation programs for people who have had heart surgery or stroke. These programs offer stress tests by exercise physiologists and a full range of exercise options to get you started in a medically supervised environment.

Stages of Exercise

The best rule for a safe workout is to listen to your body. You should not have too much fatigue, pain, or shortness of breath. Doing too much too fast can lead to injuries or even life-threatening situations. You'll want to warm up before and cool down after any exercise.

Warm Up

Warming up before you exercise reduces your risk for pulled muscles and other injuries.

- Always warm up for 5–10 minutes before any physical activity.

- Move slowly at first, using low-intensity easy movements to warm up your muscles.

- Gently stretch for 5–10 minutes, without any bouncing. For example, if you plan to walk for exercise, walk at an easy or comfortable pace for 5–10 minutes, then stop and stretch. Resume walking, and gradually increase the pace. Or if you plan on running, you could start out by walking and then stretching. Then try a brisk walk or any easy jog to take you into the aerobic phase.

> **Pace Yourself**
>
> Remember to pace yourself. Listen to what your body is telling you. The key to a safe and effective workout is to find the pace that is right for you.

Aerobic Phase

During the aerobic phase, you rev up, keep your body moving, and get your heart pumping. Your muscles will require more oxygen during this phase. Your heart beats faster and your lungs breathe deeper to deliver oxygen through your small blood vessels to muscles.

If you are starting a new exercise program, you may not be able to sustain aerobic activity for very long. That's okay. Try 5–10 minutes at first, and gradually increase the aerobic phase. An easy workout is better than none at all. Sometimes once you get going, you will feel better and will go the whole way. Eventually, you will be able to go the full 20–30 minutes. Just listen to your body and slow down when you need to.

When to Stop or Slow Down Exercise

- If you start an aerobic workout and feel increasingly worse, slow down.

- If you think you are having a hypoglycemic episode, stop and check your blood glucose.

- If it's not possible to check your blood glucose, treat your symptoms and check your blood glucose as soon as you can.

During aerobic exercise, you should be at your target heart rate. Your health care provider or exercise physiologist can advise you on the target zone that is safe for you. An exercise stress test can help determine your target heart rate. You can also calculate your target heart rate based on your age using the chart on p. 154.

How to Calculate Your Target Heart Rate

- *Resting Heart Rate.* Measure your heart rate while at rest by counting the number of beats your heart makes in 1 full minute the first thing in the morning before you get out of bed. Begin counting the first beat as zero.

- *Maximum Heart Rate.* Determine your maximum heart rate by subtracting your age from 220.

- *Maximum Heart Rate Reserve.* Subtract your resting heart rate from your maximum heart rate.

- *Lower Limit of Heart Rate.* Multiply your maximum heart rate reserve by 0.5 to determine 50% of your heart rate reserve. Add this number to your resting heart rate.

- *Upper Limit of Heart Rate.* Multiply your maximum heart rate reserve by 0.7 to determine 70% of your heart rate reserve. Add this number to your resting heart rate.

- *Voilà.* Your target heart rate range is between your lower and upper limit of your heart rate. Keep in mind that this calculation does not take into account any of your specific health conditions or medications. Check that your health care provider agrees with your calculated target heart rate.

Here's an example of how it works. If you are 40 years old, your maximum heart rate is 180 (220 − 40 = 180). If your resting heart rate is 75, then you would have a heart rate target range of 128–149 (see below), to be working at 50–70% of your aerobic capacity.

	Lower Limit	Upper Limit
HRmax − HRrest	180	180
	− 75	− 75
HRmax reserve	105	105
Limit modifier	x 0.5	x 0.7
%HRreserve	53	74
+ HRrest	+ 75	+ 75
Target HR	128	149

Be careful! This calculation does not take into account any of your specific health conditions or medications. Check that your provider agrees that the target heart rate you've calculated is safe for you.

Cool Down

A cool down allows your heart rate and breathing to slow gradually as your movement slows. No matter how tired you are, never stop exercising abruptly. This will help prevent soreness and muscle cramps.

- Keep your legs and arms moving at a relaxed pace.

- Walk around, step from side to side, walk in place, or try some easy kicks for 5–10 minutes.

- Avoid bending over so far that your head is below your heart.

- Afterward, stretch out your muscles again while they are warm. You should be able to stretch much more freely than in the warmup.

Types of Physical Activity and Exercise

You've probably heard "no pain, no gain" as a mantra of exercise. However, unless you're Rocky Balboa, you can probably find some type of activity that is beneficial and fun. The key is to pick an activity that you enjoy and do it at a pace that is comfortable for you. You'll be more likely to stick with your exercise plan if you take this approach.

There is no single perfect activity. There are some types that burn more calories, some that are particularly helpful for developing strength and flexibility, and others that are especially beneficial for your cardiovascular system.

Walking

Walking is probably the safest and least expensive form of physical activity. It can fit into almost anyone's schedule because it can be integrated into other events. For example, you can squeeze in a walk instead of driving half a mile to the post office. The only investment you need to make is in a comfortable pair of walking shoes. In exchange for this—and extra attention to foot care—you get an exercise that conditions the cardiovascular system, lungs, arms, legs, abdomen, lower back, and buttocks.

Start Walking

• You can benefit your heart and lungs by walking 30 minutes per day, five times a week.

• You don't have to walk 30 minutes all at once. You can get the same benefit by walking 10 minutes three times a day. For example, you might want to park farther from work, so you have a 10-minute walk in the morning and afternoon. You can then add a 10-minute walk at lunchtime, and you have completed your 30 minutes of exercise.

• If you are trying to lose weight, you will need to gradually increase the length of time to 60 minutes of walking per day.

Walking can be especially invigorating if you move at a brisk pace and travel over hilly terrain. Walking is a lifelong activity, and it is a good way to have a more active lifestyle. It can also help you ease into more vigorous exercise if you are newly diagnosed with diabetes or are not used to exercising.

For example, maybe you are a little afraid that exercising too vigorously will throw your blood glucose levels out of whack. After walking for a while, you will develop the confidence, stamina, and fitness level to try other activities.

Walk at a pace that is both enjoyable and invigorating for you. Some find that walking with hand weights makes for a more challenging workout, but before you do that check with your provider or exercise physiologist.

→ Pedometer

A pedometer is an inexpensive tool that counts your steps and may measure the distance and duration of your walk. You might want to purchase one as a motivating and fun way to get moving more.

About 2,000 steps are equal to a mile. Start by wearing your pedometer for two or three days to see how many steps you take with your current level of activity. Then gradually work to increase that to 10,000 steps a day.

Jogging and Running

Jogging or running will give you a more intense workout in less time than walking. But jogging is tougher on your joints and feet because each step pounds the foot with three to five times your body weight. Make sure that you discuss your running or jogging program with your provider before you start. Also, invest in a good pair of running shoes.

Avoid jogging on concrete—it's too hard. Try the track at a nearby school or park instead. Take time to develop your leg and foot muscles to reduce the possibility of injury. If you start to develop any persistent pain, especially in your joints, don't risk further injury. Rest, take a few days off, or try walking instead.

➜ Walking Pace

An experienced walker can walk a mile in 10–12 minutes. A pace of 4 miles per hour or 15 minutes per mile is a good goal to work toward. However, in the beginning, it may take you 30 minutes to walk a mile.

Good Shoes

- Try on shoes in the afternoon, when foot size tends to be a little bigger.
- Wear the socks you plan to wear while working out. You may want to try special socks designed with extra cushioning for exercise. In truth, any good athletic sock that is made with a blend of cotton and synthetic material will provide warmth and cushioning and wick perspiration away.
- Choose shoes that fit well and are comfortable from the first time you put them on. If you have nerve disease or decreased feeling in your feet, you may not be able to trust the way a shoe feels when you try it on. Consult a podiatrist or professional shoe fitter (pedorthist) to get a correct fit.
- Wear new shoes for short periods at first.
- Check your feet for red, irritated areas. You may need extra padding in some areas of the shoe to prevent friction.

Progressing from Walking to Running

- Start walking your normal route or distance.

- Walk for a few minutes and then try jogging.

- Jog for as long as you feel comfortable. If you start to feel winded or uncomfortably out of breath, switch to a brisk walk. Don't stop, but keep walking.

- When you have regained your breath, jog for a little bit. You may find that eventually you will be able to jog the whole distance.

- Of course, you may want to stick to a combination of running and walking or you may want to alternate some days running and some days walking. Do what feels good to you.

Strength Training

Almost anyone can benefit from strength training. Well-toned muscles can help in all your daily activities, whether it's carrying groceries, climbing stairs, or doing laundry. Strength training can also help prevent osteoporosis and build muscle, especially in elderly people. As people get older, they tend to lose muscle mass and tone. Lifting weights—even into your 80s and 90s—can improve strength.

Another benefit of weight training is that well-toned and larger muscles burn more calories, even when you're doing absolutely nothing. So a regular weightlifting program can help you lose fat and manage blood glucose levels in the long run, both during and between workouts.

Safe Strength Training

- Talk to your health care provider before starting any weightlifting routine. Ask them about how the routine might affect any diabetes complications or your blood pressure.

- Always do 5–10 minutes of some sort of aerobic activity, such as walking, jogging, or jumping rope, before lifting weights.

- Don't hold your breath while lifting. Instead, breathe in when lowering weights and breathe out when lifting.

- Work out with a partner or trainer who can help you if something goes wrong.

- Cool down after lifting weights.

- Always allow at least a day's rest between workout sessions or alternate between upper-body training one day and lower-body training the next.

There are several approaches to weight training. Most people combine weight training with aerobic activity for a complete workout. It can be as simple as lifting a small set of hand weights in your living room. Or you may want to join a gym or health club where you will have access to a whole array of weight machines and fitness equipment.

Most weight-training programs involve sets of weightlifting exercises. Each set consists of a series of repetitions. When you first start, perform one set each session. Eventually work your way up to three to six sets each session. As you become stronger you will also find that you can lift more weight. Add more weight, a little at a time, as your muscles become stronger.

Strength Training Goals

- If you just want to increase your endurance, choose a weight that you can lift only 15–20 times. Rest for a few minutes between each set of repetitions, also called reps.

- If you want to build both strength and endurance, choose a weight you can lift only 8–12 times. Rest for a few minutes between sets of reps.

- If you are geared toward competitive weightlifting, you might want to maximize your strength by choosing a weight you can lift only 2–6 times. Rest a few minutes between sets of reps.

Other Types of Physical Activity

Try yoga to increase your flexibility or aerobic classes if you like to dance. Community and senior centers may have equipment available or offer classes that are free or reasonably priced. Health clubs may offer free trial memberships so you can try out machines to see if there are any you would use at home.

You could rekindle your love of tennis, squash, or volleyball. Make an aerobic challenge out of washing the windows or sweeping the deck.

Your choice of activity might also take into account other factors, such as the weather. For example, if it is too hot or cold outside, consider walking inside at a local mall or around your house.

Special Precautions for Physical Activity and Exercise

You'll want to take special care of your feet when you work out, especially if you've had diabetes for a while. Most children and teens with diabetes don't need to think too much about foot complications. Check your feet daily for any red, irritated areas, blisters, corns, calluses, or ingrown toenails. If you detect a problem, don't expect it will go away on its own. Call your diabetes provider or podiatrist right away.

Certain diabetes complications might affect your choice of activity, so always discuss safe options with your doctor.

Exercising with Diabetes Complications

- *Nerve disease (peripheral neuropathy) and numb feet.* You may need to limit weight-bearing activities, such as jogging. Riding a stationary bike or walking may be a safe alternative, but you will need to take extra care to protect your feet.

- *Nerve disease (autonomic neuropathy).* Avoid certain aerobic activities that might affect your heart rate and blood pressure control.

- *Eye disease (proliferative retinopathy).* You could threaten your vision with certain motions involved in weightlifting. Ask your health care provider.

- *High blood pressure or heart disease.* Avoid activities that involve pushing against an immovable object, such as a wall, or isometric exercises, in which you keep your muscles contracted. Walking and swimming are often safe options.

- *Dialysis.* You can benefit from a gradually progressing activity program.

- *Organ transplantation.* Physical activity can be helpful for people who have had an organ transplant. Anti-rejection drugs often cause weight gain and muscle wasting. Try aerobic and strength training once you are given the okay and are ready.

Physical Activity and Your Blood Glucose

Regular physical activity is a great tool for lowering blood glucose levels. Your body uses glucose stored in your muscles and liver for fuel when you start exercising. Then, as these stores diminish, your muscles recruit glucose from your blood. So, during exercise, your blood glucose levels can fall.

If you have type 1 diabetes or you have type 2 diabetes and take insulin and a sulfonylurea, you don't want your blood glucose to get too low. Physical activity puts you at risk for hypoglycemia. Your blood glucose levels can also fall after exercise, as your body replenishes the stores of glucose in your muscles and liver. Even hours after you've stopped exercising, you need to be on the lookout for low blood glucose. Exercise-induced low blood glucose is mostly a problem for people who take insulin or some other diabetes medications.

Monitoring Blood Glucose during Physical Activity and Exercise

- Check your blood glucose level before you work out. If your blood glucose is less than 100 mg/dl, have a snack, such as a piece of fruit or a few crackers.

- Then test 15–30 minutes later. Don't start exercising until your blood glucose is above 100 mg/dl.

> **Overnight Lows after Exercise**
>
> If you exercise in the evening, you may leave yourself vulnerable to hypoglycemia while you sleep. Make sure to check your blood glucose before you go to bed and perhaps overnight.

Physical activity can also affect the action of insulin. The body absorbs insulin differently from one day to the next. Similarly, exercise can affect insulin absorption. Physical activity speeds up how fast the insulin you inject goes to work by increasing the flow of blood through your body. For example, injecting into an arm or leg involved in exercise can speed up insulin absorption. Given insulin's varying effects, make sure to check your blood glucose levels whenever you exercise.

Physical Activity and Type 1 Diabetes

The way that physical activity affects blood glucose levels in people with type 1 diabetes is a bit complicated. People with type 1 diabetes need to take extra care that blood glucose levels do not swing too widely. This includes knowing how your blood glucose responds to different types of activities. You can learn this by monitoring often— before, during, and after working out.

Lows during Exercise

- Blood glucose levels can swing too low if you exercise for long periods or on an empty stomach.

- You'll want to make sure you have taken the right amount of insulin to get the most benefit from your workout. Take the time to learn how to predict your insulin and food needs by monitoring in all types of situations.

- If you suspect a low blood glucose reaction coming on, stop exercising at once. Eat or drink some type of carbohydrate. Don't fool yourself into thinking you can last just 5 minutes longer.

- Always keep some form of glucose handy, just in case you need it while exercising. This can be a soft drink or fruit juice, which will provide sugar and replace water. Or you can use glucose tablets, raisins, or hard candy.

- Blood glucose can drop to lower levels up to 16–24 hours after exercise because the body uses glucose from the blood to replenish muscles. So make sure to monitor your blood glucose before, after, and long after exercise.

Highs during Exercise

- Blood glucose levels can also swing too high if you exercise vigorously or if your body does not have enough available insulin.

- Sometimes during vigorous exercise, the nerves signal the liver to release stored glucose, which can cause a rapid rise in blood glucose. This rise occurs even with moderate intensity if your insulin levels are too low.

- A high blood glucose level can go even higher because of exercise.

- Your body might produce ketones, and ketoacidosis can result. Check your blood glucose before and after exercising to avoid high blood glucose.

You may need to eat during or after exercising if you work out hard or for a long time. Try snacking on something that is low in fat and has 15–30 grams of carbohydrate. If you are really going at it, you may need to repeat this snack based on blood glucose levels.

Before you start exercising you may need to know which way your blood glucose level is heading. This especially true if you are about to start an activity in which you cannot easily stop (such as a long run or windsurfing). Checking your blood glucose in the middle of your activity may not be convenient or possible. Try checking 90 minutes before you start. If your monitoring shows that your blood glucose level is coming down (even if you are still in a safe range), you may want to have a snack to keep it from going any lower.

Insulin and Exercise

You'll read more about insulin in chapter 13, but here are a few things to keep in mind.

- If you have a fixed regimen of insulin taken at specific times of day, try to schedule exercise at about the same time every day.

- If you have a more flexible insulin plan, discuss with your health care provider how to adjust insulin based on your physical activity.

- Avoid exercising when your insulin is peaking, which is usually within 1–2 hours of your last injection of rapid-acting or regular insulin.

- Consider where you inject insulin in your body. Muscles involved in exercise absorb insulin more readily.

Physical Activity and Type 2 Diabetes

Regular physical activity is an important part of the management plan for people with type 2 diabetes. Many people with type 2 diabetes find their blood glucose levels are much easier to manage if they exercise regularly (because their bodies become less resistant to insulin).

Ask your doctor about any diabetes complications before you start an exercise program. However, be assured that almost everyone can benefit from some form of physical activity, as long as it doesn't increase your risk of injury.

Review your meal and exercise plan with your health care team to be sure you are getting enough vitamins and minerals and you are replacing the fluids lost during exercise. If you are on a very-low-calorie diet (fewer than 800 calories a day), your provider may closely monitor your exercise and overall health.

If you use insulin, you'll need to take steps to prevent low blood glucose. See the previous section: "Physical Activity and Type 1 Diabetes." If you take certain diabetes medications, such as exenatide, a sulfonylurea, or meglitinide, hypoglycemia is rare, but it can still occur, so know what to look for and how to treat it. People with type 2 diabetes who manage their diabetes with meal planning and exercise but without medication almost never have hypoglycemia.

> **Start Slow**
>
> Don't start a new strenuous exercise program when you're pregnant, especially if you didn't exercise regularly before pregnancy. Instead, you may be able to start a new program of low-intensity activities such as walking or swimming.

Physical Activity and Pregnancy

Pregnancy is no reason to stop working out if you have type 1 or type 2 diabetes and exercise regularly. However, you may need to lower your workout intensity. You'll need to consult your doctors about the type of workout you want to do. They will consider your medical history and advise you about whether it is safe.

Physical Activity and Gestational Diabetes

- Physical activity lowers your blood glucose level and is considered part of your treatment plan.

- Staying physically fit during your pregnancy will help you prepare for the work of labor and baby care that lies ahead.

- Working out can moderate your weight gain, increase your strength and stamina, and lower your anxiety level.

- In some cases, it may help you avoid or delay using insulin.

Most women use intensive diabetes management during pregnancy to keep blood glucose levels close to normal. If that is your goal, you'll need to be extra watchful for low blood glucose levels caused by exercise. Your glucose level can go very low very quickly. Monitoring is your way to watch out for hypoglycemia. Chances are that you'll already be monitoring frequently during pregnancy. This can help you figure out how exercise affects your blood glucose and when your levels are starting to drop.

Safe Exercise during Pregnancy

- Monitor your blood glucose levels often—before, during, and after exercise.

- Drink plenty of fluids before, during, and after exercise.

- Warm up before and cool down after exercise.

- Keep the strenuous part of your workout to no longer than 15 minutes.

- Keep your heart rate under 140 beats per minute while you exercise (about 23 beats per 10-second pulse count).

- Keep your body temperature under 100°F. Ask your provider if hot tubs or steam rooms are safe.

- Avoid exercises that involve lying on your back after your fourth month of pregnancy, straining or holding your breath, jerky movements, or quick changes in direction.

- Stop exercising if you feel lightheaded, weak, or very out of breath.

- Ask your obstetrician to show you how to feel your uterus for contractions during exercise. These contractions could be a sign you're overdoing it.

Reward Yourself

Sticking to a physical activity program is hard work. Remember to reward yourself for all your efforts. Do an easier workout, such as yoga, one day a week. Don't skip the hot tub or steam room if you really enjoy them after your workout (just ask your doctor if they are safe if you have high blood pressure or are pregnant).

Get Out There

Now that you've learned about the benefits of physical activity and exercise, it's time to get out there and get started. Keep in mind that change doesn't happen overnight. It will take several months for your new, more active lifestyle to become a habit. To keep on track, consider scheduling your workouts like you would any other appointments. You may want to find a workout partner who will keep you motivated when you are tempted to skip a workout.

Set realistic goals including long-term goals, such as walking 30 minutes a day 5 days a week, and short-term goals, such as "I'm going try strength-training today." You may want to do a variety of exercises to keep your interest piqued in working out. Track your progress by recording noticeable changes, such as your energy level, weight, belt size, and changes in medications.

Medications for Type 2 Diabetes

Some people with type 2 diabetes manage their blood glucose with changes to their diet and physical activity. However, many other people need medications, such as pills or insulin, to keep their blood glucose in the target range. There are also new injectable medications for people with type 2 diabetes. Insulin is discussed in detail in the next chapter.

This chapter will outline the basic classes of medications, uses, and warnings and precautions. You will work closely with your health care team to determine which medication is best for you. Keep in mind that the specific medication you and your health care provider choose is less important than making sure you meet your target blood glucose in a safe and effective manner. Medications change, and your needs change too, so remember to discuss any problems or concerns with your provider.

There are six classes of diabetes pills and two classes of injectable medications (not including insulin). Each drug class targets a specific problem in type 2 diabetes. Let's review the blood glucose problems that can occur in type 2 diabetes.

Review of Type 2 Diabetes

In type 2 diabetes, a number of problems can occur with both insulin resistance and insulin sensitivity. Remember, in type 1 diabetes, people eventually don't make any insulin. In type 2 diabetes, people usually make some insulin. However, people with type 2 diabetes may not make enough insulin, may become resistant to insulin, or a combination of both.

Type 2 Diabetes Basics

- Your body, including your muscle and liver, develops insulin resistance.

- Your pancreas doesn't make enough insulin to overcome this insulin resistance.

- Blood glucose stays in the blood because muscles cells won't take in glucose properly.

- Also, the liver releases glucose inappropriately.

Classes of Diabetes Pills

There are several classes of diabetes pills on the market, as well as combination pills. Some are sold under generic and brand names, and others are only sold under brand names. Each class of drug has its own target in the body, as well as its advantages and disadvantages.

Classes of Diabetes Pills

- Alpha-glucosidase inhibitors
- Biguanides (metformin)
- DPP-4 inhibitors
- Meglitinides
- Sulfonylureas
- Thiazolidinediones (TZDs)
- Combination pills

Alpha-Glucosidase Inhibitors

Alpha-glucosidase inhibitors include the medications acarbose and miglitol. Alpha-glucosidase inhibitors have been on the market for over a decade—acarbose first became available in 1996. Alpha -glucosidase inhibitors lower blood glucose by slowing the digestion of carbohydrates after meals. People take them with the first bite of each meal.

Advantages of Alpha-Glucosidase Inhibitors

- Do not tend to cause weight gain.

- Do not usually cause low blood glucose when used alone. When used in combination with another medication, glucose is required to treat low blood glucose, if it should occur.

- Can be effective in people recently diagnosed with diabetes who have trouble with post-meal blood glucose levels.

- Can be used in combination with other pills or insulin.

Side Effects and Precautions for Alpha-Glucosidase Inhibitors

- Gas, bloating, and diarrhea.

- Should not be taken if you have inflammatory bowel disease, other intestinal diseases, or obstructions.

- Can cause low blood glucose when used in combination with other medications and insulin.

- Talk to your doctor for a full list of side effects and cautions.

Biguanides (Metformin)

Biguanides include only one medication—metformin. In addition to regular metformin, there is extended-release metformin and liquid metformin. Metformin has been on the market since 1994. Metformin lowers blood glucose by putting a brake on the liver's release of stored glucose. Metformin may also lower insulin resistance in the muscles.

It is usually taken twice a day, although extended-release metformin is taken once a day.

Advantages of Metformin

- Risk of hypoglycemia is low.

- Can sometimes lower high blood lipid levels and promote weight loss.

- Can be used along with other classes of pills or insulin. Because they work in different ways, metformin and sulfonylureas are often prescribed together.

Side Effects and Precautions for Metformin

- Common, initial side effects include diarrhea, loss of appetite, and nausea. These usually subside over time.

- Lactic acidosis is a rare, but serious side effect.

- You should not take metformin if you have kidney failure or advanced heart failure, liver disease, or low oxygen from respiratory problems. You should stop taking metformin if you are in the hospital or going to have iodinated contrast X-rays.

- If you binge drink, take certain heart medications, or are 80 years of age or older, metformin may not be right for you.

- Talk to your doctor for a full list of side effects and cautions.

- People using metformin for long periods can have difficulty absorbing vitamin B2 and should have their levels checked regularly.

DPP-4 Inhibitors

DPP-4 inhibitors currently include sitagliptin and saxagliptin. The FDA approved sitagliptin in 2006. DPP-4 inhibitors increase insulin secretion and decrease the liver's release of glucose. They do this by preventing the breakdown of a compound called the glucagon-like peptide-1 (GLP-1). DPP-4 inhibitors are taken once a day.

Advantages of DPP-4 Inhibitors

- Do not usually cause low blood glucose when used without insulin or insulin secretagogues, medications that stimulate the beta-cells in the pancreas to release insulin.

- Do not tend to cause weight gain.

- Tend to have a neutral or positive effect on cholesterol levels.

Side Effects and Precautions for DPP-4 Inhibitors

- Occasional stomach discomfort and diarrhea.

- People with kidney problems may need to take lower doses.

- Acute pancreas problems have been reported with sitagliptin. The FDA continues to monitor these cases.

- Talk to your doctor for a full list of side effects and cautions.

Meglitinides

Meglitinides include the medications repaglinide and nateglinide. They lower blood glucose by stimulating the pancreas to release insulin. They may be helpful for people who have problems with high blood glucose immediately after a meal. Meglitinides are taken before each of the three meals.

Advantages of Meglitinides

- Do not cause weight gain.

- When compared to sulfonylureas, meglitinides may reduce the risk of hypoglycemia between meals and at night.

- Can be used with metformin.

Side Effects and Precautions for Meglitinides

- Can cause low blood glucose.

- People with liver problems should not take meglitinides.

• Talk to your doctor for a full list of side effects and cautions.

Sulfonylureas

Different sulfonylureas are prescribed in the United States. Some are available as brand names as well as the following generic name medications: glyburide, glipizide, extended-release glipizide, and glimepiride.

Sulfonylureas lower blood glucose levels by stimulating the pancreas to produce and release more insulin. Sulfonylureas have been used since the 1950s. The effects of sulfonylurea drugs on blood glucose levels were discovered by accident in the 1940s (they were used as antibacterial drugs during World War II). Generally, people take sulfonylureas once or twice a day before meals.

Thiazolidinediones (TZDs)

Thiazolidinediones include pioglitazone and rosiglitazone. The FDA approved them in 1999, although the first TZD, called Rezulin, was taken off the market because it caused liver problems. TZDs lower blood glucose by lowering insulin resistance in the muscles and liver. They also reduce the liver's production of glucose. They are taken once or twice a day.

→ Advantages, Precautions, and Side Effects of Sulfonylureas

Sulfonylureas can cause low blood glucose. You should not take a sulfonylurea if you are pregnant or planning a pregnancy or if you have significant heart, liver, or kidney disease. Each sulfonylurea has different side effects and precautions. Talk to your doctor about the risks and benefits of using specific sulfonylureas.

Advantages of TZDs

• If you also take insulin, you may be able to reduce your insulin dose.

• May lower triglyceride levels and increase HDL cholesterol levels.

Precautions and Side Effects for TZDs

• Can cause weight gain and fluid retention.

• Both pioglitazone and rosiglitazone have been shown to increase the risk of heart failure. Rosiglitazone (brand name Avandia) may increase the risk of heart attacks and death.

- May increase the risk of bone loss and fractures.

- Talk to your doctor for a full list of side effects and cautions.

Combination Pills

There are several combination pills available to people with type 2 diabetes. These can be more effective than a single medication and more convenient than taking three or four pills. Most combination pills combine metformin with other medications. Talk to your doctor about the advantages, disadvantages, and side effects of combination pills.

→ Rosiglitazone (Avandia) and Increased Risks of Heart Attacks

In 2007, the U.S. Food and Drug Administration (FDA) began examining rosiglitazone because research studies indicated that use of the drug might increase the risk of heart attacks and other heart-related conditions, potentially leading to death.

After reviewing the risks, the FDA restricted the use and prescription of rosiglitazone in 2010. Patients already taking rosiglitazone may continue taking the drug if they acknowledge that they are aware of the cardiovascular risks associated with it and if it is working for them. New patients will only be prescribed rosiglitazone if no other treatments have been effective in managing their diabetes. In these cases, the patient's doctor must document and prove that his or her patient would be best served by taking the drug. Further, patients must review safety information that describes the risks that come with taking rosiglitazone.

If you currently take rosiglitazone, consult with your doctor immediately about what you should do. Do not stop taking the medication on your own; uncontrolled blood glucose carries its own risks as well.

Combination Pills

- Metformin and glyburide
- Metformin and rosiglitazone
- Metformin and glipizide
- Metformin and pioglitazone
- Metformin and sitagliptin
- Metformin and repaglinide
- Pioglitazone and glimepiride
- Rosiglitazone and glimepiride

Injectable Medications

In addition to pills, people with type 2 diabetes now have the option of taking injectable medications to lower their blood glucose. There are two classes of injectable medications: glucagon-like peptide-1 agonists (GLP-1 agonists) and amylin agonists.

GLP-1 Agonists

There are two GLP-1 agonists, exenatide (brand name Byetta) and liraglutide (brand name Victoza). Exenatide is used with other diabetes medications to lower blood glucose. It is injected with a pen-like injector. Exenatide received FDA approval in 2005. Liraglutide received FDA approval in 2010. It is injected once daily and prescribed to people with type 2 diabetes. Both GLP-1 agonists work by inducing the pancreas to secrete insulin after meals, suppressing appetite, and slowing emptying of the stomach. Neither drug is insulin.

Advantages of GLP-1 Agonists

- Promotes weight loss by suppressing appetite.
- Can be used with metformin, a sulfonylurea, or a TZD.

Side Effects and Precautions for GLP-1 Agonists

- Some patients taking exenatide have experienced altered kidney function. Your health care provider may monitor you carefully for the development of any kidney problems while taking exenatide.

- During drug testing, the medicine in liraglutide caused rats and mice to develop tumors of the thyroid gland. It is currently not known if liraglutide will cause thyroid tumors or a type of thyroid cancer in people.

- Can cause low blood glucose when taken with sulfonylureas.

- Nausea, vomiting, diarrhea, dizziness, and headaches are common side effects but decrease over time.

- Rare but serious pancreas problems can occur, so talk to your doctor.

- Talk to your doctor for a full list of side effects and cautions.

Amylin Agonists

Pramlintide acetate is an amylin agonist. It is an injectable medication for people with type 2 diabetes (or type 1 diabetes) who already use insulin. In general, the medication suppresses appetite and lowers blood glucose after meals. Pramlintide acetate cannot be mixed with insulin and is available in a separate, prefilled pen or vial and syringe.

Choosing a Diabetes Medication

All diabetes medications must be prescribed by a health care professional. Your diabetes care provider will ask about your lifestyle, physical condition, insurance coverage, and personal preferences before prescribing any particular drug or combination of drugs.

Not everyone with type 2 diabetes will be helped by oral or injectable diabetes medications. Oral medications are more likely to lower blood glucose levels in people who have had diabetes for less than 10 years, who are following a healthy meal plan, and who have some insulin secretion by their pancreas. Some drugs are less effective in people who are very thin.

You may order your prescriptions from your local retail pharmacy. Or mail-ordering your medication may appeal to you. Mail order is convenient, and it could save you money. Often, when you receive your prescriptions by mail order, you pay less for a 90-day supply of the medication.

Tips for Mail-Ordering Medications

• When you start a new drug, first buy it from your local pharmacy. You may need to change the dose or type—or you may stop taking it altogether.

• Don't buy large quantities of a drug until you find the safe, effective dose for you. This is especially true if the medication is new for you.

• Buy drugs you need right away or for only a short period of time from the pharmacy. Use mail-order firms to buy drugs you use regularly.

• Ask about generic drugs. Savings offered by mail-order firms come routinely from substituting generics for brand-name drugs.

• Inspect your prescription drugs carefully when they arrive. If they look different, call your supplier to double check. Get the name of the manufacturer for your records.

• Always follow instructions when taking prescription drugs. If the instructions that arrive with your medications are different from those you remember, call your provider and ask which instructions to follow.

• Check the expiration date on each item that arrives. If you'll need the item in 6 months, make sure it doesn't expire in 2 months. Send back all items with expiration dates that are just around the corner.

Diabetes Medications and Hospitalization

During severe infections, surgery, or hospitalizations, you may need to replace your oral diabetes medications with insulin injections, at least temporarily.

- Check out other mail order and shopping tips for all your diabetes supplies in chapter 7.

General Precautions

All sulfonylurea drugs and, to a lesser extent, meglitinides, increase the risk of hypoglycemia, especially if you skip meals or drink too much alcohol. Be sure to talk to your provider about the symptoms to watch for and any precautions you need to take while on your oral medication. Teach your family and friends the warning signs of hypoglycemia. Together, make a plan of action for dealing with unexpected lows.

Oral agents can have other side effects. If you notice any changes in your behavior or your body after starting a course of oral diabetes medications, be sure to tell your provider. If you have side effects, be sure to call your provider and do not just stop taking your medication.

Drugs in Combination

Your health care provider will know which diabetes medications are safe to use in combination. Keep in mind that clinical trials are required in order to receive FDA approval for drugs to be used in combination. The list of approved drug combinations changes, so ask your doctor if you have any questions.

Drug Interactions

Tell your providers and your pharmacist about all your medications—prescription and over-the-counter. This includes vitamins and herbal products.

Sometimes, drugs that are safe by themselves can interact with each other to cause sickness or conditions that can be difficult to diagnose. Some drugs can lower or raise blood glucose levels. This must be accounted for so that your blood glucose levels don't go too low or stay too high. What looks likes hypoglycemia may really be caused by a drug interaction and can be mistreated.

Many drugs interfere with the way the body uses and eliminates oral diabetes medications. These drugs can indirectly cause high or low glucose levels.

Possible Drug Interactions to Discuss

- Are there any medicines you take when you are coming down with a cold? In bed with the flu?

- Any medications you take when getting a sudden headache?

- Do you take aspirin or thyroid, high blood pressure, or high cholesterol medicines?

In Conclusion

You may find that your blood glucose levels are consistently in the normal range after taking a diabetes medication for a while. That's great news!

Some people may be able to take a lower-dose medication if they have low blood glucose levels on a regular basis while taking the medication. Ask your health care team whether they suggest that you start a trial of taking a lower dose of your pills. During this trial period, keep monitoring your blood glucose and stay in close contact with your health care team.

There is a possibility that diabetes pills won't help you at all. Or they may help, but only for a while. Sulfonylureas stop working for 5–10% of people within a year. Eventually, they stop working for another 50% of people. If oral medications no longer help you reach your target blood glucose levels, adding insulin or other injectable medications to your diabetes care plan is usually the next step.

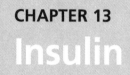

Insulin has come a long way since a young scientist named Frederick Banting first discovered it in the 1920s. Banting had a breakthrough idea to isolate pancreas cells with an odd name—the islets of Langerhans. These oddly named cells are powerhouses for making insulin in the body. Working with several scientists, Banting treated a dog and then a boy with diabetes using extracts from these cells. Medical insulin had arrived.

In 1923, Banting and his mentor J.J.R. Macleod were awarded the Nobel Prize in Medicine—and they shared their prize money with their scientific collaborators. Their discovery paved the way for the first treatments for diabetes and the foundation for technology in development today.

For many years, scientists made insulin by purifying extracts from the pancreases of pigs and cows. Now, almost all insulin is made in laboratories by inserting the human gene for insulin into bacteria, which are rapidly grown and harvested for their insulin. Although it doesn't come directly from people, it is known as human insulin.

Types of Insulin

Each type of insulin has a different action time, a term that describes the length of time it takes to begin acting and how long its effect lasts. The action times of insulin are due to the following three features: onset, peak time, and duration.

Terms for Insulin Action Time

- *Onset:* the length of time it takes for insulin to reach the blood and begin lowering blood glucose levels

- *Peak time:* the time during which insulin is at its maximum strength in lowering blood glucose levels

- *Duration:* the length of time in which insulin continues to lower blood glucose

Your insulin doses should mimic how insulin works naturally in the body. In people without diabetes, the pancreas makes and releases small amounts of insulin throughout the day and night. This is called the basal insulin. The pancreas also releases a short burst of insulin when people without diabetes eat and their blood glucose begins to rise. This is called a bolus of insulin.

Basal Insulin: An intermediate- or long-acting insulin that is absorbed slowly and gives the body a slow, low level of insulin to manage blood glucose levels between meals, thus mimicking the body's natural low-level steady background release of insulin; also called background insulin.

Bolus Insulin: An extra amount of insulin taken to cover an expected rise in blood glucose, often related to a meal or snack.

Long-acting insulins are basal insulins. Rapid-acting and regular insulins are bolus insulins. Intermediate-acting insulin may provide both basal and some bolus effect or, if taken at bedtime, provide mostly a basal effect. Most people with diabetes take both basal and bolus insulin.

Types of Insulin

Long-Acting Insulin Analogs
The two types of long-acting insulin analogs are insulin glargine (brand name Lantus) and insulin detemir

(brand name Levemir). They both start to work 2–4 hours after injection and last up to 24 hours.

Intermediate-Acting Insulin

The one type of intermediate-acting insulin is called NPH, sometimes referred to as isophane insulin (brand names Humulin N, Novolin N). It starts to work 2–4 hours after injection, peaks 4–10 hours after injection, and lasts 10–16 hours. It contains a molecule known as protamine, which slows down how fast the body absorbs insulin. It is also cloudy, rather than clear like other insulin, because it contains suspended insulin crystals.

Regular Insulin

Regular insulin is short acting and must be injected several times throughout the day. It is sold under the brand names Humulin R and Novolin R. It starts to work 30–60 minutes after injection, peaks 2–3 hours after injection, and lasts for 3–6 hours.

Rapid-Acting Insulin Analogs

Rapid-acting insulin analogs go to work almost as fast as naturally produced insulin, so it's easy to use when timing insulin with food. It gives you a lot more flexibility. For example, you can count the carbohydrates in a meal and use rapid-acting insulin to cover the exact amount. The three types of rapid-acting insulin analogs are insulin lispro (brand name Humalog), insulin glulisine (brand name Apidra), and insulin aspart (brand name Novolog). They go to work within 15 minutes, peak 1–2 hours after injection, and last for 3–5 hours.

Premixed (Biphasic) Insulin

You might be advised to mix your NPH insulin and regular or rapid-acting insulins in one injection. You can mix them yourself (discussed later in this chapter). You can also buy premixed insulins. Mixtures of intermediate and regular insulins and intermediate- and rapid-acting insulins come in various combinations that make them more convenient and easier to handle. The intermediate-acting component is sometimes referred to as "protamine."

Premixed insulins can be useful for people with eyesight or dexterity problems that make drawing different amounts of insulin from two different bottles difficult. Common mixtures of insulin are 70% NPH/30% regular, available only in vials (Humalin 70/30 or Novolin 70/30); 50% lispro protamine/50% insulin lispro (Humalog Mix 50/50); 75% lispro protamine/25% lispro (Humalog Mix 75/25); and 70% aspart protamine/30% aspart (Novolog Mix 70/30).

All insulins used for injections have added ingredients that help prevent bacteria and molds from growing in the vial. Intermediate- and long-acting insulins also contain ingredients that prolong their action times. Some people may experience allergic reactions to these ingredients. Talk to your provider if you suspect you might have an allergic reaction to your insulin.

Signs of Allergies to Insulin

- Dents under the skin at injection sites
- Redness at injection sites
- Groups of small bumps, similar to hives
- Swelling at injection sites

Buying and Storing Insulin

Insulin is sold at retail pharmacies in your neighborhood and big-box stores, mail-order pharmacies, and online pharmacies. The National Association of Boards of Pharmacy recommends buying from Internet pharmacies accredited through the Verified Internet Pharmacy Practice Sites program (VIPPS).

➔ Insulin Strength

Insulin strength is now standardized in the United States. In the past, insulin came in different strengths, which made it confusing for consumers. The most common strength is U-100, which means it has 100 units of insulin per milliliter of fluid. Some people may take U-500 if they are insulin resistant or insulin may be diluted for smaller amounts. Keep in mind that some other countries do carry insulin in different strengths, so when you travel you'll always want to bring your own insulin and syringes.

Insulins Used in the United States

Generic Name (U-100, except where noted)	Brand Name	Form	Manufacturer	Cloudy/ Clear	Action Profile		
					Onset	Peak	Duration
Rapid-acting							
insulin glulisine	Apidra	analog	Sanofi-Aventis	clear	15 min	1–1½ hours	3–5 hours
insulin lispro	Humalog	analog	Eli Lilly	clear	15–30 min	½–2½ hours	3–6½ hours
insulin aspart	NovoLog	analog	Novo Nordisk	clear	15 min	½–1 hour	3–5 hours
Regular							
regular	Humulin R, ReliOn (Wal-Mart)	human	Eli Lilly	clear	½–1 hour	2–3 hours	3–6 hours
regular	Novolin R	human	Novo Nordisk	clear	½–1 hour	2–3 hours	3–6 hours
Intermediate-acting							
NPH	Humulin N, ReliOn (Wal-Mart)	human	Eli Lilly	cloudy	2–4 hours	4–10 hours	10–16 hours
NPH	Novolin N	human	Novo Nordisk	cloudy	2–4 hours	4–10 hours	10–16 hours
Long-acting							
insulin detemir	Levemir	analog	Novo Nordisk	clear	45 min to 2 hours (depends on dose)	relatively flat	20–24 hours
insulin glargine	Lantus	analog	Sanofi-Aventis	clear	2–4 hours	relatively flat	20–24 hours

Insulins Used in the United States, *continued*

Generic Name (U-100, except where noted)	Brand Name	Form	Manufacturer	Cloudy/ Clear	Action Profile		
					Onset	Peak	Duration
Mixtures							
70% NPH/30% regular	Humulin 70/30, ReliOn (Wal-Mart)	human	Eli Lilly	cloudy	½–1 hour	dual	10–16 hours
70% NPH/30% regular	Novolin 70/30	human	Novo Nordisk	cloudy	½–1 hour	dual	10–16 hours
50% lispro protamine (NPL)/50% insulin lispro	Humalog Mix 50/50	analog	Eli Lilly	cloudy	15 min	dual	10–16 hours
75% lispro protamine (NPL)/25% lispro	Humalog Mix 75/25	analog	Eli Lilly	cloudy	15 min	dual	10–16 hours
70% aspart protamine/ 30% aspart	NovoLog Mix 70/30	analog	Novo Nordisk	cloudy	15 min	dual	15–18 hours
Less commonly used insulins							
regular (U-500 strength)	Humulin R U-500	human	Eli Lilly	clear	½–1 hour	2–3 hours	up to 24 hours

Your choice of pharmacy will depend on factors such as convenience, price, and insurance coverage. Don't assume that most pharmacies will charge the same price for insulin. Shop around, and keep these tips in mind.

> **Syringe:** A device used to inject medications or other liquids into body tissues. The syringe for insulin has a hollow plastic tube with a plunger inside and a needle on the end.

Tips for Buying Insulin

- Ask about discounts you might receive for buying in larger quantities. Check the expiration dates if you decide to buy in bulk.

- Check with your insurance company or managed-care provider to see whether they offer insulin at a reduced price for preferred pharmacies.

- Consider the convenience of the pharmacy—whether it is close by or delivers. This can be a lifesaver if you are busy, ill, or housebound.

- Consider the manner of your pharmacist. You may put a high priority on having a pharmacist who is easy to talk to or who takes the extra time to answer your questions.

- Ask questions. Check to make sure you have the desired brand and type of insulin. You may want to bring along an empty bottle to make sure you get exactly the same thing each time. Ask the pharmacist if something doesn't look quite right or if you are uncertain.

Ordering your insulin by mail may appeal to you. It is convenient and could save you money if you buy your insulin and other supplies in bulk.

Tips for Mail-Ordering Insulin

- If you live in a warm climate or order during the summer, ask how perishable items such as insulin will ship. Insulin is sensitive to heat, so overnight shipping might be best.

- When you start a new drug, such as insulin, buy it from a pharmacy. You may need a different dose or type—or you may stop taking it altogether.

- Inspect insulin vials carefully for signs of damage or crystallization on the inside vial. Call the mail-order firm immediately to report spoiled insulin.

- Check the expiration date on each item that arrives. If you'll need the item in 6 months, make sure it doesn't expire in 2 months. Send back all items with expiration dates that are just around the corner.

- Check out other mail order and shopping tips for all your diabetes supplies in chapter 7.

Storing Insulin

The basic rule in storing insulin is to keep unopened bottles in the refrigerator and opened bottles at room temperature. Insulin kept at room temperature will be more comfortable to inject than cold insulin. The expiration date on a bottle of insulin applies to bottles that have not been opened and have been stored in the refrigerator.

Tips for Opened Bottles of Insulin

- Throw away bottles that have been opened for a month and kept at room temperature, as the insulin may lose its strength.

- If you go through bottles slowly, write the date you first open the vial on the label, so you know when to toss it.

Avoid Prefilling Syringes

In general, you should draw up your insulin as close as possible to the time you want to take it. For some people, including those with vision problems, it may be helpful to have someone else prefill syringes and store them in the refrigerator for later use. If you feel that you could benefit from prefilling and storing syringes, be sure to consult with a pharmacist or your diabetes educator beforehand.

- Storage guidelines vary from 10 to 28 days for different types of insulin cartridges and pens. Read the label or package or ask your pharmacist if special storage requirements are necessary.

Avoid extreme hot or cold temperatures when storing your insulin. Generally, your insulin should be okay if the temperature is comfortable for you. Storing insulin at temperatures colder than 36°F can cause it to lose potency and clump. Make sure that your insulin doesn't come in contact with ice or become too cold if you carry your insulin in a cooler when travelling. Avoid getting insulin too hot or leaving it in direct sunlight for too long. Insulin can spoil if it gets hotter than 86°F.

Signs of Insulin Defects

- If your blood glucose values are rising, you might consider whether your insulin is working properly.

- Never use insulin if it looks abnormal.

- Regular, lispro (Humalog), aspart (Novolog), and glargine (Lantus) insulins are clear. If you use clear insulin, always check for any floating particles, cloudiness, or changes in color. This could be a sign that your insulin is contaminated or has lost its strength.

- Other types of insulin come as suspensions. This means that the material is not completely dissolved, and you might be able to see solid material floating in liquid. However, it should look uniformly cloudy. If you are using NPH, check that your insulin is free of any large clumps of material.

- Do not use any insulin if you see chunks of material floating around. These changes could mean that crystals or aggregates are forming and the insulin is spoiled or denatured. This can be caused if the insulin bottle is shaken too much or if it is stored at temperatures that are either too hot or too cold.

- If you have been instructed to dilute your insulin, use only the dilutent recommended by the manufacturer. Properly diluted insulin is good for 2–6 weeks when stored in the refrigerator.

- If you find anything wrong with your insulin right after you buy it, return it immediately.

- If the insulin looks different later, try to figure out whether you have handled or stored the insulin the wrong way. If not, talk to your pharmacist about a refund or exchange.

How to Inject Insulin with Syringes and Pens

Some people with diabetes use a needle and syringe or an insulin pen to take their insulin. Once you learn how, this will be a quick and relatively painless task. Injecting insulin today is a lot less painful than it used to be. You can choose micro-fine needles and helpful devices that make injecting with syringes possible for almost anyone. Whether you use an insulin syringe or pen, the goal is to deliver insulin into the fat that lies just beneath your skin.

Syringes

A syringe consists of a needle, barrel, and plunger. You want to consider the needle length and gauge, as well as the barrel size when selecting a syringe.

Syringe needles come in different lengths and gauges. Some people prefer a shorter length needle, particularly if you are thin and want to avoid injecting into your muscle. Syringe lengths are: 1/2", 5/16", and 3/16". Some people also prefer a thinner or higher gauge needle. Thinner needles have higher gauges. For example, a 31-gauge needle is thinner than a 29-gauge needle. You may have to try different needles to see which length and gauge you prefer.

Syringe barrels also come in different sizes. It is important to match the size of the syringe to the dose you'll take with it. You want a syringe that will hold your entire dose of insulin. For example, you would want to use a 50-unit syringe to hold your entire dose of 45 units of insulin. Make sure that you can see the markings on your

Insulin Pen: A device for injecting insulin; it resembles a fountain pen and holds cartridges of insulin; a dial is often used to set the insulin dose; some pens are disposable, and some pens have replaceable cartridges.

Tips for Selecting Syringe Size

If your dose is	Use this syringe
30 units or less, measured in ½ units	3/10 ml/cc (30 units) with ½-unit markings
30 units or less, measured in whole units	3/10 ml/cc (30 units) with 1-unit markings
31–50 units	½ ml/cc (50 units)
51–100 units	1 ml/cc (100 units)

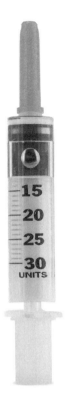

syringe. There are devices that make it easier to read the markings on the syringe, so ask your pharmacist or diabetes educator if such a product will be helpful for you.

Reusing Syringes

Some people have had success reusing syringes. It's up to you whether you want to reuse your syringes. The most important advice is to never share or borrow a used syringe. Most manufacturers of disposable syringes recommend that they be used only once. This is because syringes cannot be guaranteed to be sterile if they are reused. If you have poor personal hygiene, are ill, have open wounds on your hands, or have a low resistance to infection for any reason, you should not reuse syringes. Needles also can become chipped or dull after use. Most needles can be used several times before the tip becomes dull. Using a dull tip is more painful than using a new, sharp needle.

A 30-unit syringe with 1-unit markings.

Reusing syringes can save you money and create less medical waste to litter the environment. There is no evidence that you are more likely to become infected with something, as long as you follow some simple guidelines.

How to Reuse a Syringe

1. Carefully recap the syringe when you are finished using it.

2. Don't let the needle touch anything but clean skin and your insulin bottle stopper. If it touches anything else, don't reuse it.

3. Store the used syringe at room temperature.

4. There will always be a tiny, even invisible, amount of insulin left in the syringe. If you use glargine insulin (Lantus), be careful not to use the glargine (Lantus) syringe for other insulins.

5. Do not reuse a needle that is bent or dull because this can make the injection more painful. However, just because an injection is painful doesn't mean the needle is dull. You may have hit a nerve ending.

6. Do not clean the needle with alcohol. This removes some of the coating that makes the needle go more smoothly into your skin.

7. When you're finished with a syringe, dispose of it properly according to the laws in your area. Contact the city or county sanitation department for information.

Syringe Disposal

How you get rid of your syringe can affect anyone who might come in contact with your trash. This includes the members of your family, neighbors, your trash collector, and people using beaches and other public areas. So it's important that you do it safely.

Never toss a used syringe directly into a trashcan. Syringes and lancets and any other material that touches human blood is considered medical waste and must be handled carefully. Before deciding what you will do, you might want to check with your local health department. Some towns and counties have special laws or rules for getting rid of medical waste and may offer safe alternatives.

When traveling, if possible, bring your unused syringes home. Pack them in a heavy-duty container, such as a hard plastic pencil box. There are products specifically designed to clip and hold syringes for disposal. Check *Diabetes Forecast's* annual Consumer Guide for these products.

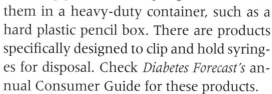
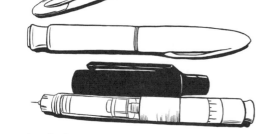

Insulin Pens.

Insulin Pens

An insulin pen looks like an ink pen. Instead of a writing tip, it has a disposable needle, and instead of an ink cartridge, there is an insulin cartridge. Always use a new needle with an insulin pen.

Insulin pens are popular because they are convenient and deliver accurate doses. You don't have to worry about filling syringes or carrying them with you when you are away from home. However, although premixed insulin is available in pens, you cannot mix insulin in pens yourself.

You can buy a prefilled pen that you throw away once the insulin cartridge is empty. A variety of insulins are available in pens. You decide the number of units you want, set the injector for that dose, stick the needle in your skin, and inject the insulin. This makes them useful for multiple-dose schedules. Pen injectors are conveniently portable because you don't have to carry around a bottle of insulin. Some are designed to make it easier for people with visual or dexterity problems to give injections.

How to Prepare Insulin Injections

Your diabetes educator or provider will explain and show you how to prepare insulin for injection. You can use a syringe or insulin pen, whichever you prefer.

Equipment

- Syringe and needle, or insulin pen
- Insulin bottle
- Alcohol swab

Instructions

1. Wash your hands.

2. Choose injection site and cleanse with alcohol swab. Do not inject insulin into a callused or hard, lumpy site. Rotate sites as instructed by your health care professional.

3. Check the bottle of insulin to make sure you are using the right kind. For an insulin pen, screw on the needle. Use a new needle every time with insulin pens.

4. For cloudy insulin, gently roll the bottle of insulin between your palms or rotate the pen slowly from end to end to mix. Make sure it is mixed thoroughly. Shaking the bottle can cause air bubbles. Do not use if it has clumps or particles in it.

5. Clean insulin syringe with alcohol swab. For an insulin syringe, hold the syringe with the needle pointing up and draw air into it by pulling down on the plunger to the amount that matches the dose to be given.

6. For an insulin pen, perform an "air shot" by pushing 1–2 drops of insulin through the needle. Set the insulin dose according to manufacturer's directions. Proceed to instructions on injecting insulin.

7. Remove the cap from the needle. Hold the insulin bottle steady on a tabletop and push the needle straight down into the rubber top on the bottle. Push down on the plunger to inject the air into the insulin bottle.

8. Keep the needle in and turn the bottle and syringe upside down so that the insulin is on top. Pull the correct amount of insulin into the syringe by pulling back on the plunger.

9. Check for air bubbles on the inside of the syringe. If you see air bubbles, keep the bottle upside down and push the plunger up so the insulin goes back into the bottle.

10. Pull down on the plunger to refill the syringe. If necessary, empty and refill until all air bubbles in the syringe are gone.

11. Remove the needle from the bottle after checking again that you have the correct dose.

12. If you need to set the syringe down before giving your injection, recap the needle, and lay it on its side. Make sure the needle doesn't touch anything.

How to Inject Insulin

Your diabetes educator or health care provider will explain how to inject insulin. Whether it's your first time or you're a seasoned pro, it's always a good idea to review the basics. It often helps to go over your injection technique with your health care team. Trying to relax before injections can help ease the discomfort because tense muscles can make the injection hurt.

Keeping your injection site clean will reduce the risk of developing an infection. You don't have to use alcohol to clean your skin before injecting the needle. Soap and water works fine. If you use alcohol before injections, make sure the alcohol dries first or the injection may sting.

Equipment

• Prepared syringe or insulin pen.

• Cotton ball or tissue, if desired, to cover the injection site for a few seconds after the injection.

• Alcohol or soap and water to clean injection site.

Instructions

1. Choose an injection site with fatty tissue, such as the abdomen (except for a 2-inch circle around the belly button), the back of the arm, the top and outside of the thigh, or the buttocks. Make sure the site and your hands are clean and dry.

2. Gently pinch a fold of skin between your thumb and forefinger, and inject straight in if you have a normal amount of fatty tissue. For a thin adult or a small child, you may need to inject at a 45-degree angle. With smaller needles, this may not be necessary.

3. Push the needle through the skin as quickly as you can.

4. Relax the pinch and push the plunger in to inject the insulin.

5. Pull the needle straight out.

6. Cover the injection site with your finger, a cotton ball, or gauze, and apply slight pressure for 5–8 seconds. Do not rub. Rubbing may spread the insulin too quickly or irritate your skin.

7. Write down how much insulin you injected and the time of day.

Mixing Insulins
If you're mixing insulins on your own, you'll mix them in a syringe. Never mix insulins without approval from your provider. Usually, only

mix insulins made by the same company. For instance, don't mix regular insulin made by Lilly with NPH made by Novo Nordisk. Never mix long-acting insulin with regular insulin, which can lead to unpredictable results. Insulin glargine (Lantus) insulin has a lower pH level and cannot be mixed in the same syringe with any other insulin. Insulin detemir (Levemir) should not be mixed as well.

How to Mix Insulin

Equipment

- Syringe, the correct size for the total units of insulin
- Bottles of insulin
- Alcohol swab

Instructions

1. Be clear on the amounts of each insulin and the total units you want. To find the total units, add the number of units of rapid-acting or regular insulin to the number of units of intermediate- or long-acting insulin.

2. Wash your hands.

3. Clean vial tops with alcohol swab.

4. For cloudy insulin, gently roll the bottle of insulin slowly between your palms to mix. Make sure it is mixed thoroughly. Do not use if it has clumps or particles in it. Shaking the bottle can cause air bubbles.

5. Draw air into the syringe equal to the intermediate dose.

6. Hold the bottle steady on the table and put the needle through the rubber stopper. Inject the air into that bottle. Take out the needle without drawing up any insulin.

7. Draw air into the syringe equal to the dose of rapid-acting or regular insulin and inject the air into the bottle of rapid-acting or regular insulin.

8. With the needle still in the rapid-acting or regular insulin bottle, turn it upside down so that insulin covers the tip of the needle.

9. Pull the correct amount of insulin into the syringe by pulling back on the plunger. Check for air bubbles in the syringe. If you see air bubbles, keep the bottle upside down and push the plunger up so the insulin goes back into the bottle. If necessary, empty and refill until all air bubbles in the syringe are gone. Remove the syringe.

10. Insert the syringe into the bottle of intermediate-acting insulin. (You have already injected the right amount of air into this bottle.) Turn the bottle upside down, so that the insulin covers the tip of the needle.

11. Slowly pull the plunger down to draw in the right dosage of intermediate-acting insulin. This will be the total units of the regular or rapid-acting and intermediate-acting insulins.

12. Do not return any extra insulin back to this bottle. The insulin in the syringe is now a mixture. Double check for the correct total amount of insulin. If incorrect, discard the insulin in the syringe and start over.

13. Take the needle out of the bottle, recap the needle, and lay the syringe carefully on a table without letting it touch anything.

14. Choose site for injection, cleanse site. (See illustration on p. 200.)

Injection Aids

Talk to your doctor or your diabetes educator if you are having problems with any aspect of insulin injections. Be sure to let them know if the injections are causing you a great deal of stress or anxiety, too. Products are available to make injections easier, such as insertion aids, insulin infusers, and jet injectors. Ask your educator if you can try out some of these insulin-injection aids before you buy anything so that you don't waste your money.

An insertion aid is an automatic injector that inserts a needle into your skin. Some automatically release the insulin when the needle hits your skin. With others, you have to press the plunger on the syringe. An automatic injector can be useful if you have arthritis or other problems that make it difficult to hold a syringe steadily. If you cringe at the thought of injecting yourself or don't like the sight of needles, an automatic injector may be for you.

How to Mix Insulin

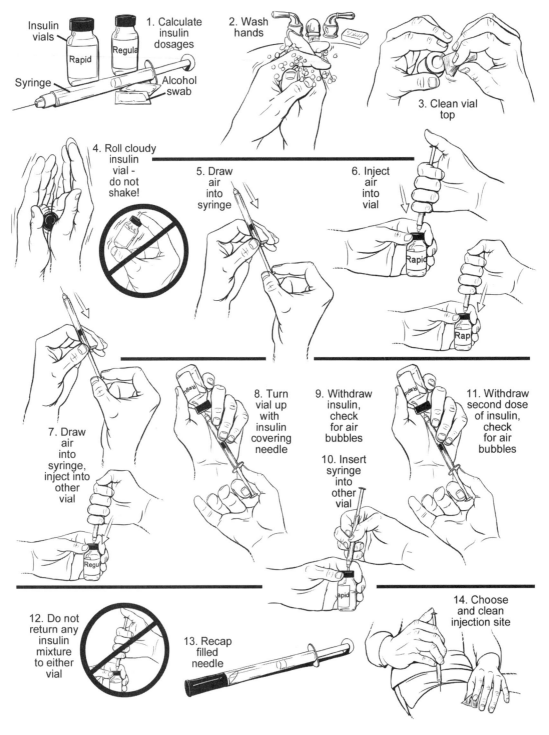

Insulin vials

Rapid
Regular

Syringe

Alcohol swab

1. Calculate insulin dosages

2. Wash hands

3. Clean vial top

4. Roll cloudy insulin vial - do not shake!

5. Draw air into syringe

6. Inject air into vial

Rapid

Rap

7. Draw air into syringe, inject into other vial

Regu

8. Turn vial up with insulin covering needle

9. Withdraw insulin, check for air bubbles

10. Insert syringe into other vial

apid

11. Withdraw second dose of insulin, check for air bubbles

12. Do not return any insulin mixture to either vial

13. Recap filled needle

14. Choose and clean injection site

An insulin infuser reduces the number of needle sticks per day. You insert a needle, called a catheter, under your skin that stays in place for 3 days. Then you inject insulin into the catheter rather than your skin. You'll need to ask your provider for training in using an insulin infuser because these devices increase the risk of infections.

Jet injectors push the insulin out so fast that it acts like a liquid needle, passing insulin directly through the skin. If you fear needles or take several injections each day, a jet injector may be an option for you.

Several products are available that make it easier for people who are visually impaired to inject insulin. Some of these aids only fit certain brands of syringes. Make sure that any aids you purchase will fit the equipment you already have.

Examples of Visual Aids for Injecting

- Dose gauges help you measure your insulin accurately—even mixed doses. Some are designed to click with every 1 or 2 units of insulin you measure. Others have Braille or raised numbers.

- Needle guides and vial stabilizers help you insert the needle into the insulin vial correctly. Some of these will also let you set a desired dose level.

- Syringe magnifiers can enlarge the measure marks on a syringe barrel. One model combines a magnifier with the needle guide and vial stabilizer. Another clips around the syringe and magnifies the scale.

Injection Sites

It is usually recommended that you rotate your injection site in order to avoid developing problems in and under your skin. You can inject insulin into your abdomen, but you can use other sites as well. Insulin works best when injected into a layer of fat under the skin, above the muscle tissue. Several areas of the body have enough fat tissue under the skin for insulin injection.

Typical Injection Sites

- The abdomen, except for a 2-inch circle around the belly button, is the most common site.

- The top and outer thighs are also common. This is best for when you are sitting.

- The backs of the upper arms, the hips, and the buttocks also work well.

- Some people, especially those with a large body size, have other options. For example, the lower back can also be a good injection site, as long as there is enough fat under the skin.

Rotating Injection Sites

Wherever you choose to inject, you will want to inject at different sites within that area so you don't develop problems in and under the skin. You may find that it works best to rotate injection sites within one general area, such as the abdomen, rather than to rotate randomly among sites in different areas of the body. However, some people achieve consistent results by doing all morning injections at one site, such as the buttocks, and all evening injections at a second site, such as the abdomen. Injecting in the same general area makes your response to insulin more predictable because insulin is absorbed at different rates in different body areas. Rotating among random sites could lead to large fluctuations in blood glucose levels.

Once you have used each injection site within a body area, you can start over in the same body area. There are many opinions on the best way to rotate injection sites. Talk to your diabetes educator about the best method for you.

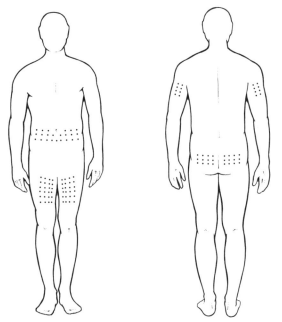

Injection Sites.

Tips for Selecting Insulin Sites

- Divide the body area into injection sites about the size of a quarter. Try to make each new injection at least a finger-width away from your last shot.

- You may need to create a way to remember where that last site was. For example, you might inject all of your morning shots on the right side and all of your evening shots on the left.

- When injecting into the arm, use the outer back area of the upper arm, where there is fatty tissue. Avoid the deltoid muscle, the large triangular muscle that covers the shoulder joint. Don't inject into muscle tissue anywhere in the body.

- When injecting in the thighs, use the top and outside areas. If you inject in the inner thighs, rubbing between the legs may make the injection site sore. Also avoid the bony area above the knees, where there isn't much fat.

- Inject anywhere there is fat on the abdomen, except for the 2-inch space around the belly button. This area has tough tissue that causes erratic insulin absorption.

- Avoid injecting too close to moles or scar tissue anywhere on the body.

Differences in Insulin Absorption

Most insulins are absorbed most quickly (and at the most consistent speed) when injected into the abdomen, more slowly when injected into the arms, and slower still when injected into the thighs and buttocks. After you have been injecting insulin into your abdomen for several weeks, you probably know how long it will take for the insulin to take effect. This predictability can help you better manage your blood glucose.

If you were to suddenly switch to injecting insulin into your thigh, you might experience a different response. You might find that it takes longer for your insulin to take effect. Then it would be more difficult to meet your target blood glucose levels without adjusting when you inject.

→ **A General Rule for Insulin Absorption**

In general, anything that increases the blood flow to an area increases insulin absorption.

Other factors, such as body temperature, food, physical activity, and level of stress, affect your body's response to insulin. Your response to insulin might even be the opposite of what you might expect, based on where you inject. For example, playing soccer for 2 hours may cause your insulin to be absorbed more quickly than usual so that your blood glucose level isn't where you expect it to be.

So what can you do? Routinely check your blood glucose level. It is the only way to make sure you are having the response you had planned. Then you'll know if your site rotation plan is working for you.

Physical Activity and Insulin Absorption

- Strenuous use of muscles near an injection site can make the insulin act more rapidly than normal because of the increased flow of blood to the exercising muscles.

- You might want to think about the insulin absorption rate if you notice that your insulin is peaking faster than expected when you exercise.

- In general, it's a good idea to avoid strenuous activity during the peak action times of your insulin. Insulin plus exercise can lead to hypoglycemia.

- When you work out, you have to decide whether to eat more or take less insulin because both physical activity and insulin decrease the amount of glucose in the blood.

- Frequent blood glucose monitoring will help you figure out these ups and downs in blood glucose and how to keep things in balance.

Skin Problems and Injection Sites

The main skin problems that can occur at insulin injection sites are lipoatrophy and lipohypertrophy. By rotating injection sites, you can avoid some of these problems.

Lipoatrophy is probably caused by an immune reaction, although its exact cause is not known. When lipoatrophy occurs, your body is responding to insulin as a "foreign" substance. This problem is not as common with human insulin or insulin analogs. Make sure you use highly purified insulin, preferably human. Injection site rotation may also help.

Lipohypertrophy is not an immune reaction, but you will need to change injection sites to avoid this. When the same sites are used over and over again, fat deposits can accumulate in the area. You may be reluctant to make changes to your insulin regimen because the injections are less painful in these areas. If you have lipohypertrophy, this may be because it can numb the affected area. On the other hand, injections can sometimes be more painful in these areas. The abnormal cell growth can limit the absorption of your insulin. Do not inject into the lumps. Insulin action can be affected because it is unable to move through the tissue. Inject away from the lumps, and remember to rotate injection sites. Ask a member of your health care team to check your injection sites periodically.

Lipoatrophy: In diabetes, fatty tissue under the skin disappears, causing dents in the skin at the injection site.

Lipohypertrophy: An overgrowth of cells, usually fat cells, that makes the skin look lumpy; can look similar to scar tissue.

Insulin Pumps

Insulin pumps are small, programmable devices that deliver a steady, measured amount of insulin under your skin. They are smaller and better than ever. They can be a great choice for people who want an alternative to multiple daily injections of insulin.

Parts of the Insulin Pump

- Most pumps consist of a refillable cartridge, which holds the insulin, and a miniature computer that allows the user

Insulin Pump: An insulin-delivering device about the size of a deck of cards that can be worn on a belt, kept in a pocket, or worn on your skin. It carries a reservoir of insulin connected to narrow, flexible plastic tubing (cannula) that is inserted just under the skin. Users set the pump to give a basal amount of insulin continuously throughout the day. Pumps also release bolus insulin to cover meals and at times when blood glucose levels are high, based on programming done by users.

> **→ Monitoring and Insulin Pumps**
>
> Pumps cannot automatically sense your body's need for insulin. They don't adjust by themselves. You still need to take blood glucose readings throughout the day.

to program the release of insulin. Wireless, disposable pumps contain insulin but are not refillable.

- Some pumps use an infusion set to deliver insulin. The infusion set includes a cannula (a needle or small tube) that is inserted beneath your skin. It has an adhesive to keep the infusion set in place for a few days. It also has small, flexible tubing to connect the infusion set to the pump.

- Several insulin pump systems don't have tubing. Instead, they are made up of two items—a small, plastic insulin holder (pod) that attaches directly to the skin and a wireless, handheld device that you use to manage the release of insulin.

Basics of Insulin Pumps

The Device
This is the insulin pump itself and is like a small computer. The device beeps if the tubing or cannula becomes clogged. It lets you know when the batteries are low. It has dosage limits to stop an accidental overdose. You can program it to change the amount of insulin to deliver in order to match your needs.

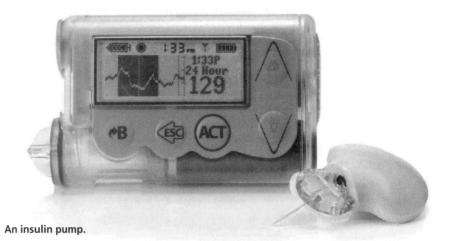

An insulin pump.

Insulin Reservoir

For most pumps, insulin is pumped from a filled syringe or cartridge inside the pump through thin plastic tubing to a needle or catheter inserted under the skin. Depending on your insulin needs, the reservoir can hold up to a 3-day supply of insulin.

Infusion Sets

The tubing comes in different lengths, but it is long enough to allow plenty of slack for normal body movement.

Basal Insulin

The insulin pump sends a continuous flow of insulin that trickles through the tube into the infusion set site at a slow, steady (basal) rate, day and night. The basal rate for pumps can be adjusted from 0.1 to 10 units per hour, depending on your needs.

Bolus Insulin

Before you eat, you push a button to deliver a desired amount of insulin, called a bolus. You can adjust the size of the bolus, depending on how much carbohydrate is in your meal. At the same time, you can deliver an extra amount of insulin to correct for higher-than-normal glucose levels, if they are present. Some new pumps ask how much carbohydrate you will eat and what your current blood glucose level is to help you calculate how much bolus insulin you'll need. Delivering a bolus of insulin is just like injecting your premeal shot of insulin when you take multiple injections—without the shot! Usually, you won't have to take an extra bolus when you eat between meals, unless the snack is large.

Choosing an Insulin Pump

A major advantage of a pump is that you don't have to stop what you're doing to fill a syringe or to prepare an insulin pen. Your insulin is delivered at the push of a button. You can do this anywhere and at any time. Pumps are also precise. You can set them to pump out as little as one-tenth of a unit (0.1 unit) of insulin per hour.

> → **Pumps Take Commitment**
>
> One of the most important factors is your level of commitment to this therapy. Using an insulin pump does take work—especially when you first begin using one—but many people find that the added flexibility and improved control are worth the extra effort.

Some Reasons for Choosing an Insulin Pump

- You're planning a pregnancy and want the tightest blood glucose control possible.

- You work odd hours at your job or don't have a regular shift, and it's difficult to adjust to a new injection schedule every weekend.

- You have had unwanted swings in blood glucose when injecting intermediate- or long-acting glucose, and you'd like to keep your blood glucose in check.

- You want an insulin plan that adapts to day-to-day changes in your lifestyle. Making a list of personal advantages and disadvantages may help you decide.

Features of Insulin Pumps

There are several insulin pumps on the market today. You can find a list of the available insulin pumps in *Diabetes Forecast's* annual Consumer Guide. Your doctor or diabetes educator may prefer one brand over another. Ask for his or her thoughts on each model. Your best bet may be to talk to other people who use pumps. Find out what they like and don't like about each model.

Features of Insulin Pumps

- Is it waterproof? Some models are waterproof and can be submerged for up to 30 minutes. Other models are splash proof or water resistant. Check to see if your pump meets your personal needs.

- Can you adjust the basal rate for different times of day? Your pump can alter the rate dozens of times a day. For example, your basal needs might be greater from 3 a.m. to 7 a.m. than your needs during the rest of the day.

- All pump manufacturers offer a 24-hour toll-free support number. You will want to talk to service people about problems when you suspect the pump isn't working correctly.

- What kind of warranty does the manufacturer offer?

- How often do you have to change the batteries? How easy are the batteries to find, and how expensive are they? Batteries usually last 2–4 months.

- Do you want a pump that will help you calculate doses based on your blood glucose level and carbohydrate intake?

- Some insulin pumps have multiple, programmable features, including alerts. Some also have larger memories than others to store boluses, insulin totals, and alerts.

- Does your pump include software that charts your progress or that you can download to your computer?

- Do you want a pump that uses dual-wave or square-wave bolus, which helps manage meals spread out over time or higher-fat meals.

- Some pumps are designed to work together with blood glucose monitors or continuous glucose monitors. For example, you may be able to program targets for correction, insulin action time, and insulin sensitivity factors. If used correctly, these features can help users do the math so they do not provide too much or too little insulin. You'll want to research your options.

Cost of Insulin Pumps

Insulin pumps can be expensive. But with a prescription and some persistence, most insurance companies can be convinced to pay for all or part of it. Monthly maintenance can run $300 or more, including insulin, infusion sets, and blood testing supplies. If your insurance company will cover them, you're all set. But some insurance companies won't pay the start-up or maintenance costs of the pump.

Getting Your Insurance to Pay for an Insulin Pump

- Pump companies have billing departments that have relationships with most insurance companies. A pump company can contact your insurance company to help you get coverage.

- Your provider can be your most convincing advocate if he or she has made an evaluation that you would do well with an insulin pump. Your health care provider may have to write a letter to your insurer. Pump companies can help prepare standardized letters to prepare for a provider's signature.

- Ask your diabetes educator to write to your insurance company as well.

- Work on writing effective, informative letters. All letters should stress how lower glucose levels can mean fewer and less severe diabetes complications in the long run, which is also less expensive for the insurance company in the long run.

- Keep asking! Keep in mind that it took many years, much research, and lots of people asking to convince insurance companies to pay for other therapeutic measures, such as prescription footwear, that have long-term health benefits.

Using an Insulin Pump

Once you've decided to go ahead with an insulin pump, your pump company will provide you with an experienced pump trainer who will teach you how to use the device properly. This will include both selecting an insertion site for the pump and programming the pump to deliver the proper amount of insulin. You will also learn what to do in an emergency and how to obtain supplies.

Insertion Sites
Insertion sites are any sites you normally use for injection. Some people choose the abdomen for insulin delivery. This area is convenient to use and gives a reliable, uniform absorption of insulin.

How you insert the insulin needle will be different for different brands of infusion sets. With some infusion sets, you use a needle to insert a catheter and then remove the needle, leaving the soft catheter under your skin. With other sets, you insert a short needle. With the pod, you insert a catheter under the skin.

You don't have to worry that it will hurt when you exercise or if someone bumps into your pump, infusion area, or pod. The needle or catheter should be comfortable at all times. If you see any redness or swelling at the infusion site, remove the needle or catheter right away and find a new infusion site. Discuss persistent problems (lasting longer than 24 hours) with your health care team.

> **Pumps Are Easy to Remove**
>
> Some pumps are easy to remove temporarily because, after connecting the tubing, you can leave part of the infusion set (the needle or flexible catheter) in place. You reattach only the pump and the tubing. Some infusion sets even have a quick-release feature.

Changing the Insertion Site

- Every 1–3 days, you'll need to replace the infusion set and move to a new insertion site. This helps you avoid infection at the insertion site or a clog in the infusion set.

- Place the new insertion site at least 1 inch away from the last insertion site on the abdomen. Just like with syringes, you need to avoid inserting the needle into scar tissue or moles and use a site-rotation schedule.

- Using the same insertion site too often or for too long can cause the same skin problems (lipoatrophy, lipohypertrophy) that develop when you don't rotate your syringe injection sites. Scarring can occur.

- Check your injection site every day to make sure insulin is not leaking out.

Programming and Wearing a Pump

A big advantage to using a pump is that you will have flexible insulin coverage for meals and snacks. You will have to spend some time at the beginning finding the best basal rates for you. You may need to adjust the basal rate during different times of the day. You will also need to figure out how big a bolus you will need for each meal.

Most people learn how to estimate the number of grams of carbohydrate in meals so they can take the needed number of insulin units. This may help you even out your after-meal blood glucose levels. You'll avoid having big changes in blood glucose levels throughout the day. Eventually, this will lead to a more flexible eating schedule.

Calculating Basal and Bolus Insulin

- Your diabetes care provider or educator will help you calculate your basal and bolus insulin doses.

- Most people learn a matching rule for giving a bolus according to the amount of carbohydrate that they would like to eat, which may be different at each meal, according to time of day.

- The total basal dose over a day is some percentage of the total daily insulin dose that you've been injecting, perhaps 40–50%.

- The other 50–60% of your daily insulin dose is divided into the before-meal bolus doses, most of it at breakfast and dinner and the remainder at lunch and bedtime.

- You will need to know how these doses were chosen, so you can learn to adjust them for fine-tuning.

➔ Unhooking the Pump

You may want to set a temporary basal level or unhook your pump during sex or other physical activities that can lower blood glucose level. How long you can keep the pump off without an injection depends on how active you are when the pump is off. Keep in mind that removing or suspending your pump for long periods can lead to clogs in the cannula when you try to start up again.

People wear the pump almost all the time. If you take the pump off, you'll need to go back to injecting insulin with either an insulin pen or a syringe and needle. However, it is possible for you to take the pump off temporarily, but not for more than 1–2 hours. Your blood glucose levels will rise quickly because you don't have any insulin. Through experience and testing, you will figure out how long you can keep the pump off before you need to put it back on or take an insulin injection.

Like all things that are worthwhile, using a pump successfully takes practice. You will most likely have problems here and there.

Unexplained High Blood Glucose on the Insulin Pump

Mysterious high blood glucose levels are some of the most common problems for people on an insulin pump. Consider these possibilities when troubleshooting your pump.

- *Insulin:* Is it expired? Has it been exposed to extreme heat or cold? Does it look clumped or is it filled with particles? Is the vial nearly empty? Have you used it for more than 1 month?

- *Insertion site:* Have you placed the catheter in or near a scar or mole or near your beltline or any other area where there's friction from clothing? Does the site hurt? Is it red or swollen? An infection could delay the absorption of insulin.

- *Infusion set or pod:* Did the needle come out? Is insulin leaking around the infusion site? Is there blood or air in the infusion line? Is there a kink in the line? Did the line come loose from the pump? Has the infusion set been in place for more than 2 days? Think about changing the infusion line.

- *Insulin pump:* Is the basal rate set correctly? Has the battery run down? Was the insulin cartridge placed correctly? Is it empty? Was the pump primed with insulin when a fresh cartridge was put in? Is the pump working correctly?

- *Alarms:* High blood glucose occurs quickly when clogged or kinked tubing or dislodged pods stop the flow of insulin and pressure builds up in the infusion line. Your pump will sound an alarm if this happens.

Insulin Plans

How often should you use insulin? There is no answer that is right for all people at all times. Different plans suit different people, depending on how easily managed your blood glucose levels are and how well you understand the way different foods, physical activity, and stress affect your blood glucose levels.

Most people with type 1 diabetes will have to start with multiple daily injections of insulin. This section begins by describing multiple daily injection plans that are appropriate for people with type 1 diabetes and some people with type 2 diabetes. Toward the end of this section, you will find less intensified insulin plans that are appropriate for some people with type 2 diabetes. First, let's review some of the basics.

Insulin and Type 1 Diabetes

- Most people with type 1 diabetes require multiple daily injections of insulin or an insulin pump and frequent blood glucose monitoring.

- The pancreas no longer secretes insulin, so the goal of insulin therapy is to mimic a normal pancreas as closely as possible.

Insulin and Type 2 Diabetes

- In some people, not enough insulin is produced in relation to how much is needed by the body. Insulin is often needed along with meal planning and exercise.

- In addition, the cells in the body resist the action of the insulin that is produced. Diet and exercise and oral diabetes medications alone or with insulin may be needed.

- Therapies for type 2 diabetes may have to take into account both lack of insulin and resistance to insulin. Some people may be able to manage blood glucose by changing their eating and exercise habits. Others will need oral diabetes medication, and still others will need insulin in addition to diet and exercise.

Insulin and Gestational Diabetes

- Some women manage the high blood glucose levels caused by insulin resistance without insulin therapy. Others need the help of insulin.

Most insulin plans try to mimic a normal pancreas. A pancreas puts out a steady stream of insulin (a basal dose) day and night. It also se-

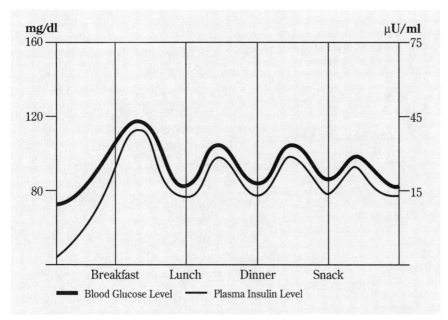

Typical changes in glucose and insulin levels over 24 hours in someone without diabetes.

cretes an extra dose of insulin (a bolus) in response to food intake (see the graph above).

If you use an insulin pump, you'll set up your basal and bolus doses of insulin to mimic this rhythm. If you choose to inject insulin, you'll use longer-acting insulin to mimic basal insulin and rapid-acting or regular insulin to mimic bolus insulin.

The type, dose, and schedule of these insulins will be up to you and your provider. You might want to refer back to "Insulins Used in the United States" (table on p. 187–188) to review when different insulins take action.

Work with your provider to come up with a plan to suit your life and schedule. If your plan is not working out for you, talk to your provider. There are usually many other plans you can try.

Multiple Daily Injections

People with type 1 diabetes must use multiple daily injections of insulin or pumps to manage their diabetes. Some people with type 2 diabetes also find that multiple daily injections of insulin or pumps work best for them.

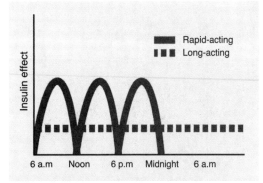

How a multiple daily injection regimen covers insulin requirements over the course of a day.

→ One Unit of Insulin

- Generally, 1 unit of insulin will lower blood glucose levels by about 25–100 mg/dl. You need to find out how it affects your blood glucose levels.

- In general, 1 unit of insulin will cover up to 20 grams of carbohydrate. You also need to find out how this applies to you.

→ Insulin Pump or Multiple Daily Injections

If you are injecting insulin multiple times a day, you may want to consider an insulin pump.

Taking multiple daily injections is sometimes called intensive diabetes management or tight control. The goal is to mimic the natural secretion of insulin from the pancreas as much as possible. The goals, advantages, and disadvantages of tight control are discussed in detail in chapter 9.

The more often you inject insulin, the more opportunities you have to fine-tune your control. You also have more freedom and flexibility with your schedule and food choices.

With this plan, long-acting insulin analogs, such as insulin glargine (Lantus) or detemir (Levemir), provide your basal dose of insulin. You then take rapid-acting insulin before a meal based on the carbohydrates you eat at that meal. The injections of rapid-acting insulin analogs provide the bolus for the three meals (see graph at left).

To make this plan work for you, you need to monitor your blood glucose frequently. You will need to adjust the amounts of rapid-acting insulin given before each meal in order to cover the carbohydrates in your meal, lower a high blood glucose level not sufficiently lowered by the previous rapid-acting insulin injection, or anticipate the rise in blood glucose caused by the next meal.

You will also have the opportunity to make adjustments during the day. If you are exercising after lunch, you might want to reduce the amount of your noon insulin dose. If you are going out to a fancy dinner where you know you'll be eating more than usual, you may want to take more insulin. Your diabetes educator can help you learn how to adjust your insulin doses.

Daily Insulin Dose

- Your starting insulin dose for either injections or the pump will be based on your weight and current insulin program. For example, for people with type 1 diabetes who are within 20% of their ideal body weight, the total daily insulin dose needed for intensive therapy is 0.5–1.0 units of insulin per kilogram of body weight. That means that if you weigh 127 pounds (1 kilogram equals 2.2 pounds), you would take about 29–57 units of insulin each day.

- Your total daily insulin dose would be at the high end of the range if you were resistant to insulin (57 units) or at the lower end of the range, if you were very sensitive to insulin (29 units).

- About one-third to one-half of your total daily dose would provide your basal insulin level, and the rest would be used to cover meals.

- Most people start out with lower doses and gradually increase the amount of insulin until they reach their blood glucose target.

- If you are pregnant, your total daily insulin dose will go up as you gain weight and develop more insulin resistance. Your insulin dose may even triple during the course of pregnancy.

Whichever formula or calculation you use, you will most likely have to make adjustments as you find the program that best suits you. You will probably have a plan for how to adjust your dose, but you will also need to be in close contact with your health care team.

You will be able to make small adjustments throughout the day to accommodate your meals and activities. If monitoring shows that your blood glucose levels are too high, you need to take extra insulin or reduce the amount of carbohydrate in your next meal.

Insulin Distribution

Here is one formula that some people find helpful as a starting point for deciding how to distribute insulin throughout the day.

- 40–50% total insulin as the basal dose
- 15–25% before breakfast
- 15% before lunch
- 15–20% before supper
- 0–10%, as needed, to cover a bedtime snack

Rapid-Acting Insulin Analogs and Meals

Knowing when and how much insulin to take at meals can be confusing. Here are some tips to get you started.

- Rapid-acting insulin is taken before meals or very big snacks to counteract the increase in blood glucose that will occur as food is digested.

- You can take your injection just before you eat.

- Rapid-acting insulin analogs begin to work in about 5–15 minutes. Taking your injection more than 15 minutes before meals may result in hypoglycemia.

One Shot a Day

A single shot of insulin can sometimes be enough to bring your blood glucose into the target range. You might be able to inject long-acting insulin, such as insulin glargine (Lantus) or detemir (Levemir), or intermediate-acting insulin, such as NPH, to provide a basal level of insulin (see graph on p. 219).

Which Type of Insulin Is Right for Me?

- Long-acting insulin provides a steady level of insulin throughout the day and night.

- Intermediate-acting insulin that is taken at bedtime might help lower fasting blood glucose levels.

→ When and How to Start Insulin?

If you have type 2 diabetes, when and how you start taking insulin is up to you and your health care provider. For example, you may take a once-daily insulin injection in addition to other medications or you may take multiple daily injections. There are many factors to consider when discussing insulin, including your current medication regimen and blood glucose goals. You'll discuss several considerations with your health care provider to develop the best insulin plan for you. Don't be afraid to ask questions.

- Intermediate-acting insulin that is taken in the morning will provide some coverage for the food you eat as well as provide a basal insulin level.

At mealtimes, there isn't always enough insulin available from one injection to lower your blood glucose. Taking one shot a day can also mean that you are locked into a schedule for your meals.

Some people with type 2 diabetes may be able to make enough insulin to cover the post-meal increase in blood glucose. For these people, providing the basal insulin helps their pancreas to do its job better. Usually, however, one shot of basal insulin does not result in optimal control because glucose rises after meals.

Another option is to take oral diabetes medications or other injectable medications along with the one injection of basal insulin. These medications can provide the coverage needed for meals.

One shot of long-acting insulin.

One shot of intermediate-acting insulin.

Two shots of intermediate-acting insulin.

More Than One Shot

You may get better coverage by splitting your one shot of insulin into two shots. These can be given in the morning and in the evening. Usually, for twice-daily injections, you'll use intermediate-acting or pre-mixed insulin instead of long-acting insulin. The morning shot will be a bigger dose than the evening shot (see graph above).

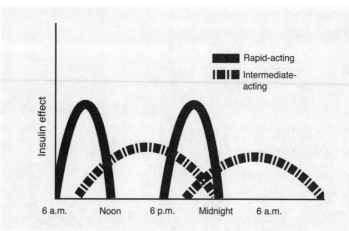

Two shots: a combination of intermediate- and of rapid-acting insulins.

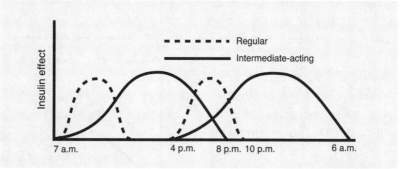

Two shots: mixed regular and intermediate-acting insulin taken at 7 a.m. and 4 p.m.

However, even with this plan, you may have a period in the early morning, between 3 and 10 a.m., when your insulin level may be low.

Another possibility is to take a combination of insulins. You can take rapid-acting or regular insulin along with your morning shot of intermediate-acting NPH insulin. This gives you a bolus of insulin to cover your breakfast meal. Additional insulin can be taken later in the day. You can either use premixed insulins or mix two types of insulin in one injection (see graphs above).

Some people choose to take a basal, long-acting insulin analog once daily and a mealtime rapid-acting insulin analog up to three times a day, rather than NPH and rapid-acting insulin.

It may take a little experimenting and consulting with your health care team to figure out how to best mix rapid-acting or regular and intermediate-acting insulins. You may have to change the ratio many times before you get the results that best suit you.

You may find it convenient to buy premixed insulin, such as a 70/30 or 75/25 mixture, or you may prefer to split and mix the doses yourself. Mixing the doses yourself gives you the flexibility to match your insulin dose to your insulin needs. This may be helpful when you are trying to account for your physical activity and meals.

With this plan, you will still need to monitor your blood glucose closely. You need to monitor your blood glucose levels before and after meals. You may need to monitor at other times as well.

Fine-Tuning Your Insulin Plan

A two-shot program gives you better insulin coverage than a single-shot plan but still keeps you closely tied to a regular meal schedule and a regular pattern of activity. Usually the three major meals have to be about 5 hours apart for optimal coverage. This is because you cannot make short-term adjustments with longer-acting insulins. Only rapid-acting or regular insulin can be adjusted to immediately respond to a blood glucose level or change in schedule.

Highs in the Morning

- You may want to move your evening insulin shot from dinner-time to bedtime so your body will have a little more insulin to cover rising blood glucose levels overnight. Make sure that your glucose levels are on target during the evening hours if you try this adjustment.

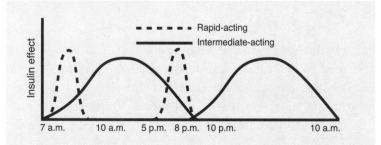

Three shots: split and mixed morning dose, rapid-acting dinner dose, and intermediate-acting evening dose.

- You may find that you have low blood glucose in the early morning (around 2 or 3 a.m.) with the two-shot plan. If this is the case, think about a three-shot plan.

- With a three-shot plan (see graph p. 221), you would give yourself a mixture of rapid-acting or regular insulin and intermediate-acting insulin at breakfast, rapid-acting or regular insulin at dinner, and intermediate-acting insulin at bedtime.

Future Prospects for Insulin Delivery

People with diabetes have more options than ever for delivering insulin. However, people are continually working toward developing better technology that will improve life for people with diabetes.

The so-called artificial pancreas (or "closed-loop system") is closer to becoming a reality every year. A closed-loop system would work as close to a real pancreas as possible—responding to glucose and delivering insulin appropriately. A truly successful closed-loop system would need to incorporate a continuous glucose monitor, a pump or other insulin delivery device, and a computer to manage the system. There may still be a role for the patient, such as confirming recommended doses.

Currently, this technology is still in the planning and development stages. However, there are several continuous glucose monitors on the market, and one company makes a continuous glucose monitor and insulin pump that specifically work together.

In Conclusion

In addition to insulin, some people with type 1 or type 2 diabetes take an injectable medication called pramlintide acetate. It is taken with meals to help reduce blood glucose levels. It can also suppress your appetite, so you feel fuller and eat less at meals. Pramlintide acetate cannot be mixed with insulin and is available in a separate, prefilled pen or vial and syringe.

Taking insulin is a big step. When you're first discussing starting insulin with your health care team, don't be afraid to take notes or ask lots of questions about anything that's not clear. Even if you have taken insulin before, you might want to review your insulin schedule on a return visit to your care provider, especially if you are experiencing any difficulties. You might also want to go over any changes in your schedule. Make sure you understand how to time injections with meals. Go step by step through a typical day. Also discuss how to adjust your insulin doses and timing for an unusual day—what happens if you oversleep, get sick, travel across time zones, or plan to be unusually active?

Before you leave your diabetes care provider's office, be sure you understand the following:

- What type of insulin you will be taking and the name of the insulin.

- Symptoms of high and low blood glucose that may indicate a problem with your insulin doses and how to appropriately treat and prevent these incidents.

- Where you should inject it.

- Whether you need to prepare any mixtures.

- How often you will take injections.

- The best times of the day to take insulin.

- How to store your insulin.

Part V
Complications of Diabetes

Diabetes Complications and Prevention

P erhaps the most difficult thing about diabetes is thinking about the complications that can arise in the future. It's true that people with diabetes have a higher risk of heart, eye, kidney, and nerve disease than other people.

However, you can take active, positive steps to reduce the risk of these problems. The best way to prevent diabetes complications is to keep your blood glucose levels as close to normal as possible. Focusing on the daily goal of controlling your blood glucose will help you stay positive about your long-term future with diabetes.

Warning Signs

A good rule is to call or visit your provider any time you "just don't feel right" and cannot explain it. Your health care providers can help you troubleshoot problems as they arise. Your problem may be something as simple as changing your exercise routine or something more serious like a complication.

Warning Signs of Diabetes Complications

- Vision problems, such as blurry or spotty vision or flashes
- Unexplained, overwhelming tiredness
- Discomfort in your legs when walking
- Numbness or tingling in your hands or feet
- Chest pain that comes on when you start to exert yourself
- Cuts or sores that stay infected or take a long time to heal

Some people have the unpleasant experience of finding out about diabetes complications soon after diagnosis. Sometimes, they may find that they already have complications when they are diagnosed. This is more likely if you're diagnosed with type 2 diabetes.

The signs of type 2 diabetes may be so subtle that you may have had high blood glucose levels for some time without ever realizing it. The damage was occurring even before your diagnosis, and perhaps the signs of the complications brought you to the doctor in the first place. In this case, you probably got a crash course in diabetes complications.

This chapter will provide background on the connection between blood glucose and complications. It will also detail some common diabetes complications, including ways to detect, prevent, and treat them.

Five Common Complications

- Cardiovascular disease and stroke
- Retinopathy (eye disease)
- Nephropathy (kidney disease)
- Neuropathy (nerve disease)
- Infections, including dental disease

Research behind Glucose Control

Luckily, we know a lot about what causes diabetes complications and how to prevent them. Two landmark studies showed that keeping blood glucose levels as close to normal as possible can help prevent or slow the progression of many complications.

The Diabetes Control and Complications Trial (DCCT) and the United Kingdom Prospective Diabetes Study (UKPDS) showed that tight control lessens the chance for eye, kidney, and nerve disease.

The DCCT showed that people with type 1 diabetes could delay or even prevent many of the complications of diabetes by tightly managing blood glucose levels. The volunteers in the DCCT's intensive management group monitored their blood more often—4–7 times each day—and injected insulin more often. They stayed in close touch with their health care team, and their hard work paid off.

They reduced their risk for developing complications by more than 50%. For example, those who kept their A1C levels closer to normal had 76% less eye disease, 60% less nerve damage, and 35–56% less kidney damage than the study group participants who used standard therapy.

The UKPDS showed that tight blood glucose control and blood pressure management could help people with type 2 diabetes delay or prevent diabetes complications. In the UKPDS, people who tightly controlled their glucose reduced their risk of complications such as eye and nerve disease by 25%. People who lowered their blood pressure reduced their risk of stroke by 44% and their risk of heart failure by 56%. Improved blood glucose control also reduced the risk of heart attacks and diabetes-related deaths.

For more information about the DCCT, the UKPDS, and intensive management, see chapter 9.

Take Action

The bottom line is that any improvement you can make in lowering your blood glucose level will benefit you. The less time you spend with high blood glucose levels, the lower your risk for developing complications.

Even if you already have some complications, it's not too late to slow the progression. Lowering your blood glucose levels can help improve most complications—even if they've already developed.

Cardiovascular Disease, Stroke, and Peripheral Arterial Disease

> **Cardiovascular Disease:**
> A disease of the heart and blood vessels (arteries, veins, and capillaries).

People with diabetes are two to four times as likely to have a heart attack or stroke as people without diabetes. It is the number one killer of people with diabetes. Therefore, it's important to understand and mitigate the risk of cardiovascular disease and stroke.

Most people associate vascular disease with heart attacks and strokes. Yet, vascular disease can affect all the blood vessels in your body. For example, blocked arteries around your heart can interrupt blood flow to the legs and cause peripheral arterial disease (PAD). This can cause painful cramping, aches, or burning sensation in your legs and feet.

Risk of Cardiovascular Disease, Stroke, and PAD

- People with diabetes are at least twice as likely to have heart disease or a stroke.

- People with diabetes tend to develop heart disease or have strokes at an earlier age than other people.

- Heart attacks in people with diabetes are more serious and more likely to cause death.

- One of every three people with diabetes over 50 is thought to have PAD.

Causes of Cardiovascular Disease, Stroke, and PAD

Blood flows through the blood vessels in your body to deliver all the oxygen, glucose, nutrients, and other substances needed to run your body and keep your cells alive. When blood can't get to cells and tissues, they can become damaged or die.

Atherosclerosis
Most of the cardiovascular complications related to diabetes have to do with a blockage or slowdown in blood flowing throughout the

body. Diabetes can change the chemical makeup of some of the substances found in blood, which can cause blood vessels to narrow or to clog up completely. This is called atherosclerosis, or hardening of the arteries, and diabetes seems to speed it up.

If you have diabetes or insulin resistance, you have a higher risk for atherosclerosis. Paying attention to conventional risk factors, such as smoking, high fats in the blood, or high blood pressure, is important for people for diabetes.

High Cholesterol

High cholesterol and triglycerides can contribute to hardening of the arteries.

> **→ Blood Flow and Cardiovascular Disease**
>
> There are several kinds of cardiovascular disease, and they are all due to problems in how the heart pumps blood or how blood circulates throughout the body.

> **Atherosclerosis:** Clogging, narrowing, and hardening of the body's large arteries and medium-sized blood vessels; can lead to coronary artery disease, resulting in stroke, heart attack, eye problems, and kidney problems.

These blood fats, also called lipids, stay in the blood and collect in the walls of the blood vessels. Keep in mind that there are several kinds of lipids. LDL, or bad, cholesterol can narrow or block your blood vessels, which can lead to a heart attack or a stroke.

HDL cholesterol is sometimes called helpful or "good" cholesterol. This lipid helps remove deposits from the insides of your blood vessels and keeps them from getting blocked. You can raise your HDL choles-

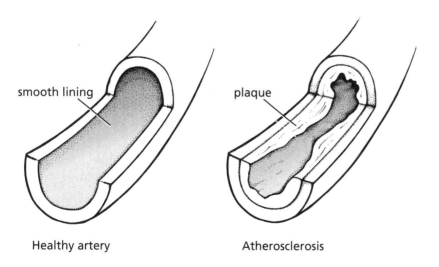

smooth lining

plaque

Healthy artery   Atherosclerosis

terol level by getting more exercise, avoiding saturated fats, choosing more omega-3 and omega-6 fats, and lowering your triglyceride levels.

Target Lipid Levels

- LDL cholesterol below 100 mg/dl.
- Triglyceride level below 150 mg/dl.
- HDL cholesterol above 40 mg/dl for men and above 50 mg/dl for women.

Lipid abnormalities are quite common in people with diabetes, especially type 2 diabetes. That has led researchers to ask whether there is a link between lipid abnormalities and obesity and type 2 diabetes. If you and other family members have severely high levels of cholesterol, you may have a lipid disorder that is not related to diabetes.

High Blood Pressure

High blood pressure, or hypertension, can also contribute to cardiovascular disease. When you have high blood pressure, blood flows more forcibly through blood vessels and makes the heart work harder than usual. This extra stress can damage the lining of your arteries, causing a type of fatty tissue called atheroma to form. Atheroma can cause your arteries to narrow or become completely blocked.

High blood pressure not only increases your risk for heart disease but also increases your risk for other diabetes complications. It can damage small blood vessels and capillaries, especially in the eyes and kidneys. People with diabetes need to be especially careful to control their blood pressure because of the potential damage to blood vessels and tissues.

Hypertension itself usually has no symptoms. If you have it, you probably won't even realize it unless you have your blood pressure checked.

Hypertension is especially common among people with type 2 diabetes. Over 70% of people with diabetes also have high blood pressure or use medicines to treat hypertension.

Hypertension: A condition present when blood flows through the blood vessels with a force greater than normal, thus straining the heart, damaging blood vessels, and increasing the risk of heart attack, stroke, and kidney disease; also known as high blood pressure.

Complications of Cardiovascular Disease, Stroke, and PAD

Blood supply to the heart, brain, and other tissues and organs can be restricted when blood vessels narrow or clog because of cardiovascular disease. If blood flow is restricted for a long time, chest pain known as angina can occur. Angina is not itself a disease, but it can be a warning sign that something is slowing the flow of blood to the heart.

A complete blockage of blood to the heart is a heart attack. A complete blockage of blood to the brain is a stroke. Another serious problem for people with diabetes is PAD. Blockage of blood flow to the feet puts your feet at risk for amputation.

One of the symptoms of PAD is intermittent claudication. The leg arteries become blocked and painful, especially when walking. The pain sometimes comes and goes.

Prevention of Cardiovascular Disease, Stroke, and PAD

There are six things you can do to prevent cardiovascular disease. All of these actions will help keep your large blood vessels open for blood to flow to all your vital organs, and you will dramatically lower your risk of developing cardiovascular disease.

Five Steps to Prevent Onset or Recurrence of Cardiovascular Disease and Stroke

- Quit smoking
- Lower your cholesterol levels
- Lower high blood pressure
- Increase your physical activity
- Ask your provider if taking aspirin will benefit you

→ ADA Blood Pressure Goals

The recommended blood pressure for most people with diabetes is <130/80 mmHg.

Heart Attack: An interruption in the blood supply to the heart because of narrowed or blocked blood vessels, causing muscle damage and sometimes death; also called myocardial infarction.

Stroke: A serious condition caused by damage to blood vessels in the brain, which stops the flow of blood and oxygen to the brain, possibly causing cells to die; may cause loss of ability to speak or move parts of the body; risk factors include diabetes, hypertension, and high cholesterol.

Peripheral Arterial Disease (PAD): A disease that occurs when blood vessels in the legs are narrowed or blocked by fatty deposits, reducing blood flow to the feet and legs; this condition puts people at increased risk of heart attack and stroke.

Quit Smoking

The role of smoking in causing lung disease is well known. But smoking is even more risky for people with diabetes. Over time, smoking damages your heart and circulatory system by hardening your blood vessels.

Narrow blood vessels can restrict the flow of blood to cells in your body. These cells can die, and the damage can lead to heart disease, impotence, and amputation. If you smoke now, talk to the members of your health care team about strategies that can help you quit.

Lower Your Cholesterol

Healthy eating can help you keep your blood glucose on target, as well as lower your cholesterol and triglycerides. Healthy eating habits are contagious, too. Your family will benefit from your healthy eating plan. A visit with a dietitian can help you make healthy food choices.

Healthy Food, Healthy Cholesterol

- Develop a meal plan low in trans and saturated fat, as well as cholesterol.

- Include whole grains, fruits, vegetables, and a moderate amount of protein in your meals each day.

- Watch the total number of calories you eat to lose or maintain your weight.

High levels of LDL cholesterol are usually treated with medications called statins.

Tips for Starting Statins and Other Medications

- Watch carefully for changes in your blood glucose levels; even if you have type 2 diabetes, you may want to monitor your blood glucose level several times each day.

- Start new drugs one at a time, if possible; some medications can interfere with the breakdown, absorption, and removal of other medicines.

- Know that many kinds of medications are used to treat high lipid levels and that side effects may occur; report anything unusual to your provider.

Triglyceride levels are closely linked to blood glucose levels. Triglycerides can usually be lowered by lowering your blood glucose levels; losing weight; increasing physical activity; eating a healthy, low-fat, high-fiber diet; or taking medications called fibrates. Consuming more omega-3 fats will help lower triglycerides too.

Lower Your Blood Pressure

High blood pressure, or hypertension, puts a strain on your body, especially your heart, blood vessels, and kidneys. In addition, high blood pressure accelerates the progression of eye and kidney complications.

You can lower your blood pressure by losing weight and working out. For some people, limiting sodium intake helps lower blood pressure. You may also take medications to keep your blood pressure at or below the recommended level.

The most commonly prescribed medications are angiotensin-converting enzyme (ACE) inhibitors and angiotensin receptor blockers (ARBs). They lower blood pressure and help protect your kidneys. Diuretics, beta-blockers, and calcium channel blockers may also be prescribed.

It will take time to figure out the best medicine plan for you. Be sure to keep in close contact with your health care team during this time and let them know if you are experiencing any side effects from these medications.

Get Moving

Physical activity helps people with diabetes in several ways. It can delay or help stop cardiovascular disease. It can help clear glucose from your blood, so that cells can use it for energy. This lowers blood glucose levels and in some individuals may lower the amount of insulin needed.

Working out also gives you a positive way to cope with stress. For people who are overweight, exercise helps with weight loss, and losing weight lowers your insulin resistance. Exercise helps your body work better. See chapter 11 on working with your health care team to design an exercise program that is safe for you.

Treatment of Cardiovascular Disease, Stroke, and PAD

Taking preventive steps can slow or stop the progression of cardiovascular disease. But sometimes, prevention alone isn't enough, especially if you have had cardiovascular disease for a while. You may need medication to reduce blood clotting, to lower cholesterol levels, or to reduce high blood pressure.

You may need surgery if your blood vessels are already blocked or significantly narrowed. Both preventive and surgical steps can also treat angina. The goal is to increase the amount of oxygen going to the heart.

Treatments for Heart Problems
Several different surgical procedures are now commonly used to remove the blockages of blood vessels. All of these procedures are performed by a cardiologist—a doctor specialized in treating people with heart problems.

Balloon angioplasty, while not performed as often as it used to be in people with diabetes, is a procedure that uses a balloon at the tip of a long tube. A cardiologist inserts the tube into the blocked artery and then inflates the balloon. This opens up the blocked vessel. A metal stent, or ring, may be left in place to help the blood vessel stay open.

Atherectomy is another kind of minor surgery used to open blood vessels. With this technique, the cardiologist bores a hole through a blocked blood vessel. Laser surgery can also be used to melt away blockages with an intense beam of light. All of these surgeries can remove smaller blockages and require little recovery time.

Stent: A metal or plastic ring inserted into a vessel to keep the previously clogged vessel open.

A more severe blockage calls for more serious surgery. Surgeons can create a detour around the blocked artery through arterial bypass surgery. Now, instead of running up against a wall, blood can flow around the blockage and through the new blood vessel.

Treatments for Stroke
Strokes are usually treated by a combination approach: treatments to lower blood glucose, lipid levels, and blood pressure; therapy to help the person recover mental and physical abilities; and medications that reduce blood clotting. Sometimes surgery is needed.

Treatments for PAD
The best treatment for PAD is regular physical activity. If you have intermittent claudication and exercise is painful, your doctor can help design an activity program. Other treatments include quitting smoking, medications, and procedures or surgery similar to that for blocked heart arteries.

People with cardiovascular disease are advised to be physically active and to eat foods that protect the heart and blood vessels. Because of diabetes, you'll also need to manage your blood glucose levels and perhaps lose weight as part of your recovery.

> **Bypass Surgery**
>
> Maybe you already know someone who has had a single, double, triple, or even quadruple bypass surgery of the heart. Surgeons can construct one, two, three, four, or even more detours, if there are multiple blockages.

Eye Problems

The most common eye disease in people with diabetes is retinopathy, a disease of the retina. The retina is the light-sensing region of the inner eye. It acts like a miniature "movie screen" in the back of your eye, on which the images you see are projected.

Risks for Retinopathy

• Diabetic retinopathy is estimated to be the most frequent cause of new blindness among adults aged 20–74 years.

• Nearly all people with type 1 diabetes show signs of retinopathy after 20 years of diabetes.

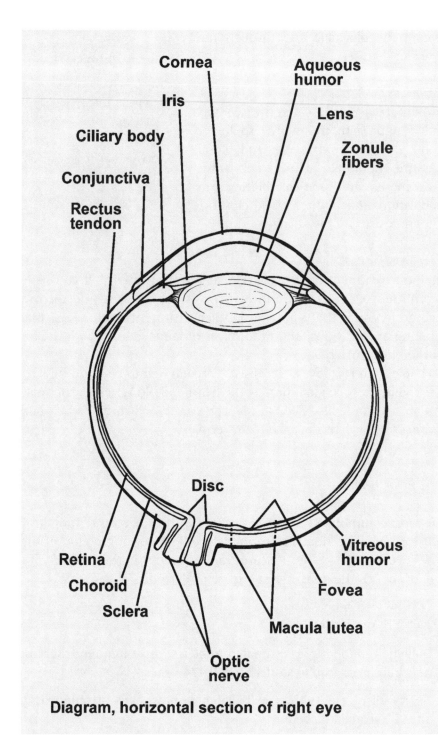

Cornea

Aqueous
humor

Iris

Lens

Ciliary body

Zonule
fibers

Conjunctiva

Rectus
tendon

Disc

Retina

Choroid

Sclera

Vitreous
humor

Fovea

Macula lutea

Optic
nerve

Diagram, horizontal section of right eye

- More than half of all people with type 2 diabetes develop some signs of retinopathy after 20 years of diabetes.

Retinopathy: Damage to the small blood vessels in the eye that can lead to vision problems; different forms include background retinopathy and proliferative retinopathy.

Causes of Retinopathy

Retinopathy is caused by damage to the blood vessels that supply blood to the retina. High blood pressure, high blood glucose, and smoking can all damage blood vessels. Retinopathy is more common among people with type 1 diabetes, but people with type 2 diabetes can also develop it.

Complications of Retinopathy

There are two major forms of retinopathy: nonproliferative and proliferative.

Nonproliferative Retinopathy

- Also called background retinopathy.
- Blood vessels can close off or weaken.
- The blood vessels leak blood, fluid, and fat into the eye.
- It can cause blurry vision, but not usually blindness.

Proliferative Retinopathy

- A more serious, although less common, form of eye disease.

- New blood vessels sprout, or proliferate, in the retina. This may seem like a good thing, but the new vessels don't grow in the way they should. Instead, they grow out of control.

- The blood vessels are fragile and rupture easily during exercise or even while sleeping, especially if you have high blood pressure. Blood can leak into the fluid-filled portion of the eye in front of the retina, which can block light coming into the eye and impair vision.

- In addition, scar tissue can form on the retina. The scar tissue often shrinks, and when that happens, it can tear the layers of the retina apart. This damages your eyesight and can cause blindness.

Ophthalmologist: A medical doctor who diagnoses and treats eye diseases and eye disorders; can also prescribe glasses and contact lenses.

Optometrist: A primary eye care provider who prescribes glasses and contact lenses; can diagnose and treat certain eye conditions and diseases.

Glaucoma, or high pressure within the eye, and cataracts occur more often in people with diabetes. If found early, glaucoma can be treated.

Macular edema can also occur in people with diabetes. Retinopathy causes swelling of the macula of the eye. Because the macula is that central portion of the retina that allows you to see fine detail, when it swells, vision can be impaired and blindness can result.

Prevention of Retinopathy

You probably won't even notice any changes in your vision when diabetic retinopathy first begins. The starting point for detection of early changes in blood vessels is a dilated eye exam performed by an ophthalmologist or optometrist specially trained in diabetic eye disease. You can read more about eye exams and your eye doctor in chapter 17.

Early detection is the key to keeping this disease from interfering with your vision. You can have retinopathy severe enough to threaten your vision without knowing it. Treatment can protect your vision. This is the reason for having regular examinations, even when you do not have symptoms.

Tips for Eye Care

- Get a yearly eye exam from an ophthalmologist or optometrist. Your eyes should be dilated for the exam. The early detection of any eye problems is critical to keeping your vision.

- Adults with type 1 diabetes need a dilated eye exam within five years after the onset of diabetes. Adults with type 2 diabetes need an eye exam shortly after diagnosis.

- Call your diabetes care provider if you notice changes in your vision, but don't panic. Highs and lows in your blood glucose level may cause temporary blurring in your vision.

- Keep your blood glucose levels close to normal. You will help prevent damage to the small blood vessels that run through your retina.

- Check your blood pressure regularly, and work to keep your blood pressure on target.

- Quit smoking.

- Discuss your physical activity with your eye doctor. Some activities can raise the pressure inside your eyes and lead to bleeding in the retina.

- If you have retinopathy, avoid taking birth control pills because they may affect the clotting of your blood or increase your blood pressure.

- Get early treatment for eye problems! Early intervention, such as laser treatment for retinopathy, cuts the risk of blindness by 90%.

The DCCT found the most striking results for the power of controlling blood glucose to prevent retinopathy. The UKPDS showed that people with type 2 diabetes who lowered their blood glucose and blood pressure also lowered their risk of retinopathy.

The bottom line, whether you have type 1 or type 2 diabetes, is that you can significantly reduce your chances of developing retinopathy or of having your retinopathy worsen.

Vision Warning Signs

- Unexplained visual problems, such as spots, "floaters," or cobwebs in your field of vision; blurring or distortion; blind spots; eye pain; or persistent redness.

- Trouble reading books or traffic signs or difficulty distinguishing familiar objects.

- Increased pressure within the eye, which could be a warning sign of glaucoma. Some physicians and most optometrists routinely test for this.

- Any retinal abnormalities. Most endocrinologists, internists, primary care practitioners, and optometrists will test for this but should refer problems with the retina to an ophthalmologist specializing in diabetic eye disease.

• Leaking of blood vessels that supply the retina, which leads to retinopathy, the main cause of blindness in people with diabetes.

Treatment of Retinopathy

The best way to treat proliferative retinopathy is with a laser procedure called photocoagulation. An ophthalmologist aims a laser beam at the retina. This creates hundreds of tiny burns in the retina. These burns will destroy abnormal blood vessels, patch leaky ones, and slow the formation of new fragile blood vessels. If you have the more serious form of retinopathy (proliferative retinopathy) or macular edema, photocoagulation can usually prevent blindness.

Photocoagulation may not be for everyone, however. It may not work if the retina has bled a lot or has detached. In these cases, a surgery called a vitrectomy can remove the excess blood and scar tissue, stop the bleeding, replace some of the vitreous humor—the clear jelly-like substance that fills the eye—with salt solution, and repair the detached retina.

If you need either of these procedures, choose an ophthalmologist who specializes in retinal disease and who has a lot of experience in treating patients with diabetes. Don't put off visiting your eye specialist. The earlier you get treated, the greater your chances of preventing blindness or further eye damage.

Kidney Disease

Nephropathy or kidney disease can occur in people with type 1 or type 2 diabetes. However, severe kidney damage is more common in people with type 1 diabetes than in those with type 2.

Your kidneys are your body's filter units. They work 24 hours a day to rid your body of the toxins that your body makes or takes in. Toxins from the blood enter the kidneys by crossing the walls of tiny blood vessels along its border.

Risk of Nephropathy

- Approximately 43% of new cases of end-stage renal disease (kidney failure) are caused by diabetes.

- Of all people with diabetes, around 30% have nephropathy.

- Native Americans, Hispanics, and African Americans are at a greater risk for developing nephropathy than whites with type 2 diabetes.

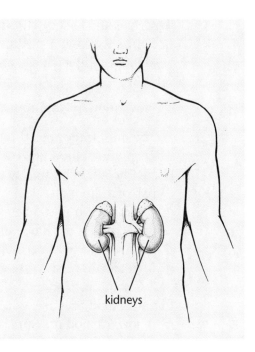

kidneys

Causes of Nephropathy

Sometimes in people with diabetes, the blood vessels on the kidneys become damaged and can no longer filter out the impurities in your blood. They begin to leak, and some of the waste products that should be removed are allowed to stay in your blood. When this happens, some of the proteins and nutrients that should remain in your blood are lost in the urine. This is called nephropathy.

The exact cause of nephropathy is unknown. However, scientists know that high blood glucose in combination with high blood pressure contributes to kidney damage. Years of high blood pressure can damage the delicate filters in the kidneys, leading to less efficient removal of waste products from the blood. The good news is that there are steps you can take to reduce your risk of nephropathy.

Complications of Nephropathy

The kidneys are so effective that noticeable problems will not appear until 80% of the kidneys are damaged. Symptoms of kidney disease may be subtle: fluid buildup, sleeplessness and tiredness, vomiting, or weakness. The complications of nephropathy are

Nephropathy: Kidney disease; high blood glucose and high blood pressure can damage the kidney; when the kidneys are damaged, they can no longer remove waste and extra fluids from the bloodstream, and protein leaks into the urine.

serious and include chronic kidney failure, in which your kidneys slowly stop working over time, and end-stage kidney disease, in which the kidneys completely fail and can no longer filter toxins from the body.

Prevention of Nephropathy

The most important thing you can do to prevent kidney damage is to keep your blood glucose levels close to normal. The DCCT showed that people who tightly controlled their blood glucose reduced their risk of kidney disease by 35–56%.

Another important step you can take is to keep your blood pressure on target. If your blood pressure is high, the delicate capillaries in your kidneys can become damaged. Two things that you can do to lower high blood pressure are to maintain a healthy body weight and to eat less sodium. If kidney damage is advanced or if you cannot reduce your blood pressure with these methods, you may need medications to lower blood pressure. ACE inhibitors and ARBs are blood pressure medications that also preserve kidney function.

Treatment of Nephropathy

The earliest sign of kidney disease is small amounts of protein in the urine, a condition called microalbuminuria. Microalbuminuria is detected using a urine test.

If you have microalbuminuria, then you may be advised to take certain steps. The first step is to bring your blood glucose levels into the target range. In the DCCT, people with microalbuminuria who tightly controlled their blood glucose cut their risk of progressing to more serious kidney disease by more than 50%. To achieve this benefit, the study participants maintained an A1C of 8.1% or lower.

Urine Tests for Nephropathy

Your urine needs to be checked once a year starting 5 years after the diagnosis of type 1 diabetes or starting at the diagnosis of type 2 diabetes. Make sure your urine is tested for microalbuminuria, not just proteinuria.

> ### Extra Proteins at Diabetes Diagnosis
>
> Nephropathy should not be confused with excess protein in your urine that can occur when you are first diagnosed with diabetes. This is usually a temporary condition, caused by unchecked high blood glucose and high blood pressure. Protein in the urine may be seen temporarily during fever, after exercise, or under other temporary conditions.

Another step is to achieve optimal blood pressure control. You may be advised to begin a diet that is low in sodium. You may also take blood pressure medications, either ACE inhibitors or ARBs. These can be prescribed even if your blood pressure is in the recommended range. ACE inhibitors and ARBs slow the progression of kidney disease.

You'll need to take more aggressive steps if your kidney disease advances. You cannot live without functioning kidneys. There are two treatment options during end-stage renal disease, when the kidneys fail. Both remedies attempt to replace the kidneys' function: dialysis and kidney transplantation.

Dialysis

Dialysis uses a machine to artificially do the job that the kidneys are no longer able to do. There are two different types of dialysis: hemodialysis and peritoneal dialysis. They both remove toxins from the blood. The illustration on p. 247 shows the differences between the two methods.

Hemodialysis

- Your blood is removed from an artery (usually in the arm), filtered through a machine, and returned to a vein.

- Most patients go to a dialysis treatment center three times a week for 2–4 hours.

- Some patients have a trained caregiver come to their home to perform hemodialysis.

Peritoneal dialysis

- A patient's abdominal cavity serves as the filtering site, instead of using a machine to filter the blood.

- A solution called a dialysate is poured through a small tube into the abdomen, where it is allowed to sit and collect waste products.

- After a few hours, the dialysate, which now contains the wastes, is drained out of the abdomen. This process can be performed manually by letting gravity carry the dialysate into the cavity and drain it out again. Or, a machine can carry out the exchange, usually overnight.

Kidney Transplantation

Transplantation is usually more effective than dialysis. A new kidney functions as well as your old ones did before disease.

However, kidneys are in high demand and transplantation requires taking drugs that suppress the immune system to prevent rejection of the new kidney. Having a genetically near-identical donor is desirable, but not essential. A relative may be willing to donate a healthy kidney, or a kidney may become available from someone who has just died. People often go on dialysis while waiting for a transplant.

Some people choose to have a pancreas transplant at the same time. Pancreas transplants are always from organ donors who have died.

Transplantation has its risks as well. It is major, expensive surgery and requires good cardiovascular health. The drugs you must take to prevent immune rejection of the new kidney may put you at a greater risk of developing infections, and the new kidney will face the same pressures as the old ones did.

Nerve Disorders

The nerves in your body are like electrical circuits. They are the wires that send and receive signals from your brain and tell other cells what to do. Your body's nervous system controls virtually everything you do and every move you make. They control your breathing, sense of feeling, blinking, and thinking, as well as move your muscles and empty your stomach.

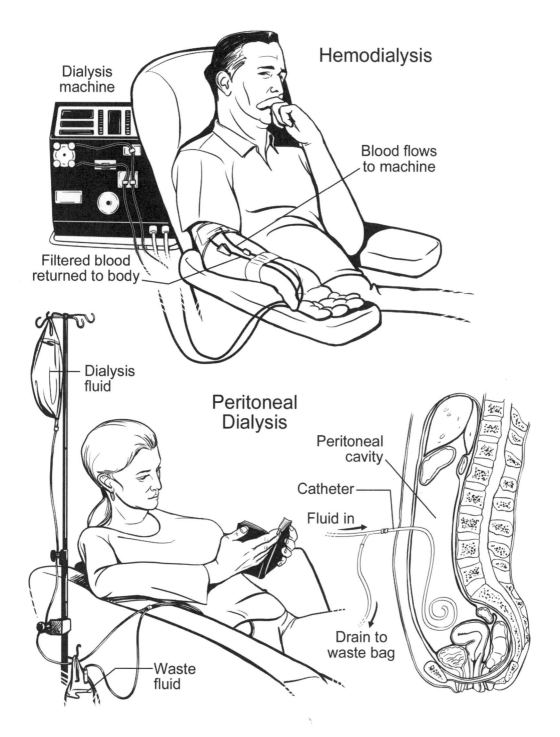

Hemodialysis

Dialysis machine

Blood flows to machine

Filtered blood returned to body

Dialysis fluid

Peritoneal Dialysis

Peritoneal cavity

Catheter

Fluid in

Drain to waste bag

Waste fluid

Neuropathy: Disease of the nervous system; a complication of diabetes; the three major forms in people with diabetes are peripheral neuropathy, autonomic neuropathy, and focal neuropathy; most common form is peripheral neuropathy, which primarily affects the legs and feet.

Diabetes usually doesn't impair the brain and spinal cord, but it can damage the nerves in other parts of the body. The nerves may be unable to send messages, may send them at the wrong times, or may send them too slowly. This is called diabetic neuropathy.

Your nerves send signals to so many places in your body that damaged nerves can have a range of effects, including pain in your feet or hands, trouble with stomach bloating or bladder or bowel control, sexual dysfunction, loss of sensation or feeling, or weakness in your muscles.

Risk of Neuropathy

- Neuropathy is more likely to affect people who have had diabetes for a long time or who have had high glucose levels for some time.

- About 60–70% of people with diabetes have mild to severe forms of neuropathy.

Causes of Neuropathy

High blood glucose seems to cause nerve damage, but no one really knows why. It may be that proteins coated with glucose cause direct damage. Or high levels of glucose may upset the chemical balance inside nerves. Or the blood supply to nerves may be cut off or constricted, and nerves may not receive the oxygen they need. The tissues surrounding them might squeeze single nerves. However, neuropathy can have causes other than diabetes.

Complications of Neuropathy

There are many types of nerve damage. Our nervous systems are so complex that it is often hard to determine exactly what type of neuropathy is present. In addition, high blood glucose levels can damage nerves in two ways: directly and by slowing down or stopping blood flow. Sometimes it's hard to know whether a problem is caused by nerve damage or by circulation problems.

Peripheral Neuropathy

Peripheral neuropathy can affect the nerves in many parts of your body, but it is most common in the legs, feet, and hands. Sensation can be either increased or decreased in peripheral neuropathy.

Some people have muscle weakness, painful cramps, and twitching. Others complain that their feet feel numb, or they lose the ability to sense temperature or the position of their feet. Some people lose all sensation in their feet, which means they need to take extra care with their feet and protect them from injury. You may also experience changed sensations in your fingers.

Autonomic Neuropathy

Some of your nerves control operations in your body that you don't ever think about, like keeping your heart beating and digesting your food. These are called autonomic nerves. Autonomic neuropathy occurs when these nerves are damaged. It is complex and can have wide-ranging effects on the body.

Autonomic Neuropathy Takes Different Forms

- *Gastroparesis.* Your stomach and intestines slow down or become less efficient at emptying, leading to feeling full after a few bites of food, erratic glucose levels, nausea and vomiting, constipation, or diarrhea.

- *Bladder Problems.* Nerves to the bladder can become damaged, causing diminished sensation of bladder fullness and an inability to completely empty the bladder. Because urine can then stay in the bladder for long periods, you are at high risk for developing urinary tract infections.

- *Erectile Dysfunction.* Men may find that they cannot have an erection even

Foot Dangers

With neuropathy, you can step on something and not feel it or burn your feet with your bath water. If you don't realize it and treat the injury, you can get an infection. If you remain unaware of the infection and don't treat that, serious problems can arise.

though they may still have sexual desire. Read more about erectile dysfunction in chapter 16.

- *Vaginal Problems.* Women may experience vaginal dryness and decreased sexual response. Read more about vaginal problems in chapter 15.

- *Blood Pressure Problems.* You may find yourself feeling lightheaded or dizzy when you stand because of a drop in blood pressure. This is called orthostatic hypotension. When you exercise, your blood pressure may go way up.

- *Skin Problems.* Nerves to the skin may cause too much or too little sweating or very dry, itchy skin.

- *Heart Problems.* Nerves to the heart may fail to speed up or slow down your heart rate in response to exercise. That is one of the reasons why it is important to get a checkup before starting any exercise program. If your heart rate doesn't respond as it should to exertion, you won't be able to use a standard method, such as counting your pulse, to find your target heart rate during and after a workout.

Focal Neuropathy

Damage to a single nerve or group of nerves is called focal neuropathy. It may develop when the blood supply to a nerve is shut off because of a blockage in the blood vessel that supplies the nerve. It could also result from a pinched nerve. Focal neuropathy can injure nerves that sense touch and pain as well as nerves that move muscles. Fortunately, it is not usually a permanent condition. It usually goes away within 2 weeks to 18 months.

Carpal Tunnel Syndrome

Carpal tunnel syndrome is a type of focal neuropathy. It occurs about three times more often in people with diabetes than in the general population and more often in women than in men. It occurs when the median nerve of the forearm is squeezed in its passageway, or tunnel, by the carpal bones of the wrists. It can cause tingling, burning, and numbness and can make you drop things you are holding without even realizing it. You might have carpal tunnel syndrome if

Charcot's Foot

Sometimes neuropathy can trigger a cascade of diabetes-related complications. Many people who have had diabetes for a long time develop a condition known as Charcot's foot.

- Affects weight-bearing joints, such as the ankles.
- It may start with a loss of feeling and thinning of bones in the feet. This can lead to a painless fracture.
- Because the injury doesn't cause pain, it can go unnoticed and untreated. You may continue walking on the fracture, making matters worse.
- Muscle shrinking (atrophy) and joint damage can occur and add to the damage, which can become severe enough to deform the foot.
- The key to treating Charcot's foot is keeping weight off the joint and wearing special footwear early on.
- If you notice any swelling in a joint, especially in your ankle or foot, see your provider right away.

you have tingling in your hands or fingers that goes away when your arms are relaxed down at your sides. Carpal tunnel syndrome is often treated with splints, medication, or surgery to remove the pressure on the nerve.

Prevention of Neuropathy

The best thing you can do to prevent neuropathy is to keep your blood glucose close to normal. The DCCT showed that people with type 1 diabetes who intensively managed their diabetes reduced their risk of neuropathy by 60%. Nerves need a constant blood supply to function properly. Keeping blood vessels healthy will protect the nerves they supply.

It's also important to stop smoking and exercise regularly to help keep the nervous system in prime working condition. Alcohol is also a direct toxin to nerves and can be another cause of neuropathy.

Treatment of Neuropathy

Each type of neuropathy calls for a different treatment. For example, treating gastroparesis is different from treating a burning sensation in your feet. Your health care provider will help you find the best treatment for your symptoms.

Treatment of Peripheral Neuropathy
The symptoms of your neuropathy will dictate your treatment. However, managing the pain caused by neuropathy is one of the most common treatments. Many people find that their pain gets better when their glucose levels are lower. Some even notice that their pain worsens when their blood glucose levels go up temporarily. Walking may help decrease calf pain. Medications may help.

Medications for Neuropathy Pain

- Nonsteroidal anti-inflammatory drugs (NSAIDs) are generally the first medications that are prescribed.

- Low doses of antidepressants and anti-seizure medications.

- Drugs designed specifically for neuropathy pain, such as duloxetine HCl.

- Medicines that contain narcotics are generally not used unless the pain is very severe.

- Lidocaine patches can be used to numb the affected area, and a high-potency, hot pepper cream (capsaicin) can be rubbed on the area.

If these therapies aren't effective, ask for a referral to a pain clinic. There are also less conventional methods to treat the pain. Biofeedback training, hypnosis, relaxation exercises, acupressure, acupuncture, and use of a TENS (transcutaneous electrical nerve stimulation) unit have all been effective for some people.

Treatment of Autonomic Neuropathy
Different types of autonomic neuropathy call for different treatments.

Gastroparesis. If you feel full or bloated, it may help to eat small frequent meals instead of three large ones. Medications, such as metoclopramide, can help food move through your stomach. There are other medications and dietary adjustments that you can use to treat constipation or diarrhea.

Bladder Problems. Incontinence, or urine leakage, can be treated with training in bladder control and timed urination using a planned bladder-emptying program. Rather than waiting until your bladder feels full, you can try urinating every 2 hours.

Men sometimes find it easier to urinate sitting down. Applying pressure over the bladder may also be helpful. If these steps don't work, oral medication may be needed. Or you may need to use a catheter or have surgery. Fecal incontinence (passing stool involuntarily) is treated in a similar way, with medicine for diarrhea and biofeedback training.

Erectile Dysfunction. There are several medications and products that men can use before sex to improve and prolong an erection. The oral medications are called phosphodiesterase-5 inhibitors. Other options include vacuum pumps, constriction rings, injections, and suppositories. Read more about erectile dysfunction in chapter 16.

Vaginal Problems. There are many causes for vaginal problems such as dryness. You may need to use a water-based cream or lubricant made especially for the vaginal area. Read more about vaginal problems in chapter 15.

Blood Pressure Problems. If you are experiencing a sudden drop in blood pressure when you stand up, there are several treatment options. If you drink alcohol or take medications, such as diuretics, ask your provider about stopping them. Other options include medications for low blood pressure, raising the sodium content of your food, or raising the head of your bed.

However, low blood pressure in itself is not unhealthy. It only becomes a problem if it makes you dizzy or disoriented. Try to stand up more slowly and avoid staying still for long periods to prevent fainting. When you get up in the morning, sit on the edge of the bed before you stand up.

Infections and Skin Problems

People with diabetes have a higher risk than other people for infection and skin problems. Skin problems and infections include everything from a scrape on the toe that gets out of hand to gum disease.

Risk of Infections

* About one-third of people with diabetes will have a skin disorder caused or affected by diabetes at some time in their lives.

* Almost one-third of people with diabetes have severe gum disease.

* People with diabetes are twice as likely to need to be hospitalized to treat a kidney infection.

Causes of Infections

During infections, your white blood cells attack the invading bacteria, viruses, and fungi. Excess glucose in your blood makes the white cells less effective. This can keep them from reaching and killing the invading germs. Extra glucose in blood can also provide food for invading pathogens and make infection even more likely.

In addition, diabetes complications can make infections worse. For example, your bladder is more likely to become infected if you have neuropathy. Neuropathy can make you unaware that you need to urinate, which increases the risk for bladder infection. Having neuropathy in your arms, legs, or feet makes you less likely to notice a cut or burn because you will not feel pain. If such a wound is left untreated, even minor skin abrasions can lead to infection.

More Infections after Surgery

People with diabetes tend to have more infections after surgery: in the mouth, ears, gums, lungs, skin, feet, and genital areas and in the incision areas.

Legs and Feet Are Vulnerable to Infection

* Neuropathy numbs legs and feet, making you unaware of injury and infection.

* Injury opens the door to infection.

- Blocked blood vessels slow blood flow to the legs and feet, impairing the healing process.

- High blood glucose disables the body's immune cells—white blood cells.

Complications of Infections

It doesn't matter where in the body an infection happens to start—the gums, vagina, skin, or feet. Infections need to be treated. They can quickly get worse and cause serious problems.

Bacterial Infections and Gum Disease

There are several different types of bacterial infections that can occur in people with diabetes. Your nails, scalp, and eyelids can become infected. Probably the most common bacterial infection among people with diabetes is gum disease.

People with diabetes are at high risk for gum disease and periodontitis. Bacteria love to feast on the areas between your gums and teeth. If bacteria set in, they can destroy the bone in your tooth socket. This can cause sores on your gums.

If gums are inflamed or infected, they will pull away from the teeth and jawbone, and the situation can get even worse. Bacteria will multiply in the newly created gap. The teeth may even become loose and fall out.

Fungal Infections

The most common cause of fungal infections is the yeast *Candida albicans,* which flourishes in a moist environment nourished by high levels of glucose. It causes an itchy rash that can sometimes have scales. Fungal infections include vaginal infections and jock itch.

Many women with diabetes find that they are susceptible to vaginal yeast infections. *Candida* or other vaginal infections can happen to women regardless of their age, sexual activity, or hygiene. Infections occur more often after menopause because estrogen levels are lower. Estrogen helps protect the vaginal lining. Infections are also more likely to occur just before your period, during pregnancy, or after you take antibiotics for another infection.

Ulcer: A deep, open sore or break in the skin.

Foot Infections

Your feet deserve special attention. No matter how much you weigh, pound for pound, your feet carry a heavy load. You never realize how important your feet are until they are injured and you suddenly find that you can't rely on them. Because the feet are vulnerable to injury, you need to check them every day for signs of injury and infection. This is doubly important if you have neuropathy, because you may not feel pain due to an injury or abnormality.

Foot ulcers can occur in people with diabetes. The word "ulcer" probably brings stomach problems to mind, but foot ulcers are more common in people with diabetes than stomach ulcers. An injured or infected area of the bottom of the foot can develop an ulcer. When you have an ulcer, layers of skin are destroyed by infection, which causes an open wound or sore to form, which allows the infection to spread further. Foot ulcers are very serious business. If you discover that you have a foot ulcer, you need to see your provider that day or go to the emergency room.

If untreated, the ulcers may go as deep as the bone and infect the bone, too. This can happen surprisingly fast. So don't underestimate the importance of daily foot care, especially if you have any loss of feeling in your feet.

Infectious Diseases

Common infectious diseases, such as influenza (the flu) and pneumonia, are often more serious for people with diabetes and are more likely to result in hospitalization.

Other Skin Problems

Besides infections of your skin, you may experience other diabetes-related skin problems. Atherosclerosis thickens arteries and creates skin problems in the feet and legs. Diabetic dermopathy causes scaly patches on the skin. Some rare skin problems occur when diabetes and blood glucose are way out of control. This can cause waxy skin, blisters, and other bumps.

Prevention of Infections

Keep your blood glucose in your target range to prevent many of the infections mentioned in this chapter. There are also specific tasks that you can do to prevent things such as gum disease and foot infections.

Prevention of Gum Disease

People with diabetes need to be extra vigilant about brushing their teeth and flossing daily. Have your teeth cleaned at least every 6 months.

Mouth Care Tips

- High blood glucose levels can cause severe gum disease and abscesses.

- Have your teeth cleaned and checked by the dentist at least every 6 months.

- Brush at least twice a day to fight plaque. Use a soft nylon brush with rounded ends on the bristles. Tilt the bristles at about a 45-degree angle against the gum line and brush gently in a scrubbing motion. Brush front and back and also brush the chewing surfaces.

- Brush the rough upper surface of your tongue.

- Use dental floss once a day to remove bacteria from between your teeth. Special floss holders and various types of floss are available to make flossing easier.

Prevention of Fungal Infections

Keeping your blood glucose close to your target range can help to prevent infections in the future. Avoiding irritating products, such as bubble bath and douches, may help prevent vaginal infections for some women. Keeping your groin area clean and dry may help reduce the risk of jock itch.

Prevention of Foot Infections

Your diabetes care provider needs to examine your feet at each visit. Taking your shoes and socks off when you go into the exam room will be a good reminder for him or her to check your feet.

Once each year, your feet should be examined more thoroughly. Sensation will be tested with a monofilament and a tuning fork, and your provider will check your reflexes and pulses.

Keeping the blood flowing to your feet is an important aspect of foot care. To do this, take steps to lower high blood pressure and cholesterol levels. If you smoke, ask your health care team for help in quitting.

Foot Care Tips

- Keep your feet clean and dry. Wash them every day with a mild soap. Dry them off carefully, especially between the toes. If the skin on your feet is too dry, apply a thin layer of lotion everywhere but between the toes.

- Inspect your feet and between your toes daily. Look for swollen, red areas and cuts or breaks in the skin. Feel for very cold areas (this could mean poor blood circulation) and very warm areas (this could mean infection).

- Never go barefoot. Although this is a good rule for everyone, it is really important for people who have lost sensation in their feet. Wear swimmers' shoes whenever you go swimming.

- Make a habit of cutting your toenails to follow the curve of your toe. This helps you avoid ingrown toenails.

- Wear only comfortable, well-fitting shoes. Don't expect to break in new shoes—they should feel comfortable right away. Shoes made of leather help your feet get the air circulation they need to stay healthy.

- Check the inside of your shoes every time you put them on. Make sure that the lining is smooth and that there are no objects inside.

- If you have a loss of sensation in your feet or have neuropathy, you may not be able to trust how a shoe feels to decide whether the fit is good for you. Find a shoe specialist who is trained to fit shoes for people with diabetes.

- Never try amateur surgery on your feet. Have your provider or podiatrist treat calluses, corns, plantar warts, and the like.

Prevention of Infectious Diseases
Flu vaccines are recommended every year for adults and children (over the age of 6 months) with diabetes. All adults need a one-time pneumococcal vaccine.

Prevention of Other Skin Problems
The number one thing that you can do to prevent skin problems is to keep your blood glucose under control. Many of the rare skin disorders are caused by extremely high blood glucose

Skin Care Tips

- Keep your skin clean. If you have dry skin, use a super-fatted soap such as Dove or Keri.

- Dry off well after washing. Be sure to prevent moisture in the folds of the skin—at the groin area, between the toes, under the breasts, and in armpits—where fungal infections are more likely. Try using talcum powder in these moist areas.

- Avoid very hot baths and showers if you have loss of sensation, because you can easily burn yourself without knowing it.

- Prevent dry skin. When you scratch dry, itchy skin, you can break the skin and open the door to bacteria. After you dry off from a shower, you may need an oil-in-water skin cream such as Lubriderm or Alpha-Keri. On cold and windy days, you may need to moisturize often to prevent chapping.

- Drink lots of water, unless your provider advises otherwise.

- Treat cuts quickly. For minor cuts, clean the area with soap, water, and hydrogen peroxide. Do not use antiseptics such as Mercurochrome, alcohol, or iodine because they irritate the skin. Only use antibiotic creams and ointments for a few days without consulting your provider.

Skin Problem Warning Signs
- Redness, swelling, pus, or pain that might indicate a bacterial infection.

- Jock itch, athlete's foot, ringworm, vaginal itching, or other signs of a fungal infection.

- Blisters or bumps anywhere, especially on the backs of your fingers, hands, toes, arms, legs, or buttocks—these are signs of high glucose levels; rashes, bumps, or pits near insulin injection site.

- Call your health care provider immediately if you notice any of these problems.

Treatment of Infections

Treating an infection depends on the area of the body that is infected as well as the level of infection. It also depends whether the infection is bacterial or fungal in nature.

Treatment of Bacterial Infections and Gum Disease

Luckily, many bacterial infections can be treated with antibiotics, either creams or pills.

Treatments for gum disease depend on the level of gum infection. In some cases, your dentist may need to scrape the plaque from your teeth and remove tissue from around the root of the tooth. In other cases, you may need to use medications (prescription mouthwash or antibiotics) or have surgery on your gums.

Treatment of Fungal Infections

You can buy antifungal products to treat infections like vaginal infections or jock itch. They usually come as creams that are placed on the problem area. They work by destroying the yeast that causes the infection. Your pharmacist can help you choose one that will work for you.

Jock itch will usually go away if you dry the affected area and apply an antifungal cream. However, talk to you doctor if the rash persists or worsens.

With vaginal creams or suppositories, it is important that you follow the product directions carefully. Be sure to use it for the entire time, even if your infection seems better. Even though it may seem to be gone sooner, the infection is more likely to return if the treatment is not completed.

If your infection is not better after using the product for the recommended period, or if it comes back right away, make an appointment to see your primary care provider or gynecologist. They can prescribe stronger medications.

Treatment of Foot Infections

If a foot or leg infection is not treated, a part of the foot or leg may need to be removed to keep the infection from spreading dangerously or to save a person's life.

Amputation is traumatic and is always the last resort. The surgeon will remove as little of the limb as possible to make walking possible. After the limb heals, you will most likely be fitted with a prosthesis. Today, prosthetic limbs are lighter and more comfortable than the clunkier models of the past.

Depression and Other Mental Health Disorders

Everyone gets the blues now and then. It's easy to feel blue when there is too much stress in your life, when sad things happen to you or your family, or when the everyday strain of living with diabetes gets you down.

However, people with diabetes are twice as likely to experience clinical depression as people without diabetes. They can also have anxiety disorders such as generalized anxiety disorder or even diabetes-specific phobias.

Risks of Depression and Other Mental Health Disorders

- Clinical depression is at least twice as likely among people with diabetes compared with people without diabetes.

- Depression also reoccurs more frequently and lasts longer.

- One study found that 14% of people with diabetes have generalized anxiety disorder.

Causes of Depression

The causes of depression and other mental health disorders are not entirely clear. However, having consistently high blood glucose can contribute to the symptoms of depression, such as fatigue. In addition, some studies have shown that depression might actually be a risk factor for type 2 diabetes. In other words, if you have depression, you are more likely to develop type 2 diabetes.

Managing your diabetes might also contribute to depression or other mental health disorders. The frustration, fear, and stress that go along with managing a chronic disease can be mentally exhausting.

Complications of Depression and Other Mental Health Disorders

It's normal to feel sad or frustrated with your diabetes sometimes. However, serious feelings of depression or anxiety disorders are nothing to ignore.

Usually, people feel relieved when they find out that depression is more common in people with diabetes. It can be comforting to know that you aren't the only out there dealing with these problems.

Depression

Depression can occur any time—when you are first diagnosed or after you have been dealing with diabetes for years. Depression can coexist with other feelings, such as denial, anxiety, or even anger. When you are depressed, it is often harder to pay attention to your diabetes.

People respond to depression in different ways. Some find that they aren't hungry at all, whereas others eat in order to feel better. Some people sleep all of the time; others can't sleep at all. People with depression often withdraw from family and friends and stop doing things that they enjoy.

Symptoms of Depression

- You no longer find pleasure in activities you once enjoyed.

- You have trouble falling asleep at night or wake up once you have fallen asleep.

- You feel tired during the day.

- You no longer enjoy eating the foods you once liked.

- You find yourself eating more or less than you used to.

- You either gain or lose weight.

- You have a hard time concentrating.

- You have a difficult time sitting still.

- You cannot seem to make even the most trivial decision.

- You experience feelings of guilt or a lack of self-worth.

- You feel that everyone else would be better off without you.

- You entertain thoughts of suicide or think of ways to hurt yourself.

It is important to recognize the symptoms of serious depression and to seek help right away. Unfortunately, when you feel depressed, you probably feel even less able to seek help. But it is the best thing you can do to get your life and health back on track.

Anxiety Disorders

Feeling anxiety is normal. After all, anxiety is a survival mechanism that gets you through a difficult situation. If you are face to face with a man-eating bear or have to give a lecture in front of 1,000 people, feeling a little anxious can help you get through the ordeal. However, for some people, their worries are more intense, frequent, or last longer than for others in a similar situation. Feelings of anxiety can coexist with feelings of depression.

There are several anxiety disorders, and together these disorders affect more Americans than any other mental illness. General anxiety disorder refers to feelings of anxiety and worry about everyday life. There are also diabetes-specific phobias that can be problematic. For example, some people have excessive fear of high or low blood glucose or fear of injecting insulin or some other medication. Other people are obsessive about tracking their blood glucose or recording their results.

Signs of an Anxiety Disorder

- You feel restless, feel irritable, and have difficulty concentrating much of the time.

- You tend to feel very worried or concerned about almost everything.

- You feel tired or easily fatigued.

- You have problems sleeping.

- You avoid people or places.

- You feel panicked or scared for no reason.

- You are not able to stop thinking about something.

- You feel like you have to do something over and over again, such as washing your hands or checking door locks.

- Your muscles feel tense or you experience frequent headaches.

If your worries or concerns are beginning to interfere with daily living or prevent you from enjoying the things you once enjoyed, it is time to seek help. First, try talking with your provider. Your anxiety may have a physical cause.

If there is no physical cause, you may be referred to a mental health counselor. Through medication, counseling, or a combination of both, your mental health counselor may help you find a way to handle or decrease your feelings of anxiety.

Dementia and Alzheimer's Disease

- People with diabetes may be at increased risk of dementia and Alzheimer's disease.

- Dementia is the term for a group of brain problems including memory loss, personality changes, and loss of daily functioning.

- One recent study showed that older people with type 2 diabetes who had a history of hypoglycemic episodes had an increased risk of dementia.

Prevention of Depression and Other Mental Health Disorders

Keeping your blood glucose levels on target will help you feel better physically and mentally. For example, people with type 2 diabetes who have blood glucose close to normal report that they feel more zest for living and experience an improved quality of life.

There may also be a physical reason for your feelings of depression. For example, you may be taking a medication that contributes to your symptoms of depression; you may need to stop or switch medications.

However, more serious physical and mental issues may require treatment. Only your health care provider can diagnose and treat a mental health disorder, so talk to him or her if you're struggling with depression or anxiety.

Treatment of Depression and Other Mental Health Disorders

Roughly two-thirds of people being treated for depression are cared for by their primary care physician. Your primary care physician is probably the first person you will talk to if you are having concerns about depression or anxiety.

It can be difficult to find the time to talk about depression in your regular checkup. After all, you probably have a number of diabetes issues to discuss with your health care provider. However, it is important for you, the patient, to take the time to bring up any symptoms of depression or anxiety.

Your primary care physician may feel comfortable diagnosing you—and then treating you—for a mental health disorder such as depression. Your health care provider can prescribe antidepressants or other medications to treat depression. However, your health care provider may also refer you (or you can ask to be referred) to a mental health professional.

You may see a psychiatrist, psychologist, psychiatric nurse, licensed social worker, family therapist, or other mental health counselor. Your counselor may recommend psychotherapy, medications, or both. Seeing a mental health professional does not mean that there is something wrong with you as a person. It simply means that you may have a medical problem that affects your emotions.

Psychotherapy

Psychotherapy, or talk therapy, can help treat your depression or anxiety disorder. There are several types of therapy that address mental health issues, such as modifying your thoughts and changing your behaviors.

Antidepressants

Many emotional problems are caused by chemical imbalances in the brain, and antidepressants can help you get back on track. Lots of people find successful relief from depression from a combination of talk therapy and medication.

Main Types of Antidepressants

- Selective serotonin reuptake inhibitors (SSRIs)
- Serotonin and norepinephrine reuptake inhibitors (SNRIs)
- Norepinephrine and dopamine reuptake inhibitors (NDRIs)
- Tricyclic antidepressants
- Monoamine oxidase inhibitors (MAO inhibitors)

Only you and your health care provider can help you find the right medication. Discuss any symptoms or improvements with new medications. Keep in mind that it can take up to 6 weeks for patients to notice significant differences.

You may need to try several different pills before you get the right one. Some experts say that the first antidepressant works well, but only half the time.

Keep in mind that your blood glucose or weight could be affected by antidepressants. You'll want to ask about any side effects of these medications as well as extra steps you should be taking to monitor or treat your blood glucose.

Dealing with Complications

Despite your best efforts, you may someday develop diabetes complications. Factors you can't control—your age, race, and genetic makeup—can affect your risk of developing complications.

If you have been taking steps to prevent complications, you may feel cheated if you develop a diabetes-related health problem. You may have many of the same feelings you had when you were first diagnosed with diabetes—anger, fear, guilt, or denial. You may feel overwhelmed that on top of dealing with diabetes and the ordinary stresses of everyday life, you now have new health problems with which to contend. You may feel tired of having worked so hard to prevent complications, only to have them develop anyway.

But there are treatments for diabetes complications, and they are getting better all the time. The earlier the signs of complications are found, the more effective these treatments can be. So be sure you are getting up-to-date information on treatments and prevention (see chapter 17 for a complete diabetes care schedule). Read all you can, and ask your diabetes care provider and other members of your health care team for updates on new treatments and research. Don't rely on hearsay from friends and relatives, who may not be up on the latest research.

Women's Health

Women with diabetes have more opportunities than ever to live healthy and full lives. Perhaps you've always dreamed of having children. Perhaps you want a richer sex life. Let's face it, every woman wants to age gracefully and go through menopause smoothly.

Your diabetes and management of your blood glucose shouldn't stop you from pursuing your goals. In fact, being more aware of your body, meal plan, and fitness could put you in better touch with your health than other women.

Read on to find tips for dealing with specific women's issues such as your menstrual cycle, pregnancy, and menopause. In addition, you'll find out about a few diseases you should have on your radar as a woman with diabetes.

Specific Risks for Women

It's no surprise that women with diabetes have specific health needs and concerns. After all, pregnancy, menstruation, and menopause are uniquely female circumstances. You'll want to consider your diabetes and your blood glucose management as you approach these different stages in your life.

Women with diabetes should also be aware of their risk for certain problems such as heart disease, obesity, osteoporosis, and depression. These disorders are common in women with diabetes. The good news is that many of these problems can be prevented or treated effectively.

Heart Disease

You've heard that diabetes makes you two to four times more likely to have a heart attack or stroke than someone without diabetes. You also know that cardiovascular disease is the number one killer of men and women with diabetes.

Yet, recent studies are shedding light on how big a problem cardiovascular disease is for *women* with diabetes—regardless of age or menopause status. Women with diabetes have a 4- to 6-fold increase of coronary artery disease, according to one study. Coronary artery disease can lead to heart attacks, heart failure, and death. This compares with a 2- to 3-fold increase in men with diabetes. In the past, cardiovascular disease was thought of as a "man's disease." Now, physicians and patients are realizing that women are at equal or greater risk for cardiovascular disease.

Preventing Heart Disease
It's important to advocate for your cardiovascular health at your regular checkups. Make sure that your health care provider checks your cholesterol and blood pressure, which are two contributors to cardiovascular health. Ask whether you are meeting the recommended goals for blood pressure and cholesterol as discussed in chapter 14.

Obesity

Women tend to be more overweight than men, so they need to take active steps to reduce and maintain a healthy weight. Obesity is a major risk factor for type 2 diabetes and cardiovascular disease.

Regular physical activity and healthy eating will help you lose weight and prevent obesity. Exercising will also help you lower your blood glucose and increase your insulin sensitivity. If you're overweight, ask your health care provider about healthy steps that you can take to lose weight and reduce your risk for cardiovascular disease and other diabetes complications.

Osteoporosis

Osteoporosis: A condition characterized by decreased bone mass and density, causing the bones to become fragile and increasingly susceptible to fractures; it can arise in men (especially elderly men) and women but is highly prevalent in women who have passed menopause.

Osteoporosis happens when your bones become weak and brittle, usually because they have lost mass and density. The most common problem is a bone fracture, which can occur even when doing the simplest of tasks.

You've probably heard that women, especially post-menopausal women, are at increased risk for osteoporosis. But older women with diabetes have an even higher risk of osteoporosis.

Risk of Fractures
Women with type 1 diabetes have four to five times the risk for fractures than other women, according to one study. In addition, women with type 2 diabetes tend to have more fractures than their nondiabetic counterparts of the same age. TZDS, a diabetes medication, may increase the risk of fractures, so women should discuss these risks with their health care providers.

Preventing and Treating Osteoporosis
Women of all ages should make sure they're getting the recommended amounts of calcium and vitamin D to promote bone health. You should also exercise regularly. Bone health starts early, so it is important to take healthy steps in your 20s and 30s, but it is never too late to become more active.

Women 65 and older should have a bone density test performed. Your doctor may recommend the test earlier if you have a family history of osteoporosis. Treatments for osteoporosis include prescription medications, such as bisphosphonates, raloxifene, calcitonin, teriparatide, denusomab, and tamoxifen.

Depression

In general, people with diabetes are more likely to experience depression. Women with diabetes are more likely to suffer from depression than men with diabetes, according to one study. Make it a point to bring up any symptoms of depression with your health care team. You can read more about symptoms and treatments for depression in chapter 14.

Menstruation

At first, you think you're just imagining it. You're going along and everything seems fine. You're in good spirits, eating well, getting regular workouts, and your blood glucose levels are on target most of the time. Then, for some unexplained reason, everything seems out of whack. Maybe your blood glucose levels are too high; maybe they're too low. Then you check the calendar. Oh, yeah—it's that time of the month.

Research behind Menstruation and Diabetes

If you have trouble keeping your blood glucose levels on target just before your period starts, you are not alone. A survey of 200 women with type 1 diabetes showed that in the week before their periods, 27% had problems with higher-than-normal blood glucose levels and 12% had lower-than-normal blood glucose levels. Another study revealed that among women under the age of 45 who were hospitalized for diabetic ketoacidosis, half were within several days of starting their periods. A survey of more than 400 women revealed that nearly 70% experienced problems with blood glucose levels during their premenstrual period. The problem was more common among women who considered themselves to suffer from the moodiness associated with premenstrual syndrome (PMS).

It's difficult to pinpoint just how many women have problems with their blood glucose levels before menstruation. Many studies are based on surveys conducted after the fact and do not take physical activity and eating patterns into account.

Menstrual Cycle

A woman's reproductive system revolves around the monthly task of ovulation—releasing an egg ripe for fertilization. This is true from the time that women begin menstruating until menopause.

Phases of the Menstrual Cycle

- The follicular phase of the menstrual cycle begins the day your period starts and lasts for about 12–14 days, until you ovulate or release the egg.

- During the early part of this stage of the cycle, the female sex hormones estrogen and progesterone are at their lowest levels.

- Another hormone, follicle-stimulating hormone, is produced, which turns on estrogen production. This prepares the ovary to respond to a surge of a second pituitary hormone called luteinizing hormone. The mid-cycle surge of luteinizing hormone causes the ovary to release an egg midway through the cycle.

- After egg release, the luteal phase takes over. Luteinizing hormone triggers the ovary to produce estrogen and progesterone. These hormones cause the lining of the uterus to thicken, in preparation for a possible pregnancy.

- If fertilization does not occur, the ovary stops making estrogen and progesterone. The sudden loss of estrogen and progesterone cause the shedding of the uterine lining, and menstruation occurs.

Causes of High Blood Glucose

Some women find that the high levels of estrogen and progesterone about a week or so before menstruation affect their blood glucose levels. Researchers aren't exactly sure why, but they have some clues.

Insulin works by binding to receptor proteins that sit on the surface of cells. Glucose can then enter the cell. When levels of progesterone and other progestin hormones are high, insulin action within cells is affected. This leads to temporary extra insulin resistance—the cells no longer respond to insulin the way they should. The result is that blood glucose levels may be higher than usual and then drop once menstruation begins.

Causes of Low Blood Glucose

Higher-than-normal estrogen levels may actually increase sensitivity to insulin by improving insulin action. When this occurs, the increased insulin action can lead to blood glucose levels that may be lower than usual before menstruation.

Other Symptoms

Not all women experience changes in blood glucose levels before menstruation. Some studies have shown no differences in blood glucose levels throughout the menstrual cycle. Some women experience bloating, water retention, weight gain, irritability, depression, and food cravings, especially for carbohydrates and fats. If you have a tendency to crave these foods, they could also contribute to high blood glucose levels before your period.

Check Your Records

You can find out for sure if you suspect that your blood glucose levels are affected by your menstrual cycle. Look at your daily blood glucose records over the past few months. Mark the date that your period started for each month. Do you see any pattern? Are your blood glucose levels higher or lower than normal during the week before your period? If you are not recording your blood glucose levels, now may be a good time to start.

Troubleshooting Your Blood Glucose during Menstruation

You can get things back on track if you find your blood glucose levels harder to manage on a monthly basis. Changes in blood glucose levels could be due to normal changes, PMS, or both. Some women find that they need to adjust their insulin dose before their period and again once the period starts.

Think about charting your symptoms along with your glucose levels. It will also help to note how you are feeling throughout the month, not just before your period, to see whether you can detect any sort of pattern.

Here are some specific strategies to try depending on whether you tend to have high or low blood glucose around your period. Try one strategy at a time, so you know which one is the most effective.

Strategies for Highs before Your Period

- If you use insulin, gradually increase your dose. Work with your health care team to add small increments, so that insulin levels are higher the last few days of your cycle, when blood glucose levels normally rise. One to two additional units of insulin may be all it takes. It will take a little trial and error to figure out the right dose for you. As soon as menstruation begins, estrogen and progesterone levels drop. When this happens, return to your usual dose of insulin to lower your risk of hypoglycemia.

- Eat at regular intervals, when possible. This will keep your blood glucose levels from swinging too much. Large blood glucose swings could contribute to some of the emotional and physical symptoms of PMS, which may in turn make variations in blood glucose levels worse.

- Try to avoid eating extra carbohydrates. Keep a handy supply of crunchy veggies—for example, celery, radishes, or cucumbers—and dip them in fat-free salsa.

- Cut back on alcohol, chocolate, and caffeine. They can affect both your blood glucose levels and your mood.

- Be especially careful about your sodium intake, which causes bloating. Use pepper, fresh or powdered garlic, lemon, cayenne pepper, or scallions to add some zing to food.

- Try to be more physically active. Many women find that regular exercise diminishes mood swings, prevents excessive weight gain, and makes it easier to manage blood glucose levels.

Strategies for Lows before Your Period

- If you use insulin, work with your health care team to gradually decrease the amount of insulin you take a few days before your period starts. A decrease of 1 or 2 units of insulin may do the trick.

- Reducing diabetes medications may help, especially if you are concerned about having to take extra food. Ask your provider about the safest way to go about this.

- Try spreading your carbohydrate intake over the course of the day. Multiple small meals can help even out your glucose levels.

- Eat a small amount of carbohydrate before you work out.

If your periods are irregular and your blood glucose swings are unpredictable, try to chart your ovulation to see whether you can tell when your period will occur so you can adjust your treatment plan. If you are taking insulin, you may want to try intensive diabetes management, perhaps with an insulin pump. This may give you the flexibility you need to deal with changes in blood glucose levels on a daily basis.

Polycystic Ovarian Syndrome

Polycystic ovarian syndrome (PCOS) is common in women with diabetes. Roughly 5–10% of American women have PCOS. It can cause abnormal menstrual cycles and is the most common cause of infertility. No one knows exactly what causes PCOS, but some people think there may be a link to insulin.

Polycystic Ovarian Syndrome:
A hormonal disorder that affects young women of reproductive age and can cause infertility in some patients; many patients with this disorder also have insulin resistance.

Symptoms of PCOS

- Abnormal menstrual cycles
- No periods
- Irregular periods
- Heavy or prolonged bleeding
- Painful periods
- Infertility
- Acne
- Facial hair

- Waist measurement greater than 35 inches or a waist bigger than hips (apple shape).
- Acanthosis nigricans: darker patches of skin in neck folds, armpits, folds in the waistline, or groin.

There are treatments for the symptoms of PCOS, so talk to your health care provider if you experience any of the above problems.

Menopause

Menopause is a natural process, not an event. It proceeds slowly, often lasting 8–10 years. It begins when your body slows down its production of estrogen and progesterone, the hormones that set the stage for pregnancy.

Ovulation and menstruation become irregular. Some months you may ovulate and have a period; other months you may not. You may also experience other symptoms, such as vaginal dryness, weight gain, and mood swings—problems that you may initially attribute to your diabetes.

It can begin before you turn 40, but many women continue to menstruate well into their 50s or 60s. The average age for U.S. women having their last period is 51. Your mother's age at menopause is highly predictive of yours.

Menopause and Blood Glucose

Menopause can throw your diabetes management plan out of balance. That's because you may have learned to adjust your plan around your normal hormonal fluctuations. The hormones that keep your menstrual cycle going—estrogen and progesterone—can also affect blood glucose levels.

In some women, high levels of progesterone and other progestin hormones may decrease the body's sensitivity to insulin. High levels of estrogen tend to improve insulin sensitivity. As you start the transition of menopause, you'll want to pay close attention to the effects it will have on your blood glucose levels.

> ### Weight Gain during Menopause
>
> Some women find that they gain weight during menopause. This can increase the need for medications. Many women find that they need to eat less and exercise more to maintain their weight.

Menopause can be a very positive time in life for women. They are free from some of their responsibilities and can spend more time taking care of themselves.

Complications of Menopause

Menopause changes the amount of estrogen and progesterone in your body. These hormones have protective effects that can be diminished during menopause. This can put you at risk for heart disease, osteoporosis, and yeast infections. These risks are particularly pertinent for women with diabetes, who already have a greater risk for these problems.

Heart Disease
You will be more sensitive to insulin during menopause. That's good news. But losing estrogen can increase your insulin resistance. The lack of these hormones can also cause other changes, some of which can affect diabetes complications.

Diabetes increases your risk for heart attack and stroke two to four times above the general population. Women without diabetes are protected against cardiovascular disease until menopause. This is not the case for women with diabetes. Diabetes overrides the protective effect of estrogen. If you have diabetes, your risk for heart attack and heart disease is six times that of a woman without diabetes.

Total cholesterol levels tend to rise and levels of "good," or HDL, cholesterol tend to drop after menopause. For some women, hormone replacement therapy may increase triglycerides, a common problem in type 2 diabetes. High blood glucose levels can make this situation even worse. Keeping your blood glucose, blood pressure, and cholesterol levels on target can help.

Osteoporosis
Estrogen also helps to maintain strong bones. As estrogen levels fall, your bones can lose some of the minerals that hold them together. This can lead to osteoporosis, a condition in which bones are brittle and easily broken.

Eating calcium-rich foods, taking calcium supplements, and participating in regular weight-bearing exercise, such as walking, can help. Hormone replacement therapy can increase bone density and lower your risk of osteoporosis. Other medications to combat osteoporosis are available.

Yeast Infections

Many women with diabetes find they are more prone to vaginitis and yeast infections once they enter menopause. Yeast and bacteria can irritate the vaginal lining if they grow out of control. They thrive in warm, moist places with a good supply of food (glucose).

Even before menopause, you are more likely to develop yeast infections when your blood glucose levels are high. After menopause, the risk increases. That's because estrogen normally nourishes and supports the vaginal lining. Without it, yeast and bacteria have an easier time growing. These infections are not related to sexual activity or personal hygiene.

Treatments for Menopause

Hormone replacement therapy is a complicated issue. On one hand, estrogen can decrease the risk of osteoporosis and vaginitis and alleviate hot flashes. On the other hand, it can increase the risk of breast and uterine cancer, heart disease, and stroke.

Hormone Replacement Therapy

- The current recommendation is to take the smallest dose of hormone replacements for the least amount of time possible to control symptoms.

- Reevaluate your treatment plan every six months.

- Women with breast cancer, heart disease, or a history of blood clots should avoid hormone replacement therapy.

Whether you decide to use hormone replacement therapy is up to you. Many factors can influence your decision, like whether diseases like cancer, heart disease, and osteoporosis run in your family.

As a woman with diabetes, you need to play an active role in your overall health care throughout menopause and beyond. You have more at stake during this time in your life than women without diabetes. As with other issues related to your sexual health, it's important that you discuss concerns with your provider and other health care team members.

Important Tests for Women Taking Hormone Replacement Therapy

- Have your A1C tested two to four times a year. This test tells you about your blood glucose levels over the long term.

- Have your cholesterol and triglyceride levels checked as recommended by your provider.

- Have yearly eye exams and kidney function tests.

- Have a yearly mammogram to detect breast cancer.

- Have a yearly Pap smear and gynecologic examination to detect cancer of the cervix, uterus, endometrium, and ovaries.

Sexual Health

Diabetes can affect sexual function and fulfillment for both men and women. The good news is that sexual health is getting more attention, and there is more help available.

If you are having any problems related to sexual issues and you want help, talk to your health care team. If you don't feel comfortable talking with your provider, perhaps you need to find a health care professional with whom you do feel comfortable discussing personal matters.

Your provider will evaluate your concerns and help you sort out the causes. There are many factors that can result in sexual difficulties, including medications, hormonal changes, problems caused by diabetes, and your emotional health.

Your Sexual Health

- If your sexual problem appears to be due to a physical cause, you may be referred to a gynecologist or urologist.

- If stress or anxiety is contributing to your problem, a visit with a mental health professional may be in order.

- Depression, which is more common among people with diabetes, can also contribute to problems with sexual fulfillment and performance.

Problems with Arousal

Many women with diabetes at one time or another experience some sexual difficulties. In fact, one study showed that 30–40% of women with diabetes reported that they have problems with sexual function, refrain from sexual relations, and are generally not satisfied with sex. But for women, long-term blood glucose levels and diabetes complications don't appear to have a direct effect on sexual functioning. For most women with diabetes, the problem is caused by lack of arousal.

There is a very strong link between mind and body. If a woman does not feel in the mood for sex, then her body does not respond the way it needs to in order for her to enjoy it. If she is not emotionally ready or interested in sex, then she will be less likely to enjoy it physically.

Common Causes of Lack of Arousal

- Vaginal infections that affect how you feel physically and how sexy you feel
- Bladder infections that can cause painful intercourse
- Hormonal changes due to your menstrual cycle or menopause
- Vaginal dryness
- Lack of sexual desire
- Fear of pregnancy
- Depression and medications used to treat depression

Vaginal Infections

Vaginal infections (yeast infections, vaginitis) are more common among women with diabetes. Blood glucose gives the bacteria an excellent medium in which to grow. These infections do not have anything to do with how clean you are, your age, or sexual activity. Although vaginal infections do not directly affect your sexual health, they can affect how sexy and desirable you feel.

You can buy over-the-counter antifungal products to treat these infections. If the infection does not clear up within a week, contact your health care provider for stronger medicine.

Urinary Tract Infections

Women with diabetes are also at risk for bladder or urinary tract infections (UTIs) for the same reason. Signs of a bladder infection include feeling like you need to go to the bathroom more often, painful urination, painful intercourse, and blood in the urine.

If you think that you have a bladder infection, call your health care provider right away. These infections usually respond quickly to antibiotics. Some women find that cranberry juice helps treat or prevent these infections. Choose artificially sweetened cranberry juice or purchase a bottle of cranberry pills.

Hormonal Changes

Many women find that during their menstrual cycle, and especially around the time of their period, their blood glucose levels are erratic, and they have less energy for everything, including sex.

During menopause, hormone levels change, and some women find that their blood glucose levels go up and down. Mood changes and hot flashes are also common during this time. Although menopause does not affect sexual desire, some women find that they have vaginal dryness that can make sex painful or uncomfortable. You can buy lubricating gels (e.g., water-soluble jelly) that can help. You can also ask your provider about estrogen creams.

Lack of Sexual Desire

Some women find that they are just too tired. They are coping with busy lives, caring for children and grandchildren, working, and trying to find some time for themselves. Diabetes adds more stress and work to their lives. High blood glucose levels add to feeling tired and run down. Because of nerve changes related to diabetes or simply due to getting older, some women find that they need more stimulation to fully enjoy sex.

Depression is more common among people with diabetes. Depression usually causes people to feel less interested in sex. In addition, some of the medications used to treat depression can affect sexual desire.

Women with either type 1 or type 2 diabetes may feel less desirable or that their bodies are less attractive as they get older and perhaps heavier. Diabetes complications can also cause you to feel less desire, both emotionally and physically.

Tips to Increase Your Desire

- If you have dryness, infections, or are worried about getting pregnant, talk with your diabetes care provider or your gynecologist.

- If you are worried about your blood glucose levels, do a quick blood glucose check before having sex. Knowing that you are not likely to have a reaction can help you relax and enjoy yourself. You may also want to keep something to treat a low glucose nearby so that if you do go low, you won't have to interrupt things too much. See more about avoiding lows during and after sex in chapter 8.

- If you feel sad and blue or if your sadness is affecting your desire for sex, talk with your provider. There are medicines that will work for depression that do not affect your desire for sex.

- Help set the stage to get into the mood. Take time for yourself and your partner. Let your partner know what will help you feel more romantic and in the mood.

Birth Control

Practicing birth control and safe sex are important for anyone, but especially for women with diabetes. You don't want to be caught off guard. Instead, you want to plan and prepare for a pregnancy as much as possible to ensure optimal health for you and your baby.

Why It's Important

Choosing and using an effective form of birth control allows you to plan your pregnancies. This will help you get your blood glucose on target before you become pregnant.

Blood Glucose and Early Pregnancy

- High blood glucose levels can interfere with the early development of a baby, and the baby has a greater chance of a birth defect.

- A baby's organs are formed in the first six weeks after conception. Most women are not even sure that they are pregnant during this critical time.

- Also, when blood glucose levels are high, the risk of spontaneous miscarriage may double in early pregnancy.

- You increase your chances for a healthy child when you plan your pregnancy and have an A1C level that is as near to normal as possible before you.conceive.

- In fact, when blood glucose levels are close to normal, the risk for birth defects is about the same as for women without diabetes.

Types of Birth Control

Women with diabetes have the same birth control options as other women. The pill, intrauterine device (IUD), barrier methods, and spermicides are all ways to reduce the risk of unplanned pregnancy.

The rhythm method, in which women predict ovulation and avoid intercourse during fertile times, is generally not a sufficiently reliable method of birth control for women with diabetes. A tubal ligation may be an option if you are sure you never want to become pregnant, because it is nearly impossible to reverse.

Many birth control methods work by altering hormone concentrations. The methods of birth control that rely on hormones, such as birth control pills and the IUD that releases progesterone, can affect your blood glucose levels. Birth control methods that don't rely on hormones are not likely to change your blood glucose levels.

Which method you choose will depend on your own personal and family health history and your individual preferences. If you have any special concerns, be sure to bring them up with your health care team.

Birth Control Pills and Other Devices
Oral contraceptives ("the pill") are the most popular and effective birth control method available. Hormonal methods of birth control prevent pregnancy by preventing ovulation. They are available as pills, patches, vaginal rings, and by injection. Hormonal contraceptives are about 95–99% effective. But whether the pill is right for you depends on many factors.

Types of Birth Control Pills

- Some pills contain estrogen and progesterone.

- Other pills contain only progesterone (called mini pills).

- Another pill is taken for three months straight, and a woman only gets her period four times a year.

Other Types of Hormone Delivery

- The patch contains both estrogen and progesterone. You leave it on for 21 days and then remove it for seven days.

- The vaginal ring is a small circular device that contains estrogen and progesterone. You insert it deep into your vagina and leave it there for 21 days.

- An injection called Depo-Provera contains only progesterone. It is given at your provider's office every three months. Before committing to any long-lasting method, you may want to try a progesterone-only pill, which you can stop at any time, to see how you respond.

- Progestin implants are surgically implanted beneath the skin and work for several years. The Norplant implant was taken off the market, but other implants are available.

In general, hormonal methods of birth control are safe for women with diabetes. If you are over 35 and smoke or if you have a history of heart disease, stroke, high blood pressure, peripheral blood vessel disease, or blood clots, these methods may be risky for you.

If you've found that your insulin sensitivity varies at certain times of the month, being on the pill, patch, ring, or injections may help smooth out your blood glucose levels. By providing a steady dose of hormones, blood glucose swings can be kept to a minimum.

Some women find that oral contraceptives increase insulin resistance. If your blood glucose levels are affected, your insulin or your dose of oral diabetes medication can be adjusted. Taking the lowest possible dose or the mini pill can also help.

Pill Precautions

- Check your blood glucose levels frequently, especially during the first couple of months.

- Some women need to slightly increase their insulin dose. By keeping complete records, you and your health care team can decide whether you need to make changes in food, activity, or diabetes medication.

- Have your A1C, blood pressure, cholesterol, and triglyceride levels checked three months after you go on the pill and then as often as recommended.

IUD

The IUD is a small T-shaped object that is placed into the uterus by a provider. IUDs prevent sperm from reaching the egg or from implanting in the uterus. One type contains copper, and others contain progesterone. IUDs can remain in place for one, five, or ten years, depending on the type.

IUDs are generally recommended for women who have had one or more children. When properly inserted and retained, IUDs are 95–98% effective in preventing pregnancy.

Diaphragm

The diaphragm is a shallow rubber cup that fits tightly over the cervix, the entrance to the uterus. It prevents sperm from entering the uterus. The diaphragm is coated with spermicidal jelly before you insert it. The diaphragm is put into place just before intercourse and needs to be kept in place for at least 6 hours after intercourse and then removed.

It is 80–94% effective for preventing pregnancy. The effectiveness depends on the user's ability to place the device correctly, use of spermicidal jelly, and leaving it in place for the full time. Your gynecologist will fit your diaphragm and teach you how to place it properly and check to be sure it is covering the cervix.

Sponge

The sponge contains spermicidal jelly and is placed into the vagina over the cervix to prevent sperm from entering the uterus. It can be inserted up to 24 hours prior to intercourse and needs to be left in place for 6 hours afterward. Sponges are 80–91% effective.

Cervical Cap

The cervical cap is a small, thimble-shaped barrier device that fits tightly over the cervix to prevent sperm from entering the uterus. It is used with spermicidal jelly.

Condom

The condom, a thin sheath that is placed over the penis before intercourse, is a common form of birth control. It prevents the sperm from entering the woman's vagina. When used correctly and along with a spermicide, the condom is 85–90% effective in preventing pregnancy. The condom should be put on before intercourse and can be removed soon afterward. Condoms also help prevent the spread of several sexually transmitted diseases, including gonorrhea, chlamydia, and AIDS.

Female Condom

The female condom is another barrier method of contraception. It is a larger type of condom that you insert into your vagina up to eight hours before intercourse. You remove it afterward, taking the sperm with it. It can also help protect against sexually transmitted diseases. It is 74–79% effective.

Spermicides

These work by killing sperm and can be purchased without a prescription. There are several types: foam, gel, cream, suppository, or tablet. They can be used alone or to increase the effectiveness of barrier methods. They are 72–90% effective.

Sterilization

If you are sure you never want children or don't want any more children, you may want to consider surgical or nonsurgical sterilization. With the surgical method, the fallopian tubes are tied off to prevent eggs from reaching the uterus. With the nonsurgical method, tiny spring-like coils are placed into the fallopian tubes. Material embedded into the coils irritates the lining of the tube, causing scar tissue to grow. After about three months, there is enough scar tissue to block the tubes.

Done correctly, these methods are almost 100% effective in preventing pregnancy. In very rare cases, a fertilized egg may reach the uterus, resulting in pregnancy, or may grow outside the uterus, resulting in an ectopic pregnancy. You'll need to be certain about your decision to be sterilized, because it is nearly impossible to reverse.

Pregnancy

In the past, it was common for women with diabetes who became pregnant to experience serious problems, such as miscarriage, stillbirth, or a baby with birth defects. Today, it is very common for women with diabetes—either type 1 or type 2—to have safe and healthy pregnancies.

Although women with diabetes and their unborn children face additional risks because of diabetes, these can be kept to a minimum through careful blood glucose management, before and during pregnancy, and intensive obstetrical care. For this reason, all women with diabetes need to plan ahead before becoming pregnant.

Before Pregnancy

The first step is to meet with your health care team to consider the specific challenges you may face during your pregnancy. You need a complete evaluation of your overall health and any diabetes complications. It's important to get a good idea of how much extra work and expense may be involved before you become pregnant.

You may have specific questions for your health care provider. You may be concerned that your baby could develop diabetes. You may be worried for your own health. Your glucose levels may also be an issue.

Baby's Risk for Type 1 Diabetes

You may have concerns about your child someday developing diabetes. A child born to a parent who has type 1 diabetes is at slightly greater risk of developing type 1 diabetes than children of parents without diabetes. The risk is slightly higher when the father has type 1 diabetes.

Researchers have identified genes that could play a role in type 1 diabetes. However, there is no genetic test for predicting whether your baby will develop type 1 or type 2 diabetes.

- A baby has a 1% risk of developing diabetes if the baby is born to a mother who is age 25 or older and has type 1 diabetes.

- A baby has a 4% risk of developing diabetes if the mother is younger than age 25 when the child is born.

- A baby has a 6% risk of developing diabetes if the father has type 1 diabetes.

- Each of these risks is doubled if the parent with type 1 diabetes developed it before the age of 11.

- If both parents have type 1 diabetes, the risk is not known but is probably somewhat higher.

- A baby born to parents who do not have diabetes has a 0.3% risk of developing the disease.

Baby's Risk for Type 2 Diabetes

Type 2 diabetes tends to run in families. You can inherit genes that increase the chances you will develop type 2 diabetes. Studies of twins have shown that genetics play a very strong role in the development of type 2 diabetes. However, scientists do not yet have tests that can predict which genes cause diabetes.

Lifestyle also influences the development of type 2 diabetes. Obesity tends to run in families, and families tend to have similar eating and exercise habits.

If you have a family history of type 2 diabetes, it may be difficult to figure out whether your diabetes is due to lifestyle factors or genetic susceptibility. Most likely it is due to both. However, don't lose heart. Studies show that it is possible to delay or prevent type 2 diabetes by exercising and losing weight.

Ask your provider to refer you to a medical geneticist or genetic counselor if you have concerns about your baby's risk for diabetes. They are trained to assess the contributions of genetic and environmental factors in causing many diseases, including diabetes. They will know the results of the latest diabetes and genetics studies and studies to prevent diabetes in high-risk individuals.

Pre-Pregnancy Exam

You'll need a thorough physical exam before you become pregnant to assess any problems that could jeopardize your health or that of your baby.

Pre-Pregnancy Checkup

- An assessment of any complications, such as high blood pressure, heart disease, and kidney, nerve, and eye damage. If you have any of these complications, they need to be treated before you try to conceive. Even kidney transplant recipients who are otherwise healthy have had babies.

- Your A1C level will be measured.

- If you have type 1 diabetes, your thyroid function will be measured.

- In addition, your exam will include a review of all the medications, herbs, and supplements you are taking to make sure they are compatible with a safe pregnancy.

Diabetes Complications and Pregnancy

In rare cases, diabetes-related problems may be so serious that it's safer to avoid pregnancy. For example, you'll need to think carefully about pregnancy if you have untreated high blood pressure, cardiovascular disease, kidney failure, or crippling gastrointestinal neuropathy. Pregnancy can make these conditions worse.

Heart Disease. Your doctor may recommend an electrocardiogram if you have any signs of heart disease, such as chest pain during exertion.

Neuropathy. Signs of nerve damage will also be checked. If the nerves that control heart rate or blood pressure have been damaged, this can affect how you will respond to the physical stresses of pregnancy. Neuropathy can also affect how well your body nourishes you and your growing baby, so tell your provider if you have had persistent problems with nausea, vomiting, or diarrhea.

Kidney Disease. Your pre-pregnancy exam will also include an evaluation of your kidneys. In women with high blood glucose levels and untreated kidney disease, kidney function can worsen during pregnancy. Fortunately, pregnancy does not appear to have long-lasting effects on kidney function. If you have kidney problems, you need to be prepared for a potentially more difficult pregnancy. This can include problems with edema (swelling) and high blood pressure.

Retinopathy. You will also be referred to an ophthalmologist, who will examine your eyes, especially the retina—the part of your eye that senses visual images. Your pupils will be dilated so that the back of the retina can be checked for damage caused by diabetes. Untreated diabetic retinopathy may get worse during pregnancy and should be treated and stable before you become pregnant. You will continue to get your eyes examined throughout the pregnancy.

→ ACE Inhibitors, Statins, and Pregnancy

You will need to change your medication if you have been taking ACE inhibitors or ARBs for kidney disease or high blood pressure. Taking these drugs during pregnancy can cause kidney problems for the baby. Likewise, if you take a statin to treat your cholesterol levels, you will also need to discontinue those before becoming pregnant.

Ideal Pregnancy Health Care Team

- Diabetes care provider

- Obstetrician experienced in treating pregnancy complicated by diabetes

- Pediatrician experienced in the care of infants of mothers with diabetes

- Registered dietitian

- Diabetes nurse educator experienced in teaching women how to intensively manage their diabetes

Managing Your Blood Glucose before Pregnancy

Birth defects occur in 1–2% of all babies born to women without diabetes. These problems include abnormalities of the central nervous system, heart, and kidneys.

Women with diabetes have a higher risk of birth defects in their babies, but they can lower the risk to the same level as mothers without diabetes by keeping blood glucose levels on target. This means keeping blood glucose levels as close to normal as possible before and during the first trimester of your pregnancy. Keep in mind that pregnant women without diabetes have lower blood glucose levels than non-pregnant women.

Why is well-controlled blood glucose important before conception? Because you want your blood glucose levels to be as favorable to your developing baby as possible. All of the baby's major organs are formed during the first 6–8 weeks of pregnancy, which may be before you know you're pregnant.

Research behind Tight Control and Pregnancy

In several studies, women who had an A1C that was 1% above normal levels before conception lowered their baby's risk of birth defects to 1–2%, the same as women without diabetes. Normal A1C is less than 7%. Babies of mothers who began intensive diabetes management *after* conceiving were more likely to have birth defects.

Planning ahead of time will ensure that you find a diabetes management plan that will work for you. This takes some trial and error as well as patience. It may take too long if you wait until you are pregnant.

Tips for Pre-Pregnancy Blood Glucose Management

- Before you become pregnant, you probably will intensify your daily diabetes care.

- If you have type 1 diabetes, you will begin or fine-tune your plan by using several insulin injections each day or switching to insulin pump therapy.

- If you have type 2 diabetes, using oral diabetes medicines may not be recommended.

- You will probably need to begin insulin therapy. Many women with type 2 diabetes find that they need to use insulin during pregnancy.

Health Care Expenses
Having a baby is a major financial investment for any parent. Your pregnancy will include the added expenses involved in tight blood glucose management. It used to be worse. Before self-monitoring of blood glucose, a woman could easily spend half of her pregnancy in the hospital. Now the major expenses are fetal monitoring and blood glucose monitoring instead of hospitalizations.

Before you conceive, check with your insurance company to find out what is covered. Your insurance plan may cover more during your pregnancy if you have the appropriate documentation.

Extra Expenses and Doctor Visits

- You will need to see both your obstetrician and your diabetes health care provider frequently—perhaps every week or every 2 weeks for most of

A1C before Pregnancy

Your A1C level will be measured frequently. It is recommended that your A1C level be as close to normal as possible before you stop using birth control.

your pregnancy. You will learn to make adjustments to insulin doses based on blood glucose values. This requires time, practice, and lots of support from your health care team.

- Your health care should include nutrition counseling with a registered dietitian and diabetes educator. You will likely learn how to count carbohydrates and adjust insulin doses.

- You'll need to check blood glucose values often to make sure you are within your target ranges. Many pregnant women do seven or more checks each day. Test strips are the big expense in monitoring.

- You may need to do ketone monitoring each day. This will protect you against surprise ketoacidosis as well as starvation ketosis, which can occur after a low blood glucose value, when carbohydrate intake is very limited, or when calorie intake is lower than needed. This means buying ketone strips.

- If you treat your type 2 diabetes with oral diabetes medications, you may need to switch to insulin before you become pregnant. This means paying for insulin pens or syringes and insulin, plus training from an educator on how to give insulin and to adjust your dose.

During Pregnancy

Your pregnancy is one of the most important times to take good care of yourself and your diabetes. You'll want to create the healthiest environment possible for your growing baby. Women with diabetes can deliver perfectly healthy babies with the right care, planning, and management.

Managing Your Blood Glucose

The first step is to choose blood glucose targets for your pregnancy. Talk to your health care team about how to personalize blood glucose target ranges to your health and your lifestyle.

Sample Target Blood Glucose Ranges during Pregnancy

- Before meals: 60–99 mg/dl
- One hour after meals: 100–129 mg/dl
- A1C less than 6%

In the first trimester, targets are designed to help you minimize the risk of birth defects or miscarriage. In the second and third trimesters, the targets will help prevent your baby from growing too large. If you have trouble staying in the target range, or if you have frequent or severe hypoglycemia, talk to your health care team about revising your treatment plan or your targets.

Insulin during Pregnancy

- Women with type 2 diabetes usually need to use insulin during pregnancy.

- Many women with gestational diabetes need to use insulin.

- Women who use insulin will find that they need to increase their insulin dose over the course of the pregnancy to reach these targets.

- You may also need to make adjustments in the kind of insulin you take and how often you inject.

- Usually, the amount of insulin you take increases with each trimester. Some women need to increase their insulin dose by as much as two or three times, especially in the last trimester.

You'll probably need more insulin throughout your pregnancy because the hormones of pregnancy, which increase in effect over time, create more and more insulin resistance. This does not mean that your diabetes is getting worse. You and your provider need to decide together when and how to make any changes in your insulin schedule or dose.

Monitoring Your Blood Glucose

You will probably need to check your blood glucose levels several times each day. If you take insulin, you may monitor before and after meals and at bedtime. If you have type 2 or gestational diabetes and

Hypoglycemia Unawareness during Pregnancy

Some women develop hypoglycemia unawareness during pregnancy (chapter 8), and your early-warning signs of hypoglycemia may change. You may have less shaking and sweating and more rapid development of drowsiness or confusion.

are managing it through meal planning and regular exercise, you will need to check more frequently than usual.

When to Monitor

- Once before each meal
- 1–2 hours after each meal
- At bedtime
- During the middle of the night, around 2 a.m.

If you take insulin and keep your blood glucose levels near normal, you are more likely to have episodes of low blood glucose. During pregnancy, blood glucose of 70 mg/dl or lower is considered hypoglycemia.

Monitoring frequently helps you know whether you are close to being low. There is no evidence that hypoglycemia is dangerous for the baby. But, a hypoglycemic episode can be dangerous for the mother-to-be.

In addition to checking before and after physical activity, always check your blood glucose before you drive. Be prepared for severe low blood glucose by carrying a glucagon kit and training several people (whom you see daily) how to use it (chapter 8).

Food, Physical Activity, and Exercise

You may need to change your eating habits during pregnancy to help stay on target. You will also want to make sure that you are eating foods that provide adequate nutrition for you and your baby. You will probably want to visit your dietitian even before you become preg-

Common Weight Goals for Pregnancy

If your pre-pregnancy weight is...	Then gain...
Underweight (BMI less than 18.5 kg/m^2)	28–40 lb
Normal (BMI 18.5–24.9 kg/m^2)	25–35 lb
Overweight (BMI 25–29.9 kg/m^2)	15–25 lb
Obese (BMI 30 kg/m^2 or higher)	11–20 lb

nant. In general, choose nutritious foods that are part of any healthy eating plan.

Eating five or six small meals a day may help your efforts to stabilize your blood glucose. Women with gestational diabetes may be able to manage their blood glucose levels more effectively by limiting their carbohydrate intake to 35–40% of calories.

Ketone Testing

Checking your urine for ketones each morning may be recommended. It will help you know if you are getting the carbohydrates and insulin you need.

Eating small meals may also help with "morning sickness," which is often worse when your stomach is empty. Morning sickness is not limited to mornings, and nausea can occur day or night, often accompanied by vomiting.

If you have morning sickness, there are some dietary steps you can take to feel better. It can help to keep some starch, such as Melba toast, rice or popcorn cakes, or saltines or other low-fat crackers, close at hand to eat if you become nauseated. Some women find it helpful to eat a small snack at bedtime or before they get up in the morning to prevent morning sickness.

Help with Nausea

- Eat dry crackers or toast before rising.

- Eat small meals every 2½–3 hours.

- Avoid caffeine.

- Avoid fatty and high-sodium foods.

- Drink fluids between meals, not with meals.

- Take prenatal vitamins after dinner or at bedtime.

- Always carry food with you.

- Talk with your health care team. They may have helpful suggestions. Also tell them about any herbs or supplements you may be using. These may make nausea worse.

It is important to maintain physical activity during pregnancy, as long as your overall health permits it. Being fit prepares you for the physical stress of labor and delivery and the busy days that follow. It is usually safe to continue with any exercise you were doing regularly before pregnancy. But pregnancy is not the time to take up any new, strenuous activities (see chapter 11).

Doctor Visits

You'll need more frequent visits to your obstetrician, perhaps every two weeks for the first part of your pregnancy and weekly during the last month. The reason for these visits is to make sure that your baby is developing as expected and that you stay in good health.

Common Tests during Pregnancy

- You will be screened for neural tube defects early in pregnancy (around weeks 15–18) by measuring the concentration of alpha-fetoprotein in your blood.

- You'll need an ultrasound test early in your pregnancy (to show when your baby was conceived) and several more throughout your pregnancy to follow the baby's growth.

- A fetal echocardiogram may be done around the middle of your pregnancy.

- Other monitoring includes counting your baby's movements for an hour each day and fetal movement and heart rate monitoring during the last 6–12 weeks of pregnancy. These tests help ensure your baby's well-being and will assist your health care team in deciding when to deliver your baby.

Birth

In the past, babies born to women with diabetes tended to be large. This problem, called macrosomia, was the baby's response to the extra amounts of glucose in the mother's blood. To reduce the risk of delivery problems or stillbirth, these babies were usually delivered by inducing labor or by cesarean section (C-section) before or during the 37th week of a 40-week pregnancy.

Now, because more women are able to manage their diabetes more intensively and better tests are available to monitor the baby's health, most women can deliver close to their due date.

Macrosomia is less common now, but sometimes the baby is too large or the woman's pelvis is too small for a safe vaginal delivery. Trying to deliver a too-large baby vaginally can result in shoulder damage or respiratory distress for the baby. In this case, a C-section is performed.

What to Expect during Birth

Your blood pressure will be checked frequently throughout your pregnancy. High blood pressure can be a sign of preeclampsia, a serious condition that occurs more often in women with diabetes. Preeclampsia may also lead to early delivery, often by C-section.

Labor is work, and usually you will not be able to eat. You will probably get an intravenous catheter so that fluids or calories can be given as needed. Your blood glucose levels will be monitored frequently during labor. You can be given insulin either as injections or intravenously. Many women don't need insulin during active labor.

After Delivery

Once you deliver your baby, both you and the baby will be watched closely in the hospital. It's a time of celebration and recovery. You'll have new challenges in managing your diabetes with a little one to nurture and feed. Taking care of yourself—and your diabetes—is one of the most important things that you can do to take care of your new baby.

Baby's Health

Your baby will be closely watched after birth. He or she is at risk for hypoglycemia and will have frequent blood glucose monitoring during the first 24 hours after birth. Hypoglycemia occurs because the baby has been producing enough insulin to cover the high glucose levels in the uterus. This does not mean your baby has diabetes.

Jaundice is also common and may require therapy with lights. If your baby was delivered early or is very large for his or her age, your baby will also be evaluated for respiratory problems. It is not unusual for these babies to be in an intensive care nursery for a short time so that they can be watched very closely.

Mother's Health

If you have type 1 diabetes, you may require less insulin for the first few days after delivery. Your health care provider may check for postpartum thyroiditis. If you have type 2 diabetes, you may not need insulin at all during this time. Your insulin needs will gradually go back to your pre-pregnancy level in about 2–6 weeks. If you had gestational diabetes, your blood glucose levels will most likely return to normal after delivery (see chapter 5).

The postpartum period may be one of unpredictable swings in blood glucose. Your hormones and body chemistry are in flux. You are recovering from a major physical challenge. You are probably exhausted from caring for your baby, too. If you find that keeping your blood glucose on target poses a greater challenge, try not to get too discouraged.

If you find that you feel overwhelmed by trying to care for a new baby and diabetes or if you are feeling depressed, contact your health care team. They can help you find support or make a referral for evaluation or counseling. It's not a sign of weakness if you need help at this time. Your baby needs a healthy mother!

Don't forget that you can become pregnant again soon after you give birth. Even if you have not had a period, you can still ovulate. Breast-feeding does not necessarily prevent you from becoming pregnant. So, before you resume having intercourse, be sure you are using effective birth control.

Although virtually every aspect of your life may seem turned on its head after the birth of a new baby, the four basic management tools remain the same: insulin or other diabetes medication (oral diabetes medications cannot be used while you are breast-feeding), blood glucose monitoring, meal planning, and physical activity.

Working out may be the last thing you are thinking about after the baby is born. But as soon as you feel well enough and you have your doctor's okay, taking your baby along on a daily walk can help you feel better and more relaxed.

Highs and Lows

Hormonal changes, emotional shifts, irregular sleep patterns, and fatigue may hide or change your symptoms of high or low blood glucose. You may find it hard to tell the difference between "after-baby" blues, such as unexplained crying or moodiness, and low or high blood glucose. Fatigue, feeling spacey, weakness, or forgetfulness can be caused by both high and low blood glucose and by lack of sleep. If you're not sure, play it safe and check your blood glucose.

Avoiding Lows

- Check often.

- If you feel hypoglycemia coming on, treat it right away, regardless of whether you can check.

- Keep items such as glucose tablets, hard candy, or regular soda handy in several rooms.

- Make sure that those around you know how to spot your signs of low blood glucose; teach them what you want them to do if you don't seem like yourself.

- Keep a glucagon kit on hand, and be sure that your family members know how and when to use it.

If you have had hypoglycemia unawareness in the past, be vigilant not to let your blood glucose get too low when you are alone with your baby. Get help with middle-of-the-night feedings, or make it a habit to eat a snack then. Take care to check before you get into the car to drive. Don't nap or sleep on an empty stomach. Remember that your best protection is still frequent blood glucose monitoring and regular snacks and meals.

Having a new baby can affect your diabetes care habits, especially if you have to care for other children. You may find that your baby's unpredictable schedule and your own erratic sleep patterns make it difficult for you to eat or snack when needed. Using multiple injections may make your life easier and give you more flexibility. Although it is tempting to put your infant's needs before your own, taking care of yourself is important for both you and your baby.

Breast-Feeding

The ideal food for your baby is your own breast milk. Some studies have shown that breast-feeding may help protect your baby from developing type 2 diabetes later in life. You will need to take in about 300 additional calories per day while breast-feeding, so you may want to schedule another visit with your dietitian. Your hunger level may change, and you may need some help with balancing your meals and your baby's meals with your insulin doses.

The extra energy your body uses to make breast milk can cause your blood glucose levels to become erratic. Throughout the time you breast-feed, continue checking your blood glucose level often.

Tips for Breast-Feeding and Blood Glucose Management

- Keep a source of fast-acting carbohydrate, such as glucose tablets or orange juice, handy when breast-feeding.

- When your baby is ready to nurse during the day, eat your own snack or meal, plus a glass of water or low-fat milk, while you feed your infant. It helps to have the snack or meal portion ready so you don't have to prepare your food while the baby is waiting to be fed. This provides your body with fluids and helps prevent low blood glucose.

- During nighttime feedings, have a snack yourself. Otherwise, you might have a low blood glucose reaction, especially if you have been up several times in the night.

Listen to Your Body

As a woman, you have so many possibilities in life. Having diabetes should not stop you from pursuing them. One of the most important things that you can do for your health is to listen to your body. Listening to your body will help you take care of yourself and communicate with your health care team.

Men's Health

Historically, men have not discussed their health as much as women. However, times are changing. Men are encouraged to talk about their physical and emotional health as much—if not more—than women.

Men with diabetes are in a position of power to advocate for their health. After all, you probably have a health care team in place—or you are assembling one at the moment. Your health care providers are there to help you prevent and treat diabetes complications. In this chapter, you can find out about the conditions that specifically affect men and how to discuss them with your health care provider.

Male Sexual Health

Many men are not comfortable with the idea of discussing their sex life with a doctor or nurse. But the truth is that diabetes can affect your sexual performance and how you respond to aging and sex. It is important to open the lines of communication with your health care team. They will not be shocked by your questions, and there are ways of coping with any problem you might face.

For men with diabetes, the major concern is erectile dysfunction (ED). Men with diabetes can also have low testosterone. Other important topics in sexual health are birth control and safe sex.

Don't face these important issues alone just because they concern your sexual life. Sex is a part of each of our lives as humans and belongs in a healthy life.

Erectile Dysfunction

Among men, the diagnosis of diabetes brings with it the concern about impotence or ED. But, are problems with erections really more common in men with diabetes than in men without diabetes? Because so many men suffer from this condition in silence, it's difficult to count how many men with and without diabetes actually have a problem.

ED Facts

- ED is age related. It is primarily a problem among men over 40, with and without diabetes.

- Of all men with diabetes over the age of 50, it is estimated that 50–60% have some degree of ED.

- Some studies have suggested that the risk of ED is much higher in men with diabetes.

- ED has a range of severity. The above statistics include all types of ED, from occasional to complete. Complete ED (the complete inability to have an erection) occurs much less often.

So just what is ED? Having ED means that most or all of the time, the penis fails to become or stay hard enough for sexual intercourse. If you have ED, you can't achieve or maintain a satisfactory erection.

Erectile Dysfunction (ED): The inability to get or maintain an erection for sexual activity; a complication of diabetes that is usually treated with medication; also called impotence.

If, on occasion, you fail to maintain or achieve an erection, you do not have ED. You also do not have it if you experience a decrease in sexual desire, have premature ejaculation, or if you fail to ejaculate or reach orgasm.

Causes of ED
Physical or psychological factors—or both—can cause ED. Figuring out why ED occurs can be complicated. Sexual desire begins in the brain, and signals are sent through the nervous system to the blood vessels to trigger an erection. The male sex hormone testosterone is also involved in sexual desire and achieving erections.

The most common causes of ED in men with diabetes are blood-vessel and nerve-related damage. Neuropathy and cardiovascular disease put you at risk for ED.

Blood vessel damage is a common cause of erection problems in men with diabetes. When blood flow to the penis is reduced, the penis can no longer become erect.

Tests for ED

- A frequently used test for blood-vessel damage is an ultrasound study of the penis. Sound waves are used to measure blood flow through the arteries and veins.

- Another test involves injecting a drug or mixture of drugs into the penis to cause an erection. The drug is injected in such a way that it bypasses the penile nerves. If the injection causes you to have an erection, damaged blood vessels are not the cause. If you don't have an erection, it means there may be some damage to your blood vessels.

Nerve disease is also a culprit in ED. When the nerves that signal the penis are damaged, erection can be impaired. You may be referred to an urologist to find out if the nerves in your penis are affected.

ED caused by physical problems usually comes on slowly and worsens over time. Early symptoms include a less rigid penis during sexual stimulation and when you wake up. Over time, men with ED may not be able to sustain firm erections long enough to enjoy sexual intercourse.

Psychological factors, depression in particular, are also common culprits in

Low Testosterone and ED

In rare cases, low amounts of testosterone can cause ED. If it is too low, your problem may be caused by a hormonal problem not related to diabetes. See more about low testosterone in the next section.

men with diabetes. You can read more about depression and its treatment in chapter 14.

Fears that Contribute to ED

- Expecting ED to happen if you know you are at increased risk because of your diabetes may lead to ED.

- You may be unable to have an erection if you feel pressure to perform.

- You may develop a great deal of fear and anxiety after a single erection problem, which can eventually lead to ED.

- Worry and stress can decrease your brain's response to testosterone.

Also be aware that certain medications can cause temporary ED. Tell your provider about all the medications you are using—even over-the-counter remedies. Drugs frequently used to treat high blood pressure, anxiety, depression, and peptic ulcers can all be factors.

If you have signs of trouble and suspect that it may be related to a new medication you are using, tell your provider. There may be other medicines you can use. But don't stop taking the medicine. Smoking and alcohol consumption can also contribute to erection problems.

Prevention of ED
The way to reduce your risk is to keep your blood glucose levels as close to normal as possible. In addition, it will help to quit smoking, decrease your alcohol intake, and keep blood pressure near normal.

Treatments for ED
There are several treatments available. In choosing a treatment, find the one that is most compatible with the needs and desires of both you and your partner.

Medications. There are several drugs available for treatment, and many men with diabetes have found them to be effective. Sildenafil and vardenafil can help stimulate and maintain an erection 30–60 minutes after taking a pill. Tadalafil is similar but lasts for up to 36 hours.

Ask your provider about these drugs if ED is a problem for you. Side effects include headache, indigestion, hearing or vision loss, and an erection that won't go away. Some people with heart problems, blood pressure problems, eye problems, or a history of stroke may not be able to take these medications. Some medications such as nitrates can be dangerous if taken with ED medications.

Penis Injection. Another option is to inject a form of the drug alprostadil directly into the penis. This induces an erection that lasts about 30 minutes to 1 hour. Side effects include bruising and prolonged erection. Some men also develop scarring in the penis, which occasionally results in a permanent curvature during erection.

Vacuum Pump. Another option uses a vacuum pump to create an erection. A cylinder is placed around the penis. A small vacuum pump pulls air out of the container, creating a vacuum. This causes blood to flow into the penis, triggering an erection. To maintain the erection, the container is removed and replaced with a constriction ring. This provides an erection for about 30 minutes. The ring can cause bruising if kept on for more than 30 minutes. Separate constriction rings and external support devices are also available.

Implant. You can also have a pump device with a penile prosthesis surgically implanted into your body to produce erections. Your best bet is to visit a urologist with experience if you are interested in this type of implant. Be sure to ask about the risks, which can include infection and the need for further surgery in case the device doesn't work correctly.

Testosterone. Testosterone injections or patches can be prescribed if a low hormone level is the problem. The injections are usually given every 3–4 weeks. Men should not take testosterone unless they have abnormally low levels and have been evaluated for prostate cancer.

Psychotherapy. It may also help for you and your partner to work with a therapist who knows how to deal with sexual issues.

All of the treatments for ED have risks or drawbacks. You may decide to seek no treatment. Some men and their partners choose to express their sexuality in ways that do not involve intercourse. If you do want to consider treatment, you need to tell your provider, even if you are not asked about your sexual life. Your provider can only help you if you let him or her know about your concerns.

Low Testosterone

Testosterone is the most important male hormone and promotes the development of male characteristics. It is also tied to sexual desire and mood. Low testosterone is twice as common in men with diabetes as in men without diabetes. It can cause a range of problems, from ED to disinterest in sex to depression. It is estimated that 5 million American men have low testosterone.

Symptoms of Low Testosterone

• Decreased sexual desire
• ED
• Reduced lean body mass
• Depressed mood and lack of energy

Causes of Low Testosterone
Aging is associated with less testosterone. However, just because you are older does not mean that you will have low testosterone or little interest in sex. Low testosterone can be caused by problems with your hypothalamus, pituitary gland, or testes. Some medications such as morphine also contribute to low testosterone.

Treatments for Low Testosterone
You can ask to be referred to an endocrinologist or urologist who specializes in treating men with low testosterone. A simple blood test can be used to detect low testosterone.

Low testosterone can be easily treated with testosterone injections, patches, or gels. Patches and gels can cause skin irritation. Women and children should not touch the applied area. Men with prostate or breast cancer or heart or liver disease may not be able to use testosterone replacement therapy.

Birth Control

Another aspect of men's sexual health is preventing sexually transmitted diseases and pregnancy. Birth control options are more limited for men than women. Yet, there are still several options.

The most popular is the condom, a thin sheath that is placed over the penis before intercourse. It prevents the sperm from entering the woman's vagina. When used correctly and along with a spermicide, the condom is 85–90% effective in preventing pregnancy. The condom should be put on before intercourse and can be removed soon afterward. Condoms also help prevent the spread of several sexually transmitted diseases, including gonorrhea, chlamydia, and AIDS.

Men who are certain they do not want to father any or any more children can opt for a vasectomy. This is a simple procedure that prevents the release of sperm into the seminal fluid. When the man ejaculates, the semen contains no sperm, but men still experience the full pleasure of intercourse.

However, it is very difficult and expensive to reverse a vasectomy, and you'll need to be certain about your decision. Some men opt to store some of their sperm before vasectomy for possible in vitro fertilization or artificial insemination, should they decide they want children at some later time.

Low Blood Glucose during and after Sex

Sex, like any physical activity, can lead to low blood glucose. If you use insulin, you'll want to monitor and manage your blood glucose with this in mind. Taking steps beforehand can also help you enjoy and feel more relaxed during sex. See more about avoiding lows during and after sex in chapter 8.

Talk about Your Sexual Health

Diabetes can affect sexual functioning and fulfillment for both men and women. The good news is that sexual health is getting more attention, and there is more help available.

If you are having any problems related to sexual issues and you want help, talk to your health care team. If you don't feel comfortable talking with your provider, find a health care professional with whom you do feel comfortable discussing personal matters.

Your provider will evaluate your concerns and help you sort out the causes. There are many factors that influence your sexual health, including medications, hormonal changes, your diabetes, and your emotional health.

Sleep

Everyone knows it's important to get your zzzz's. But if you're like many Americans, you're probably not getting enough sleep. Sleep disorders are more common than you think. The Institute of Medicine estimates that 50–70 million Americans have a sleep disorder. Many men with diabetes have sleep disorders such as sleep apnea.

Sleep Apnea

Have you ever been accused of loud snoring? Have you ever been woken up by your own snoring? Loud snoring is a symptom of sleep apnea. Sleep apnea is the most common sleep disorder. It occurs when breathing is briefly and repeatedly interrupted during the night. It is more common in men than women.

Sleep apnea can make you tired during the day, and it can also lead to more serious complications such as cardiovascular disease. Talk to your health care provider if you have difficulty sleeping, are drowsy during the day, or your family members complain about your snoring.

Preventing and Treating Sleep Apnea
Weight is a major risk factor for sleep apnea. So losing weight is one of the best ways to prevent sleep apnea.

Sleep Apnea: A disorder in which you briefly stop breathing or breathe very shallow, usually for 10–20 seconds.

Continuous positive airway pressure (CPAP) is one of the most common treatments for sleep apnea. At night, you wear a mask that is hooked up to a machine that circulates air through the nose and mouth. Surgery can also be used to open the airways.

Cardiovascular Disease and Obesity

Having diabetes makes you two to four times more likely to have a heart attack or stroke than someone without diabetes. Cardiovascular disease is the number one killer of men with diabetes.

Therefore, it's important to advocate for your cardiovascular health at your regular checkups. Make sure that your health care provider checks your cholesterol and blood pressure, which are two contributors to cardiovascular health. Ask whether you are meeting the recommended goals for blood pressure and cholesterol (as discussed in chapter 14).

Roughly one-third of American men are obese. Obesity is a major risk factor for type 2 diabetes and cardiovascular disease. If you're overweight, ask your health care provider about healthy steps that you can take to lose weight and reduce your risk for cardiovascular disease and other diabetes complications.

Getting regular physical activity and eating a healthy diet will help you lose weight and prevent obesity. Exercising will also help you lower your blood glucose and increase your insulin sensitivity. Read more about physical activity in chapter 11.

Quitting smoking and drinking less alcohol will reduce your risk for cardiovascular disease, ED, and a host of other health problems.

Talk to Your Health Care Provider

In general, men are less likely to seek medical advice from their health care providers than women. However, men with diabetes should have more reason than anyone to reverse this trend. There are real ways to prevent and treat men's health issues such as cardiovascular disease, ED, and sleep apnea. Listen to your body and talk to your health care providers about your concerns.

Unhealthy Habits: Smoking and Drinking

Men are more likely to smoke, and men are more likely to drink alcoholic beverages than women. Twenty-three percent of American men (over 18) smoke, and 31% of American men had 5 or more drinks per day during the past year.

Part VI
Diabetes and Health Care

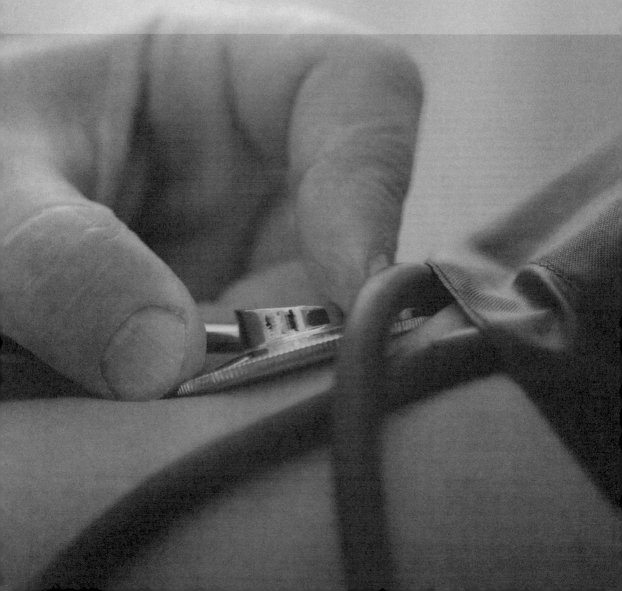

CHAPTER 17

Your Health Care Team

Covered in This Chapter

- Diabetes Care Provider
- Visits with Your Diabetes Care Provider
- Diabetes Care Schedule
- Other Health Care Providers
- Communication
- Second Opinions

Your health care team is one of the most critical facets of your diabetes care. Your team includes your primary care provider, and specialists such as a diabetes educator, registered dietitian, eye doctor, podiatrist, pharmacist, and others. Of course, your health care team also includes you.

Sometimes, diabetes professionals will already practice together in a center that specializes in diabetes care. Or your diabetes care provider may routinely work with some of these professionals. If not, you may have to assemble your own group. If your provider doesn't have a diabetes nurse educator or dietitian on staff, ask him or her to recommend one, as well as other professionals you should have on the team. It may be helpful to think of your diabetes care providers as a team and yourself as the team captain.

Your choice in providers will depend on your personal needs and preferences, as well as cost and insurance coverage for different services or providers. This chapter will give you tips in selecting a primary diabetes care provider and specialists—as well as background about what to expect during your medical visits. You should keep in mind that assembling a team and developing a plan may take some time.

Endocrinologist: A doctor who treats people who have endocrine gland problems, such as diabetes.

Your plan will need fine-tuning along the way. Try to choose providers who are easy to reach and willing to adapt to changes along the way.

Diabetes Care Provider

A diabetes care provider is often an endocrinologist, although it could also be a primary care physician or internist who has experience treating people with diabetes.

Your diabetes care provider is responsible for providing certain basic care, such as a yearly physical exam, complete medical history, and A1C tests every 3 months. What you can expect during these basic care visits will be discussed in more detail in the next section.

Your diabetes care provider should also be available on an as-needed basis to discuss problems, changes in your blood glucose management or other diabetes care, or any other concerns.

Choosing a Diabetes Care Provider

Take the time to select a diabetes care provider who is right for you. You will have your own needs in terms of your health, insurance coverage, and convenience, as well as your preferences in style and demeanor. Keep in mind that your diabetes care provider is your primary contact, so you'll want to select someone whom you respect and with whom you feel comfortable talking openly.

Schedule an Interview
You may want to schedule an appointment to talk with several candidates before you choose a provider. Some health care professionals may charge an "interview fee," so be sure to ask about this ahead of time.

Come to your interview with questions you would like answered. Write them down in advance, and don't be afraid to look at them during your interview. Write down answers to your questions during the interview, if need be.

Sample Interview Questions for Providers

Education
- Where did you go to school?

- Are you board certified in endocrinology or internal medicine?

- Do you hold professional memberships in associations such as the American Diabetes Association (ADA), the Endocrine Society, or the American College of Physicians?

Diabetes Experience
- Do you see a lot of patients with diabetes?

- Are they mostly patients with type 1 or type 2? How many patients like me do you see each month?

Insurance
- What insurance do you accept?

- Are you a provider in my Preferred Provider Organization (PPO) plan?

- If I require a referral to a specialist, do you have colleagues who also participate?

Basic Care
- How often will regular visits be scheduled? What tests are conducted routinely?

- Who covers for you on your days off?

- What procedures should be followed in the event of an emergency? What conditions indicate an emergency?

- How do I know whether I should call you?

- How hard is it to get an appointment?

Other Team Members
- Are you associated with a nurse educator, dietitian, or other health care professionals so that I can benefit from a team approach?

- Are you likely/willing to try new approaches/therapies to diabetes management, or do you prefer to wait until new methods have stood the test of time?

Office Considerations

- Is the office neat and clean?

- Is the staff polite?

- Are you accommodated at your scheduled appointment time or are you kept waiting?

- Are educational materials on display?

- Is there someone you can call with questions or concerns?

Consider Your Needs

After you've met with a provider, take time to reflect on the interview. You'll want to consider how you felt about the physician's philosophy, demeanor, and experience. Think of yourself as a customer.

Sample Questions for Yourself

- How did the visit with your health care provider feel?

- Were you comfortable with the practitioner?

- Did he or she seem concerned about you as an individual?

- Was the provider willing to work with you to achieve your health goals?

- Did you feel free to express your feelings?

- Did you feel that he or she was listening to you? Were you given sufficient time to get all your questions answered or did you feel rushed?

- Did the provider seem likely to tell you what to do or more likely to work with you to reach your goals?

Ask Other Patients and Providers

If the idea of scheduling an interview seems daunting, you may start by asking other patients for recommended providers. For example, recommendations from members of a diabetes support group could be helpful. You may also want to ask other health care providers (whose opinion you trust) for advice. If you like and trust your eye doctor, then you could ask him or her to recommend an endocrinologist.

You'll also want to consider the location and convenience of the office. Maybe the closest endocrinologist is 50 miles away and you would like someone closer. In that case, you might want to find an internist or primary care practitioner with expertise in treating patients with diabetes.

You can also contact the ADA for a list of recognized providers (www.diabetes.org). Your local hospital or community health organization may also provide referrals. Professional medical societies may provide recommendations as well.

Visits with Your Diabetes Care Provider

Yearly physical examinations are important for everyone as a preventive health measure, but they are especially important for people with diabetes. People with diabetes have a greater risk for developing diabetes complications, including damage to the eyes, kidneys, nervous system, heart, and circulatory system. You are also more susceptible to developing infections. That's why a thorough examination is needed to make sure your whole body is functioning properly. You'll also discuss your blood glucose management, so don't forget to bring your meter, logbook, and any medications you're taking.

Medical Questionnaire

If you are seeing your diabetes care provider or other health care professional for the first time, you will most likely be asked to provide a medical history. The forms and questionnaires may vary, but all will want the same basic information. It is important to answer honestly and trust that your health care team will maintain confidentiality.

Most histories include questions about the health of your close relatives. Think about the general health and specific conditions that have arisen in your family, especially your mother, father, grandparents, sisters, and brothers.

> ➜ **Fill Out the Questionnaire in Advance**
>
> Ask that that your provider mail a medical questionnaire in advance. That way, you can answer all of the questions more accurately and at a leisurely pace. You'll want to provide the most complete and accurate picture to get the best health care.

You will also be asked to provide a general inventory of your past and present health problems, such as back pain, appendicitis, headaches, and depression. Do not deny or hide any illnesses, such as psychiatric disorders or AIDS.

Dig out a record of your immunizations. You may even need to call past health care providers for dates and names of procedures.

Sample Medical History Questions

- What medications are you currently taking?

- Do you smoke? Have you ever smoked? If so, how much and for how long?

- Do you have any allergies?

- Have you ever been pregnant? What was the outcome?

- When were your last chest X-ray, eye exam, and dental exam?

- Have you ever been treated by a psychiatrist?

- Have you recently lost or gained weight? What was your maximum weight? What did you weigh at the diagnosis of diabetes?

- Have you ever been rejected for health insurance or employment for a medical reason?

- Do you use alcohol or any street drugs?

Some medical questions may be difficult to answer. You may not remember or you may not want to be reminded. Make an attempt to overcome your fears of being judged harshly by what you put on the form. A concerned health care professional will use this information to provide you with the best possible care—not to criticize you. What is important is achieving good health.

Physical Exam

After taking a medical history, your diabetes care provider will give you a complete physical exam. In fact, you need a complete physical once each year.

It will include a close examination of all the parts of your body, from head to toe. Your provider is trained to detect small problems and prevent them from becoming bigger problems and will examine all of the following, and perhaps more.

The Physical Exam

- *Weight or Body Mass Index.* Talk to your provider about the body weight that you think is best for you and whether you have any difficulty maintaining that weight.

- *Blood Pressure and Pulse.* Ask what your current readings are and whether these fall within the recommended range. If not, ask what levels are best for you to achieve and how to go about it.

- *Eyes.* Your eyes will be checked for problems, and you will be asked about any changes in your vision. Make sure to keep your provider aware of any changes that have occurred, even if you are also seeing an eye care specialist.

- *Heart and Lungs.* Your provider will most likely listen to your heart and lungs through a stethoscope. Sometimes an electrocardiogram or stress electrocardiogram may be performed to detect symptom-free heart disease. Such tests measure the electrical activity and pumping of your heart muscle and can detect many subtle abnormalities.

- *Feet.* Removing your shoes and socks each time you visit—not just during your yearly physicals—will remind your diabetes care provider to check your feet. You will be checked for dry, cracked spots; calluses; infections; and sores. Using a monofilament to check for sensation, your provider will also look for any loss of feeling that could indicate neuropathy. A tuning fork may also be used for examining changes in sensation.

- *Skin.* Your skin will be examined by sight, with special attention to insulin injection sites.

- *Nervous System.* Your reflexes and your sensitivity to the sharpness of a monofilament or pin or the light touch of cotton or a brush will be checked. If you are experiencing any persistent problems, such as dizziness on standing, pain, burning sensation, numbness in your legs or arms, constipation, diarrhea, difficulty urinating, or difficulty with erections or sexual satisfaction, make sure to mention them.

- *Mouth and Neck.* Your provider will examine your gums, teeth, mouth, and throat. She or he will feel for swelling in the glands in your neck and ask you about your brushing and flossing habits. The function of your thyroid gland will also be assessed during your initial physical examination.

- *Blood.* A sample of blood will be drawn to test for glucose levels and A1C. A fasting lipid profile, which measures cholesterol and triglycerides, will be performed to determine the levels of these fats in your blood. Your urea nitrogen and serum creatinine concentrations in the blood will also be measured to assess your kidney function. Your microalbumin-to-creatinine ratio should be reviewed, too.

- *Urine.* Testing urine for ketones, glucose, and protein also assesses kidney function. People with diabetes are more likely to have urinary tract infections because of the high concentrations of glucose in urine and the loss of the sensation of knowing when the bladder is empty or full because of neuropathy. If you have any symptoms of infection, a urinary culture may also be performed.

- *Vaccinations.* People with diabetes are more likely to develop complications from the flu or pneumonia. You need a pneumonia vaccine once in your lifetime and a flu shot each year.

- *Other Tests.* Other members of your health care team may perform some tests. For women, this includes a Pap smear, mammogram, and gynecological and rectal exam. Contraception and pregnancy planning should also be discussed. Men should receive prostate and rectal exams. Both men and women should have their stool samples tested for blood to detect colon cancer. Men may receive a prostate cancer test.

Your examination will also include a discussion of your health, such as a review of your blood glucose measurements, insulin therapy and other medications, eating habits, and physical activity.

Keep your provider up to date on any changes you have made in lifestyle or habits. Maybe you just quit smoking or started an exercise program. If you feel a need to consult one of the other professionals on your team, now is the time to ask about it. If you feel that there are any parts of your treatment plan that are not working, tell your provider. Also keep your provider informed of what treatment options are successful.

A1C Test and Blood Glucose Management

Beyond the yearly physical, your A1C should also be checked every 3 months. Measuring your A1C tells you how well your treatment program is working. You need this test whether you use insulin or not. You may hear your results reported as estimated average glucose or eAG. Estimated average glucose is a different way to report A1C results using the same units as your blood glucose meter (mg/dl). You can use your A1C or eAG results to compare with your own self-monitoring records.

Be sure to discuss your blood glucose readings at every visit. Always bring your logbook, meter, and medications to your exam. If your daily blood glucose tests are in range but your A1C is too high, you and your provider need to discuss ways to better manage and monitor your blood glucose levels. It is important to understand why your tests might show good blood glucose readings when your overall blood glucose measure is too high.

Other Topics

You may be asked about any unusual concerns you may have, such as a sore shoulder or abdominal pain. If you are experiencing any sexual or personal problems, don't be afraid to bring them up.

Ask about what to do on sick days. Even a mild cold can throw off blood glucose levels, usually by making them higher than normal. Ask what symptoms to be on the lookout for and when you should call

Thyroid Test

If you have type 1 diabetes, you have a five times greater risk of also someday developing thyroid disease, which is another type of autoimmune disease. Make sure you have a blood test to detect thyroid disease.

> **Children's Height**
>
> Children whose blood glucose levels are often high sometimes are slow to grow and mature. Height should be measured at every visit, not just the first one. The progress of sexual maturation should also be checked.

your diabetes care provider. What precautions should you take when you feel under the weather?

Changes in your health may result in more frequent trips to your provider. If you're just starting insulin or are changing your dose and your glucose is out of range, you may need to talk by telephone or see your provider as often as every day for a while, until your blood glucose is in range. If you are trying to manage high blood pressure, you may need to monitor your blood pressure often and keep records of the readings.

Diabetes Care Schedule

Each person with diabetes has unique health care needs. You may make several office visits a month when you are experiencing difficulties or making changes to your regimen. Or you may go through periods where you only see your provider every 3 months. In any case, it's good to keep some general guidelines in mind for your schedule.

Having a general idea of your diabetes care schedule will help you know what to expect at each visit. Your health care provider may provide you with your own schedule or you can use the schedule below for guidance.

Diabetes Care Schedule

Every visit
• Blood pressure
• Weight
• Foot check

Every 3 months
• A1C test
• Regular visits to your diabetes care provider

Every 6 months
- Regular visits to your dentist

Every year
- HDL, LDL, triglycerides, total cholesterol: for average reading; more often if high levels are being treated
- Kidneys: microalbumin measured
- Eyes: examined through dilated pupils
- Feet: more often in patients with high-risk foot conditions (neuropathy, vascular disease)
- Flu shot
- Review meal plan
- Update with diabetes educator

Every 2 years
- HDL, LDL, triglycerides, total cholesterol: if last reading indicates very low risk.

Once a Lifetime
- Pneumococcal vaccine

Other Health Care Providers

Diabetes is a complicated disease that affects many different organ systems in your body, so it is no surprise that you may need multiple providers as part of your health care team. The type and number of providers on your team depends on your health and needs. Some people may have an endocrinologist, dietitian, eye doctor, and dentist, whereas other people may have eight or more different specialists.

The best resource for recruiting other team members is your diabetes care provider or certified diabetes educator. It is important not only that your provider communicates with other members of your team, but also that team members are able to communicate with each other about any changes that may arise in your diabetes management plan.

It's a plus if the members of your team are comfortable communicating with each other, which is often the case if they are recommended by your provider. However, you should also pick team mem-

> **Keeping Everyone Connected**
>
> Make sure all your providers have the phone numbers, fax numbers, and e-mail addresses of other members of the team.

> **Diabetes Educator Credentials**
>
> The initials CDE (for certified diabetes educator) indicate that the professional has experience caring for people with diabetes, has passed a national exam in diabetes education, and is up to date in diabetes care treatments.

bers with whom you feel comfortable. Don't be afraid to shop around a little and find the team members who best suit your needs.

Diabetes Educator

A diabetes educator is usually a registered nurse (RN), registered dietitian (RD), or pharmacist (RPH) with a special interest and training in caring for people with diabetes. However, physicians, physician assistants, and other health care specialists may also be diabetes educators.

Diabetes educators often work in locations where people with diabetes are treated, such as doctors' offices, hospitals, and pharmacies. The American Association of Diabetes Educators can also provide local referrals.

A diabetes educator can answer many of the concerns or questions you may have about diabetes. Diabetes educators may give you background information about the biology of diabetes, teach you how to take insulin or check blood glucose levels, explain how to handle sick days and pregnancy, discuss the effects of various habits on blood glucose levels, and help you learn to cope with stress, and how to choose, set, and reach goals.

In addition to meeting with a diabetes educator, you may also want to participate in a diabetes education program. Your local American Diabetes Association office can refer you to a program that has been recognized as meeting its national standards. This means that it can provide you with quality diabetes education. These programs are covered by Medicare and many insurance plans.

Topics in Diabetes Education Programs

- General information about diabetes and its treatments

- Adjusting psychologically to managing diabetes

- Setting goals and solving problems

- Understanding your meal plan and incorporating it into your life

- Incorporating physical activity into your life

- Checking and recording your blood glucose and urine ketones accurately and using the results to manage your diabetes

- Medications

- Managing sick days

- Preventing, detecting, and treating long-term complications

- Managing diabetes before and during pregnancy

Dietitian

A registered dietitian is a member of your health care team who has training and expertise in food and nutrition. A balanced meal plan is critical for anyone with diabetes. You and your dietitian can develop a meal plan that includes foods you enjoy and that will help you balance your food and physical activity.

You may want help in adapting your diet to special goals, such as losing weight, reducing dietary fat or sodium, or complementing a regular exercise program. Your dietitian can help ensure that your diet achieves these goals and that it accommodates your likes and dislikes, culture, schedule, and lifestyle.

It is recommended that you see a dietitian whenever you are having problems reaching your blood glucose targets. It is a good idea to see a dietitian once a year, even if you aren't having problems with diabetes care.

Dietitian Credentials

In choosing a dietitian, look for the initials RD (registered dietitian). This indicates that the dietitian has passed a national credentialing exam. Many states also require a license, and you may see the initials LD (licensed dietitian) after a dietitian's name. Some dietitians are also CDEs.

Meal Plan Tune-Up

If you can answer, "yes" to any of the following questions, then your meal plan may need a tune-up.

- Has it been more than a year since your dietitian reviewed your meal plan?

- Is your blood glucose level or body weight more difficult to manage than usual?

- Are you bored with your meals?

- Are you planning to start or have you already started an activity program or changed your insulin regimen since your last nutrition checkup?

- Have you decided to aim for blood glucose levels that are closer to normal?

- Have you been diagnosed with high blood pressure, high cholesterol levels, or kidney disease?

- Are you planning to or have you recently become pregnant?

- Are you entering menopause?

What to Expect from a Dietitian

During your first visit, your dietitian will assess your nutritional needs, a process that generally takes an hour or more. Follow-up visits usually take 30 minutes. Follow-up visits allow for sharing further helpful information, progress checks, and adjustments to your meal plan. Even though your diabetes management may seem to be on target, don't neglect periodic follow-up visits with your dietitian.

Topics for Your Dietitian

- How to use meal planning and carbohydrate counting guides, such as those published by the American Diabetes Association and the American Dietetic Association

- How to count dietary carbohydrate and fat and make adjustments to your insulin dose

- How to read food labels

- How to handle eating out

- How to make choices when grocery shopping

- How to handle holidays and other special events

- How to prepare and include foods that are important and meaningful for you and your family

Dietitians may also provide you nutritional resources, such as cookbooks and other reading materials, so that you can learn how to prepare easy, nutritious, and satisfying meals for your whole family.

How to Afford a Dietitian
The best way to afford your visit to the dietitian is obvious: get your health insurer to pay. More and more plans are covering services by a dietitian. Medicare now covers medical nutrition therapy provided by a Medicare-certified dietitian. Medicaid covers it in some states.

Tips for Dietitian Reimbursement

- Call your insurer first. You may have an insurer who provides this benefit. If so, ask what paperwork you will need to submit.

- Only a doctor can refer you to a registered dietitian for medical nutrition therapy.

- Submit a claim after each visit to the dietitian. Include a written referral from your doctor. The referral should not prescribe "nutrition counseling" or "nutrition education," but language such as "medical nutritional therapy for diabetes management."

- If you are turned down, resubmit your claim. This time, document how your visit to the RD can save the insurer money. Ask the dietitian for supporting documentation to get the visit covered. For example, you can cite the Diabetes Control and Complications Trial, which proved that complications can be prevented or delayed with near-normal glucose levels.

- If you are turned down, ask for your claim to be reviewed. Many insurers will tell you "no" at first, only to eventually cover some or all of the claim.

- In writing, ask for your disputed claim to be reviewed. Follow up with phone calls. Write down the names and titles of the people you call and the dates when you spoke. It pays to be persistent, so continue to write letters and make phone calls until either you or your insurer decides to pay for treatment.

Exercise Physiologist

It's hard to know how to start an exercise plan. For example, you may not have been very active in the past or you might want to learn how to integrate a favorite sport or exercise into your diabetes plan.

A professional trained in exercise science and safe conditioning techniques is in the best position to help you design a fitness program. To find a qualified exercise physiologist, ask your diabetes care provider or other members of your diabetes care team.

Exercise physiologists can help you develop a tailor-made fitness program, set realistic goals, and offer tips for staying motivated to stick with your routine. Whatever your goals—to improve cardiovascular fitness, lower blood glucose levels, lose weight, lower blood pressure or cholesterol, or develop muscular strength and flexibility—your exercise physiologist can help you achieve those goals.

Even if you have arthritis, are overweight, have diabetes complications, or have been sedentary and want to become more active, an exercise physiologist can develop an exercise program to accommodate your specific needs. But before embarking on any new exercise program, make sure to clear it with your diabetes care provider. Also make sure that your provider and exercise physiologist are in contact with each other.

➡ Exercise Physiologist Credentials

Look for someone who holds a master's or doctoral-level degree in exercise physiology or a licensed health care professional with graduate training in exercise physiology. You may want someone certified by the American College of Sports Medicine to ensure that your exercise physiologist has the skills necessary to design a safe, effective fitness program to suit your needs.

Mental Health Professional

In addition to creating physical and metabolic problems, diabetes affects a person's thoughts and feelings. Sometimes these feelings can become overwhelming. Mental health professionals can help people deal with some of the personal and emotional aspects that are inevitably associated with diabetes. Mental health professionals include social workers, family therapists, psychologists, or psychiatrists.

Types of Mental Health Professionals and Credentials

- A *social worker* should hold a master's degree in social work (MSW) and have training in individual, group, and family therapy. Social workers can help you cope with many concerns related to diabetes, including problems within the family, coping with workplace situations, and locating resources to help with medical or financial needs.

- A *marriage and family therapist* should hold a master's or doctoral degree in a mental health field and have additional training in individual, family, and marriage therapy. These therapists can help you with personal problems in familial and marital relationships and with problems on the job.

- A *clinical psychologist* usually has a master's or doctoral degree in psychology and is trained in individual, group, and family psychology. You may visit a clinical psychologist to help you through a particularly stressful period over the course of several weeks or months or on a longer-term basis to work through depression, anxiety, or other problems.

- A *psychiatrist* is a medical doctor with training in the relationship between physical well-being and mental health. Psychiatrists with expertise in treating people with diabetes can help you understand how the physical problem of diabetes can also affect your mental health. Psychiatrists prescribe medications or hospitalization for emotional problems, if needed.

If you feel that you need some help coping with the emotional burden of diabetes, don't be afraid to talk to your diabetes care provider, who can recommend an appropriate health care professional.

> → **Children with Diabetes**
>
> Having a child or teen with diabetes can be a challenge. Make sure your child's health care team includes a mental health professional. This team member will work with you and your child to identify the developmental, behavioral, emotional, and social issues confronting your child and to offer support and help for the whole family.

Eye Specialist

Eye care is a priority for anyone with diabetes. You can preserve your eyesight by keeping your blood glucose level close to normal.

An eye specialist monitors changes in your eyes, especially those changes associated with diabetes. He or she then determines what those changes mean and how they should be treated. For example, changes in the tiny blood vessels that supply your retina—the part of the eye that detects light and thus visual images—could be an early sign of diabetic retinopathy. If left untreated, diabetic retinopathy can lead to blindness.

Your diabetes care provider will look at your eyes during the course of your yearly physical examination, but you also need to have them more thoroughly examined by a trained eye specialist. Your eyes need to be dilated for this exam.

Eye Exam Schedule

- If you are an adult, have a thorough eye exam (including dilation) at the time of diabetes diagnosis and yearly thereafter.

- If you are 10 or older and have type 1 diabetes, you should have a comprehensive examination 3–5 years after you are diagnosed with diabetes and yearly thereafter.

- Also, if you notice any changes in your vision or you are planning a pregnancy, you should be examined.

When to See Your Eye Doctor

- Your vision becomes blurry
- You have trouble reading
- You see double
- One or both of your eyes hurt
- You feel pressure in your eye
- You see spots or floaters
- You lose vision

> ### Types of Eye Specialists and Credentials
>
> *Ophthalmologists* are medical doctors (MD) qualified to treat eye problems, both medically and surgically.
>
> *Retina specialists* are ophthalmologists with further training in the diagnosis and treatment of diseases of the retina.
>
> *Optometrists* are trained to examine the eye for certain problems, such as how well your eyes can focus. While they can prescribe corrective lenses, they do not perform laser surgery to correct retinopathy.

Choosing an Eye Doctor

The right eye doctor is an important aspect of your health care team. You may want to schedule an interview with a potential eye specialist before choosing one. Here are some questions and topics to discuss.

Interview Questions for Eye Specialists

- Do you see many patients with diabetes?

- Do you have experience treating patients with diabetic retinopathy?

- Do you perform eye surgery? (This is usually limited to ophthalmologists.)

- Are you a retina specialist? (This is important because eye disease in people with diabetes affects the retina, the part of the eye that detects visual images.)

- Will you send regular reports and keep in touch with my diabetes care provider?

Podiatrist

Foot care is especially important for people with diabetes because they are prone to poor blood circulation and nerve disease in the extremities. In addition, people with diabetes are likely to develop infections that often appear in the feet. Even small sores can turn into serious problems quickly.

People with diabetes should see a foot doctor called a podiatrist. Your diabetes care provider or podiatrist should check any foot sore or callus. Don't try to treat any foot problems yourself.

Podiatrists treat corns, calluses, and foot sores to prevent more serious problems from developing. They can also show you how to correctly trim your toenails and how to buy shoes that fit properly. To find a podiatrist, ask your diabetes care provider for a referral, or check with local hospitals

> **Credentials for Podiatrists**
>
> Podiatrists graduate from a college of podiatry with a Doctor of Podiatric Medicine (DPM) degree. They also complete residencies in podiatry and can perform surgery and prescribe medication for your feet.

or your local American Diabetes Association office. During your initial visit, ask what percentage of his or her patients have diabetes.

Get early treatment for foot problems! Call your doctor or podiatrist if you have any of these problems: an open sore (ulcer) on your foot; a cut or blister that is slow to heal; any infection in a cut or blister; a red, tender toe; any change in feeling, such as pain, tingling, numbness, or burning; and any puncture wound, such as if you step on a nail or thorn.

Pharmacist

A pharmacist has a wealth of information on medicines: what's in them and how they interact with each other. Pharmacists are highly trained professionals who must know about the chemistry of the products they dispense and what effects, both good and bad, medications have on the body. Therefore, they can also give advice on whether and how any medication you take for your diabetes or other conditions could or will affect your blood glucose levels.

It is important to find a pharmacy you like and to stick with it. This way, the pharmacist can keep an accurate and up-to-date profile of your medical history, allergies, and medications.

Pharmacists do more for you than fill your prescriptions. They alert you to the potential common or severe side effects of any drug you are going to take. With each new prescription, they can review your medication profile to see if any of your current medications might interact with your new prescription.

So, in addition to asking your diabetes care provider, you can ask your pharmacist to recommend over-the-counter medicines for colds or other minor illnesses. For example, if your pharmacist knows you take a sulfonylurea, he or she may recommend a cold medicine with little or no alcohol to avoid any possible interaction between the two medications.

Pharmacist Credentials

Pharmacists are required to have their PharmD degree. They must also pass an exam in the state where they practice pharmacy.

Dentist and Dental Hygienist

People with diabetes are at higher risk for gum disease and mouth infections. To prevent gum disease, see your dentist or dental hygienist every 6 months for a thorough teeth cleaning. Make sure your dentist knows that you have diabetes, and ask him or her to observe your brushing and flossing techniques to make sure you're doing all you can.

Call your dentist if you find any of the following: your gums bleed when you brush or eat; your gums are red, swollen, or tender; your gums have pulled away from your teeth; pus appears between your teeth and gums when the gums are touched; any change in the way dentures or partial plates fit; any change in the way your teeth fit together when you bite; or persistent bad breath or a bad taste in your mouth.

Some medications may cause dry mouth, so tell your health care provider, dentist, or hygienist if you experience this problem. They can offer suggestions.

Dermatologist

High blood glucose can cause dehydration, which causes dry skin. Diabetes also increases your risk of developing skin infections, especially if your glucose levels are often above normal. For instance, staphylococcal skin infections can cause itchy spots on the buttocks, knees, and elbows.

> **Dermatologist Credentials**
>
> Dermatologists are medical doctors (MD) with special training in skin disorders.

Your best weapon against dry skin is to keep your glucose within your target ranges through healthy eating, exercise, and medication. If you develop a skin problem, you'll need to see a skin doctor—a dermatologist. Your diabetes care provider or local ADA office can provide a referral for a dermatologist, if needed.

Communication

You've chosen your health care team. Now what? Your diabetes care provider may already use a team approach and may already be in contact with other team members. If they are not already in touch, make sure all team members know about everyone else on your team.

Ask your health care team to consult with each other whenever appropriate. Be sure that they have each other's phone numbers, e-mail addresses, and mailing addresses. If you are making any lifestyle adjustments—quitting smoking, starting a weight-loss diet, or taking up jogging, for example—make sure you notify all team members.

Professional	Degree	Look for	Consult for
Physician (primary care, internist, endocrinologist)	MD or DO	Specialization in diabetes, such as board certification in endocrinology	Medical management of diabetes, including oral agents or insulin, and the detection and treatment of complications
Nurse practitioner or physician assistant	APRN, BC-ADM, PA	Specialization in diabetes, such as board certification in advanced diabetes management (BC-ADM)	Management of diabetes, including oral agents or insulin, and the detection and treatment of complications
Nurse	RN, BSN, MSN, APRN	Certified diabetes educator (CDE)	Counseling on diabetes self-care, including medicines, blood glucose monitoring, managing sick days, stress, coping, and behavior change
Dietitian	RD	CDE is desirable	Helping you to develop or alter your diabetes meal plan, lose weight, or manage health problems (such as cutting dietary sodium or fat)
Eye doctor	MD specializing in ophthalmology, or an optometrist	Familiarity with diabetic eye disease	Detecting and treating diabetic eye disease such as retinopathy; ophthalmologists treat eye disease with laser therapy or eye surgery

Remember, your health care team is there to help you manage your diabetes. They can provide a wealth of information and the resources you need to make the decisions that affect your health. But you are the one who ultimately makes the decisions and puts your health care plan into action.

To work together as a team, you must be able to communicate with your fellow health care team members. It's not always easy to communicate, especially when you're feeling nervous, worried, or under pressure. Sometimes people can feel intimidated by health care professionals. However, just remember that they are there to help you. To best help you, they need to know what is on your mind. Only you can tell them how you are feeling and what special concerns you might have.

Tips for Talking with Providers

- Plan for your visit. Write down questions or concerns you want addressed. Bring your blood glucose logbook, a list of your medications, and anything else your diabetes care provider needs to know.

- Share the conversation. Begin the visit by telling your provider what you hope to accomplish and what you want him or her to know. Your provider cannot read your mind or guess what problems you may have.

- If the vocabulary becomes too technical or the concepts too complex and you don't understand, speak up. Ask for an explanation of anything you don't understand. Don't worry about feeling "stupid" or worry that this is something you should already know.

- Write down any information or instructions. It is important that you thoroughly understand everything that your health care professional is telling you.

- Consider bringing a spouse or support person to sit in on the visit.

Your emotional health is critical to your well-being. Let your provider know if you are struggling. Don't be afraid to bring up sexual or personal topics. Your team members are professionals and are prepared to help you deal with even the most sensitive topics.

Don't be afraid to discuss money. Health care professionals realize that financial worries can contribute to patient anxiety, and most will be willing to discuss payment options. Tell your provider if you are having trouble paying for your medications or diabetes care supplies, even if you are not asked.

If you don't feel comfortable with any member of your health care team or feel that you are not communicating effectively, consider interviewing other professionals until you find someone with whom you feel at ease.

Second Opinions

No matter how much you trust your doctor and other health care professionals, there may be times when you would like a second opinion. This could occur when surgery, long-term medication, or other treatments that will drastically affect your lifestyle are recommended. You may also want a second opinion if your health care provider says you have a problem for which there is no known therapy or your provider calls the problem you have incurable.

Check with your insurance company to determine whether medical costs for a recommended procedure are covered. Also ask whether they cover the cost of a second opinion and whether they pay only their own recommended consultants. Some insurance companies insist on a second opinion before they will fully cover certain treatments.

When searching for a physician to provide a second opinion, first ask your physician or a health care professional you trust. Look for a doctor who is board certified in the field in which you are seeking information, such as cardiology, surgery, or endocrinology. One option is to call the appropriate department of a major medical center or teaching hospital and ask for the name of a specialist in the field.

Sometimes insurance companies require a second opinion. Ask your insurer what costs for the recommended procedure are covered and whether they will cover the cost of a second opinion. Also ask if they pay only if you see one of the consultants they recommend.

Be sure to tell the physician about your diabetes. If the problem is diabetes related, or you suspect that it is, call the American Diabetes Association for the names of specialists in your area (see Resources). For problems not related to diabetes, try calling the appropriate department of a major medical center or teaching hospital and asking for the names of specialists in the field.

Questions to Ask When You Get a Second Opinion

- What is the diagnosis and how was it determined?

- What treatments are available and which are most effective? Most risky? Most commonly used?

- What treatment do you suggest and why?

- What is the success rate for this treatment?

- Is the condition reversible?

- What are the potential side effects and complications of the treatment and how likely are they?

- Is the problem or treatment likely to affect my blood glucose levels?

- Will the treatment require hospitalization? For how long? Will I need follow-up care?

- Are there any additional costs associated with this treatment, such as repeated blood tests, physical therapy, or postoperative nursing care?

- Is this an experimental treatment? Will I be participating in research? Will I be part of a placebo/control group or will I receive treatment?

- If this is the case, you may need to evaluate the potential risks and make sure they do not outweigh the benefits. If this is a research protocol, are more conventional treatments available should this one fail?

Team Approach

Assembling your health care team will not happen overnight. It can take time and persistence to find the right people to take care of you.

You're not alone. Your primary provider and diabetes educator are excellent resources for finding specialists in various fields of diabetes treatment. After all, treating diabetes is a team effort and you may need several experts to help keep things running smoothly.

As in all matters of our health, you are the most important advocate. Trust your instincts and try to choose providers who have your best interests at heart.

CHAPTER 18

Health Care System

As a person with diabetes, you will probably learn more about the health care system than many other people. You will see multiple health care providers and purchase various medications, equipment, and supplies.

Making the most out of the health care system takes diligence. In this chapter, you'll find an introduction to navigating your health insurance. The chapter includes background information on some of the most common types of health insurance as well as benefits and costs to look out for with your diabetes. You'll also find tips on dealing with denied insurance claims, preparing for hospital stays and surgery, and finding an assisted living facility or care in your home.

Health Insurance 101

Medical care is expensive, and costs continue to rise every year. Diabetes can make health care even more expensive—even if you have insurance. Not only do you have to pay for routine care, but you also have to be prepared for the unexpected. Getting the best insurance coverage possible is critical, not only for your pocketbook, but also for your health.

Why It's Important

People with diabetes should be especially diligent about understanding and maintaining health insurance because managing diabetes can be expensive and having adequate insurance can improve the affordability and accessibility of your health care. Losing or letting your health insurance lapse can be problematic and expensive.

Before you leave your old insurance—or the employer who is supplying it—be sure you understand the steps you have to take to protect your current coverage or obtain new coverage. The important thing is not to get caught without insurance, even briefly. Insurance is like having an umbrella in case it rains. The day you forget your umbrella, you can be sure it will rain.

Throughout the course of your life, your career, and your diabetes, you'll need to periodically evaluate your health insurance situation to make sure it is still appropriate for your health care needs. It's a good exercise to go through before you make any major changes.

Evaluating Your Health Insurance

- Ask yourself if your health care needs are being met.

- Ask yourself if your health care costs are affordable.

- If you are unhappy with your current situation, evaluate the options.

- Arc there changes you want to make that could affect your health insurance? For example, do you want to switch jobs, retire, get married or divorced, or move out of state?

Whatever your answers, don't be too quick to jump ship. Any change in your health insurance coverage requires careful evaluation. You need to make sure that any new situation provides the health care coverage you need.

New laws make it easier for people with diabetes to obtain and keep the coverage they need for appropriate treatment. Some of these laws are federal laws that affect all U.S. residents, but others are state laws that vary from state to state.

Affordable Care Act of 2010

On March 23, 2010, the Affordable Care Act was signed into law. The act includes many reforms to our health care system, including prohibiting discrimination due to preexisting conditions, changes to dollar limits on insurance coverage, and new options for obtaining health insurance. The following sections outline the most significant changes for people with diabetes. For more information on the new health care reforms visit www.healthcare.gov or www.diabetes.org.

Tips for Changing Jobs or Insurance Companies

• Talk to your new employer's benefits coordinator or the insurer.

• Read all you can, and make a list of questions.

• You should be prepared to ask for details on the cost of monthly premiums, copayments, deductibles, coinsurance, and coverage (including non-dollar limits on benefits) for diabetes-related care and supplies like test strips, diabetes education, durable medical equipment, and so on.

• Also be sure that your policy covers office visits (including specialists), laboratory tests, hospitalizations, and preventive care.

• Be prepared and be persistent to get all of your questions answered.

Types of Health Insurance

You can obtain health insurance in several ways. If you are employed or if your spouse is employed, you can often obtain insurance from an employer. If you leave

→ Preexisting Conditions

Beginning in 2014, insurance companies will no longer be able to refuse to sell or renew policies because of a preexisting condition such as diabetes. Higher rates based on preexisting conditions will not be allowed in the individual or small-group marketplaces. For children under 19, insurance companies cannot deny policies due to preexisting conditions as of September 2010.

your job, you can purchase transitional coverage, such as COBRA or state continuation coverage, or you can purchase coverage through a conversion policy.

If you are unemployed or self-employed, other insurance options include individual coverage or coverage through the federal or state high-risk pool programs. People who are over 65, disabled and unable to work, or have a very low income may have other insurance options, such as Medicare and/or Medicaid. It is worthwhile to investigate all of your insurance options because you may not realize that you are eligible for certain programs. For example, the Affordable Care Act expands eligibility for Medicaid.

Employment-Based Insurance

You may have the option of joining a group policy offered by your employer. These are often called group policies because you join a large pool of insured customers, which can help drive costs lower for the entire plan and broaden the range of available benefits. Group policies are usually open to all employees, regardless of their health. Many policies will also cover your spouse and/or children for an additional fee.

Employer-sponsored health care is considered a tax-exempt expense, so if you pay a fee or premium for health care coverage, you may have it deducted from your paycheck before taxes are taken out.

COBRA

If you are laid off or choose to quit your job for whatever reason, you may need insurance coverage while you make the transition from job to job or from work to retirement. Fortunately, a federal law called the Consolidated Omnibus Budget Reconciliation Act (COBRA) may help you.

COBRA: The Consolidated Omnibus Budget Reconciliation Act (COBRA) requires that an employer with more than 20 employees allow you and your dependants to keep your same health insurance policy with equal coverage for 18 months (sometimes longer) after you leave your job.

COBRA Facts

- Under COBRA, you will have to pay for the total cost of your coverage (including the share your employer previously paid on your behalf) and may be charged up to 2% more than the rate the insurance company was charging your employer for coverage.

- Once you have been laid off, voluntarily leave your job, or are not eligible for coverage on your parents' health plan, you have 60 days to accept COBRA benefits.

- Employers with fewer than 20 employees, the federal government, and churches are exempt from COBRA requirements.

State Continuation Insurance

If you work for an employer with fewer than 20 employees, state continuation coverage may be an option for you when you leave your job. Available in most states, state continuation coverage is similar to COBRA in that it allows you and/or your dependants to continue receiving the health care coverage you had as an employee.

State Continuation Insurance Facts

- You will have to pay both your share of the monthly premium as well as what your employer paid toward your health coverage while you were employed, plus an administrative fee that varies from state to state.

- In most states, the continuation coverage policy has the same types of benefits as were available under the group plan. However, for some states, the coverage is limited to hospital, surgical, or major medical benefits only and might not include certain group policy benefits, including dental care, vision care, prescription drugs, and similar supplementary benefits.

- Not all states offer continuation coverage, and the states that do offer it vary widely in how to sign up for coverage and how long coverage lasts.

- To find more information on state continuation coverage, contact your state's Department of Insurance.

State Continuation Coverage: A state plan allowing you to keep your health coverage by transitioning your employer group coverage to an individual health coverage policy.

Conversion Insurance and HIPAA

When your group health insurance ends, many states require employers to offer you a conversion policy regardless of your health or physical condition. When you convert your policy, you remain with the same insurer but begin paying for your own insurance. This is called a conversion plan because you convert from a group to an individual plan.

Conversion coverage is almost always more expensive than the group plan you may have had while employed, and it usually provides fewer benefits. However, it may be your only choice for coverage and is preferable to going without insurance.

Conversion Insurance Policy Facts

- Conversion policies are not available in all states.

- In some states you must use up any COBRA or state continuation coverage that you are eligible for before purchasing a conversion policy.

- In other states, you can buy a conversion policy immediately after losing or leaving your job.

- If at all possible, be sure to explore all insurance options as far in advance as possible, including the application process.

HIPAA Facts

- HIPAA policies must be offered without preexisting condition exclusions to anyone who has had continuous coverage in a health plan for the previous 18 months (without significant breaks in coverage), the last day of which must have been under a group health plan.

HIPAA: The Health Insurance Portability and Accountability Act (HIPAA) of 1996 ensures that insurers and employers may not make insurance rules that discriminate against workers because of their health. The act makes it easier for people with diabetes to get and keep health insurance.

- HIPAA is available to people not currently eligible for coverage under any group plan, Medicare, or Medicaid.

- People must first use up any COBRA or state continuation coverage available to them.

Individual Insurance

If you are self-employed, unemployed, or do not receive health insurance as an employment benefit, you may not be eligible for any form of group insurance coverage. Finding an affordable policy under these circumstances may be difficult. If at all possible, don't forfeit health insurance altogether. Having diabetes makes health insurance an absolute necessity. Individual policies are contracts between individuals and an insurance company. You'll want to be especially careful to review the policy for costs and coverage.

High-Risk Pool

If you have been turned down for insurance due to your health status, you might want to consider high-risk pool health insurance. This kind of insurance is offered in over 30 states to people who have lived in the state for 6–12 months and are ineligible for group or individual coverage due to a preexisting condition. Coverage is generally adequate; the costs can vary widely among the different states that offer it. Some states have waiting lists to buy into the pool. Some states may impose an exclusion period for coverage of certain health conditions.

The Affordable Care Act established a new temporary federal high-risk pool program (the Pre-Existing Conditions Plan or PCIP) that operates in every state. To qualify for coverage in PCIP, you must have been uninsured for at least 6 months and have been denied health coverage because of a preexisting condition. The PCIP is a transitional coverage program until January 1, 2014, at which point exclusion for coverage due to preexisting conditions will be prohibited. Coverage in PCIP is comprehensive and may be less costly than coverage in the traditional state high-risk pool, although those costs vary from state to state. For more information, go to www.pcip.gov.

Be sure to inquire about all the high-risk pool coverage options in your state.

Medicare

The federal insurance program Medicare covers a portion of hospital bills, provider fees, and other expenses for people over the age of 65 and for some people with disabilities who cannot work. Even if you get Medicare, you may still have to pay for a portion of your medical bills.

Most people over the age of 65, those with end-stage renal disease, and those with certain severe disabilities are eligible for Medicare. However, some people who have worked at state or local government jobs may not be eligible for Medicare. If you are unsure about your eligibility for Medicare, contact your local Social Security Administration office or the Medicare hotline at 1-800-MEDICARE (1-800-633-4227).

Medicare coverage for people with diabetes has improved dramatically in recent years thanks to the efforts of the American Diabetes Association. You can sign up for Medicare 3 months before the month of your 65th birthday. For more information, contact your local Social Security Administration office, listed under the United States Government listing in your telephone book. Bring your birth certificate when you apply.

Medicaid

If you have a low income, you might be eligible for Medicaid, a joint federal and state health care program. Medicaid eligibility varies from state to state, so you will have to contact the Medicaid office in your state to find out whether you qualify. The Affordable Care Act requires that in 2014, all states' Medicaid eligibility levels be set at 133% of the Federal Poverty Level.

In general, prior to 2014, to qualify for Medicaid you must meet certain income limits as well as other criteria. For example, in most states, in addition to having income below a certain level, you must also be a child under age 19, elderly or disabled, a parent, or pregnant. Ask about what health expenses will be covered. If you have questions, a social worker can help you with this.

The health care provisions under Medicaid can change as states exercise their discretion in distributing funds. Most states provide coverage for essential diabetes care, but some states are trying to reduce this coverage due to state budget difficulties. For more information about how these changes may affect you, contact your local Social Security Administration office or call 1-800-772-1213.

CHIP

The Children's Health Insurance Program (CHIP) is available to children and some pregnant women and some parents whose income may be too high for Medicaid but who cannot afford other health insurance options. It is also sometimes called S-CHIP. Each state varies in its eligibility requirements for this program. To find information on CHIP in your state, go to www.insurekidsnow.gov or contact 1-877-KIDS-NOW.

Health Insurance Exchanges

Exchanges are new marketplaces that will be established in each state to offer health insurance coverage to individuals and small businesses. Established by the Affordable Care Act, the state exchanges will go into effect in 2014 and will grant Americans the ability to choose among a variety of health insurance plans based on benefits, costs, provider networks, and more.

Types of Coverage with Private Insurance

However you are covered, there are different agreements between insurers and providers as to how services will be provided. If you have insurance through your job, some employers may offer an array of health plans and service options. Other employers may have settled on a single insurance company offering a single type of service.

The major types of insurance plans are fee-for-service and managed-care plans. You'll need to consider your diabetes care needs when comparing and selecting a health insurance plan. Coverage under Medicare will be discussed in the next section.

Fee-for-Service Plans

These plans require you to pay a certain amount—a deductible—before your insurance pays benefits. Usually, you can choose your own providers among a wide range of health care professionals and hospitals with whom your insurer is affiliated.

Basics of Fee-for-Service Plans

- You must first pay an out-of-pocket deductible for your health care.

- Once you have met your yearly deductible, your insurance company will pay for the remaining expenses during the year, according to the particulars of your contract.

- Often, insurance companies will also require that you pay a portion of the cost of visits or health care (the copayment) and/or a percentage of your expenses (coinsurance), even after the deductible is met.

- However, most plans have out-of-pocket limits. Check the plan for a description of these limits.

- Check to see whether preventive health care, such as mammograms, Pap smears, or well-child visits, is covered by your plan. The Affordable Care Act requires that, after September 23, 2010, all new or renewed health plans must provide free access to certain preventive services. For information about which preventive services must be available without cost sharing, visit www.healthcare.gov.

Changes to Limits under the Affordable Care Act of 2010

Some insurance policies have annual dollar limits for covered services. Under health reform law, insurers will have restrictions placed on their ability to establish annual dollar limits. In 2014, annual dollar limits on essential benefits will be completely banned. Lifetime dollar limits on essential benefits such as hospital stays will be prohibited for new or renewed health plans after September 23, 2010.

HMO, PPO, and POS Managed-Care Plans

Under managed-care plans, you or your employer pay a fixed premium and you typically receive a comprehensive care

→ **Comparing Policies**

Pay special attention to what you may have to pay as a deductible, copayment, coinsurance, out-of-pocket limits, and annual limits. There may be a separate deductible for pharmacy benefits. Plans with lower premiums usually have higher deductibles and/or copayments, or may limit benefits.

package, ranging from routine office visits and preventive care to hospitalization. The three main types of managed-care plans are preferred provider organization (PPO), health maintenance organization (HMO), and point of service (POS).

Basics of Managed-Care Plans

- Your cost is generally lowest if you seek care from the network of participating providers and hospitals.

- You generally have lower deductibles to satisfy and limited paperwork to process.

- You also may *not* be expected to pay large out-of-pocket amounts for services.

Limited-Benefit Plans

Sometimes, insurers will offer limited-benefit plans for consumers. They are sometimes called bare bones, mandate-light, or minimum benefit plans. They offer more limited coverage than most other

→ Types of Health Care Plans

PPO: The insurance company has a contract with hospitals or doctors to provide care at a discounted rate. You may have more flexibility in your choice of in-network providers or specialists without the need for a referral from a primary care provider. However, if you choose to see an out-of-network provider, you may pay more.

HMO: The insurance company has a contract with a network of providers that will provide your care. Generally, you'll need to see a primary care provider first for a referral before seeing specialists, and your choice in doctors may be limited. The HMO may not pay for care from out-of-network providers or if you see a doctor without a referral.

POS: You'll see a primary care provider first, just like an HMO, but you may have more flexibility about seeing providers out of network. However, if you see an out-of-network provider, you may pay more in the form of a separate deductible, copayment, or portion of the total bill.

health plans and may have restrictions on the type of care covered, including items and services essential for people with diabetes.

Covering Your Diabetes Needs

Obtaining insurance coverage is only the first step. What is covered is just as important for people with diabetes. Today, thanks to the efforts of the American Diabetes Association and its allies, 46 states and the District of Columbia require that state-regulated insurance plans provide comprehensive coverage of diabetes supplies, equipment, and education.

But be careful—only about one-half of the private plans in any given state are regulated by the state. The other plans are regulated under federal law and are exempt from state-mandated benefit laws.

Your insurance policy is a contract between you and the insurance carrier that outlines the services covered. Like any contract, you need to read it carefully to make sure it meets your health care needs.

Coverage of Diabetes Care

Your plan may include coverage for office visits and annual or semi-annual physical exams and laboratory tests. Some insurance companies will only provide partial coverage or will require a copayment for each visit. Others may not always cover routine physical examinations but will pay for a specific medical problem or medical emergency.

Tips for Coverage of Diabetes Care

- Check to see that your carrier considers routine diabetes care (e.g., diabetes supplies, visits with your dietitian) part of the treatment for diabetes and provides coverage.

- Check to see if there are any limits on how many visits are allowed.

- Check to see how much you will have to pay per visit.

- Ask if your plan includes diabetes self-management education and medical nutrition therapy.

- Find out if visits to other members of your health care team are covered and under what conditions. Some carriers will provide coverage for routine physicals but will not cover visits to a dietitian, for example.

- You may recognize that treating your diabetes is a team effort, but not all insurance carriers provide coverage that supports this.

Coverage of Medical Equipment

If your health insurance covers durable medical equipment, it may pay for a blood glucose meter, a fingerstick device, pens, pen needles, syringes, a pump, infusion sets, a continuous glucose monitor, and/or an insulin injector. Some insurance plans may cover some or all of these supplies under the prescription drug benefit. As there may be differences in copayment or coinsurance depending on how your diabetes supplies are covered, be sure to check your insurance policy for clarification.

Tips for Coverage of Medical Equipment

- Many insurers cover blood glucose meters and strips, often under a separate coverage agreement. Read the policy and talk to your human resources department or your insurer to be sure.

- Today, more and more plans will pay for an insulin pump if it is prescribed by your provider as "medically necessary."

- Check your policy to see that none of these items is specifically excluded.

- Your provider may have to write a letter explaining why each of these items is necessary. This serves as your "prescription" for these items.

Coverage of Medication and Supplies

If your insurance covers prescription medications and/or medical supplies, it usually will pay for insulin, lancets, syringes, pens, glucose meter strips, and insulin pump supplies, if you have a prescription for them.

Tips for Coverage of Medication and Supplies

- Purchases of prescription drugs and supplies may require a copayment and/or a separate deductible.

- However, if your coverage includes prescription drugs, always ask your provider to write a prescription for insulin. Most insurance plans will reimburse you for insulin with a prescription.

- It is a good idea to ask the insurance company in advance what is covered. What medications are covered? Is there a prescription plan to reduce costs? How often can prescriptions be refilled? Is copayment required for each prescription? Which pharmacies accept your health insurance?

- Always keep a record of the name of the person who answers your questions along with the date, in case you need this information to appeal a denied claim.

Other Things You Should Know about Your Plan

- What mental health benefits are covered? The services of a social worker or psychologist can help you through the rough spots in coping with diabetes.

- Does the plan cover the services of specialists, such as an endocrinologist, podiatrist, eye doctor, or dentist, whose care is very important to people with diabetes?

- What kind of home health care coverage is included? Are there any limitations?

Diabetes Coverage with Medicare

Medicare coverage can be complicated. You'll need to do some research to find the best options for your situation and what benefits are covered. This section provides an overview of the major parts of Medicare that cover diabetes care, medication, equipment, and supplies.

Keep in mind that the two main parts of Medicare coverage are Part A and Part B. There are also Medigap plans, Medicare Advantage Plans, and Prescription Drug Plans.

Part A

Part A helps to pay bills for medical care provided in hospitals, skilled nursing facilities, hospices (for people who are terminally ill), and, in some cases, your home. Generally, people covered by Medicare get Part A. You will pay deductibles and coinsurance.

Part B

Part B helps to pay for health care provider services, ambulance services, diagnostic tests, outpatient hospital services, outpatient physical therapy, speech pathology services, home health services, and medical equipment and supplies.

It is critical for people with diabetes to purchase Medicare Part B. You can get Part B by paying a monthly fee. Part B also has deductibles and coinsurance amounts that you pay.

Part B and Diabetes Screening, Care, Equipment, and Supplies

Medicare Part B coverage includes:

- Diabetes screening test per 12-month period for beneficiaries with identified risk factors (for the specific risk factors, go to www.cms.gov/DiabetesScreening).

- Blood glucose meters, lancets, test strips, and other supplies for the meter, whether you are on insulin or not.

- Insulin pumps and supplies (including insulin) for people who meet certain qualifications.

- Diabetes self-management training and medical nutrition therapy.

- Medicare will help pay for annual podiatry checkups, therapeutic footwear and shoe inserts, checks for diabetic retinopathy, and kidney dialysis.

Your health care provider must certify in writing that you need all of these items to manage your diabetes, that is, that they are "medically necessary." Make copies of your provider's written statement. Give a copy of it to your pharmacist each time you purchase these supplies so that it can be submitted along with your Medicare claim.

Medicare Parts A and B Don't Cover

- Diabetes pills, insulin if you are not using an insulin pump, or syringes.

- Regular eye exams, prescription sunglasses, or contact lenses.

- Routine foot care, such as nail trimming or removal of corns and calluses.

- Custodial care provided in a nursing home or private home when that is the only kind of care needed. Custodial care includes help in walking, getting in and out of bed, bathing, dressing, eating, taking medicines, and other activities of daily living.

For more information on Medicare, call the Medicare hotline at 1-800-MEDICARE (1-800-633-4227). For a more detailed explanation of Medicare, ask for a free copy of the *Medicare & You* handbook and check out the Medicare Plan Finder at www.medicare.gov.

Medigap

Even in its present state, Medicare does not cover everything you need for your diabetes care. To fill gaps in your coverage, you can choose from the many Medigap plans available from private insurance companies.

Medigap plans pick up some of the charges that Medicare won't cover. These Medigap plans are standardized and regulated by state and federal law. There are a number of different Medigap plans that provide different benefits.

A particular plan's benefits are the same, regardless of which private insurance sells it. However, the costs may vary. Be sure to compare plans between insurance companies before purchasing a Medigap plan.

The booklet "Choosing a Medigap Policy: A Guide to Health Insurance for People with Medicare," written by the Centers for Medicare

and Medicaid Services (CMS) of the U.S. Department of Health and Human Services and
the National Association of Insurance Commis-
sioners (NAIC), is updated every year and is
available at www.medicare.gov or through any
insurance company.

Ask for it, or call Social Security to have it
sent to you. It will be very helpful in face of the
changes that regularly occur in Medicare. It
contains the federal standards for Medigap policies and general information about Medicare.

> **Medigap Tip**
>
> You cannot be denied Medigap
> coverage if you apply within the
> 6-month period beginning the first
> day of the month when you are
> 65 years or older *and* enrolled in
> Medicare Part B.

Medicare Advantage Plans

Medicare Advantage Plans are another option to help pay for care and
medications not provided under Medicare Part A and B. If you choose
to purchase a Medicare Advantage plan, you will not need to purchase a Medigap policy.

Medicare Advantage plans provide Medicare Part A and B benefits
and may cover other services, such as prescription drugs. They are like
HMOs and PPOs, and you usually see an assigned or network provider instead of choosing your own physician.

Medicare Advantage plans are not available everywhere, and you
may have to pay a monthly premium for these policies.

Prescription Drug Plans (Part D)

Medicare works with private companies to offer optional prescription
drug plans as part of Medicare Part D. These plans were introduced
when the Medicare Modernization Act (MMA) was enacted in 2003.

Under these plans, you will have a member card that gives you discounts on prescription drugs. The cost of plans and availability vary by
state. Some have annual deductibles and monthly drug premiums.

If you have a lower income, you may be eligible for one of the prescription drug subsidies available to some beneficiaries under Medicare. For information on whether you qualify for a subsidy, contact
Medicare directly at 1-800-MEDICARE for more information.

➜ **Gap in Drug Coverage or "Donut Hole"**

The "donut hole" is a gap in the Medicare drug benefit that appears when a Medicare beneficiary surpasses the prescription drug coverage limit. When this happens, seniors are required to pay the full cost of their medications out of pocket until they reach the catastrophic coverage limit, at which point Medicare Part D then pays the full cost of the medications for the remainder of the year. Starting in 2011, seniors who reach the donut hole will receive a 50% discount on brand-name prescription drugs and a discount on generic drugs. The Affordable Care Act includes a provision focused on completely closing the donut hole by 2020. Visit www.medicare.gov or call 1-800-MEDICARE (1-800-633-4227) for the latest information.

Denied Insurance Claims

Having a claim denied is bound to happen at some point. Just when you think you've done all of your homework and think you know just what is and what is not covered by your health insurance, you receive a claim marked "DENIED."

To resolve the situation fairly and efficiently, it will help if you have all the paperwork on hand to support your claim.

Tips for Denied Claims

➜ **Other Drug Assistance Programs**

Some states offer assistance for medications. In addition, some pharmaceutical companies offer drug assistance to qualifying individuals. You can visit www.rxassist.org for a list of statewide drug assistance and pharmaceutical company assistance programs.

- When your claim is denied, you will receive an explanation of benefits from your insurance company, which should include a reason for the denial of your claim.

- If you do not understand the reason for the denial, you may want to call an insurance company representative for a thorough explanation.

- Make sure to ask for and record the name of the person with whom you are speaking.

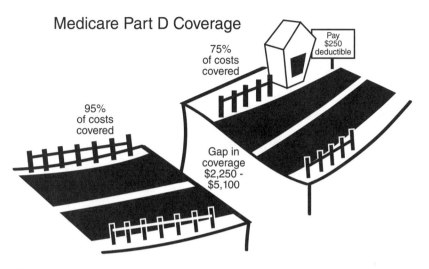

Medicare Part D Coverage

75% of costs covered

Pay $250 deductible

95% of costs covered

Gap in coverage $2,250 - $5,100

The "Donut Hole".

- Understanding what the problem is may help you better organize the papers and documents you need to support your claim.

- Contact your human resources department if your policy is through your employer. They can often explain why it wasn't covered or help you work through the system more quickly.

- You will have a certain period of time in which to appeal the denied claim. State laws vary on the amount of time allowed to appeal, so make sure to check the law in your state or contact your state's department of insurance.

Double-check that the claim form has been completed correctly. If it has, get the rest of your paperwork in order. Make sure you have a prescription for every piece of equipment you need, even if it does not require a prescription at the pharmacy. Sometimes, just submitting the prescription and receipt will be enough. Some companies may also want a letter of explanation from your health care provider.

> **Copies Only**
>
> Never send any original documents to your insurance company. Make copies of everything you plan to submit and keep them in a safe place. Send in the copies, and keep the originals. Send all pertinent paperwork by registered mail so you have a record that they have been received.

Tips for Appeals

- Write to the claims manager of your insurance company, explaining what is wrong. It helps to address the claims manager by name.

- Point out the items that have been denied payment and ask for a written response to your request.

- Give your address and phone number and that of your provider.

- Also, send your provider a copy of your appeal request for his or her records.

- State that you will call the insurance company on a certain date if you have not received a response by that time. On that date, call the claims manager and discuss your case. Two or three weeks is a reasonable period of time to wait.

Sometimes claims are denied for simple reasons. Maybe a clerk was unfamiliar with the newest equipment for diabetes care. Requesting an appeal moves the decision out of the clerk's hands and into those of people who should have greater familiarity with blood meters, test strips, and other equipment.

If you work for a company that is self-insured (which many larger employers are), appeal directly to your human resources manager or to the head of the company first. Often they can easily remedy the situation.

State Insurance Commissioner
Write to your state labor department if your claim is still denied. Your state insurance commissioner acts as a consumer complaint department. Do not hesitate to contact this office. They can also provide you with an opportunity for a hearing. This is where your paperwork is most important.

→ Don't Give Up

Even if you are denied again, don't give up! Request an insurance hearing.

Tips for Writing the State Insurance Commissioner

- Include the name of your insurance company.

- Detail the coverage provided in your policy as you understand it, along with a copy of your policy.

- Describe what happened (this should include copies of all letters or details of phone conversations between you and the insurance company).

- Specifically request a hearing to determine the insurance company's responsibility for payment.

An insurance hearing is like a court hearing in many respects. Both you and the insurance company will be allowed to state your case. You must also submit copies of all the documents you sent to the commission. Some people represent themselves, whereas others have lawyers.

A decision may be made right away or within the ensuing few weeks. If you are dissatisfied with the decision, you still have the option of taking your case to small-claims court.

Check with your local small-claims court, because each system has a different way of handling cases. You can find a listing in the city or county government section of the telephone book. The judges there understand that most people represent themselves. The judge will want to hear your side of the story and see copies of your documents.

Diabetes Care in the Hospital

At some point, you may need to stay in the hospital. A hospital stay doesn't always mean that there is a life-threatening problem—it can include anything from routine elective surgery to a life-threatening emergency.

When you are admitted to a hospital, you may feel that you are no longer in charge. All of a sudden, your daily routine is disrupted, and you may have to face a recovery period that lasts from days to weeks or even months.

As unpleasant as it seems now, taking time to plan for how to handle hospital stays will pay off in the long run. You can take steps that will help get you the best possible care, whether you face an emergency situation or one for which you can plan ahead. Because, the truth is, the people who get the best care are the ones who take a proactive role in their health care, are well informed, and know what questions to ask.

→ **Health Insurance in the Hospital**

Ask your health insurance company which hospital services they cover and for how much. Also, many insurance companies require you to notify them in advance for any service, except emergencies, so they can pre-approve your treatment. It is important to understand which services require pre-approval because it will determine whether a service is covered.

Evaluate Local Hospitals

You'll want to learn about your local hospitals when planning ahead for hospital stays.

There are three types of hospitals: city or county hospitals, private community hospitals, and hospitals that serve as teaching centers, usually affiliated with a medical school. But these types of hospitals are not mutually exclusive. A county or private hospital can also be affiliated with a medical school.

General Hospital Considerations

• Which hospitals are accepted by your health insurance?

• Does your primary care provider and/or specialist have privileges at a particular hospital?

• If he or she has privileges at several local hospitals, which is preferred?

• Are there advantages or disadvantages to a particular hospital depending on the situation?

Talk to your diabetes care provider to learn about a hospital's general reputation, as well as its reputation for treating people with diabetes. Discuss the steps you should take in the event of an emergency and agree on which hospital to use. Ask your provider where he or she would go or would send a family member.

You may want to ask any friends, neighbors, or relatives who have had recent hospitalizations. You can also check with your diabetes educator or support group for further input.

How to Evaluate a Hospital's Reputation

- Are there endocrinologists on the staff?

- Does the hospital have diabetes education and dietitians with expertise in diabetes on the staff? Are they available to both inpatients and outpatients?

- Is there a diabetes education program within the hospital or affiliated with the hospital?

- What other types of support services are available to people with diabetes?

- What is the protocol for managing blood glucose levels in the hospital? Will you be able to do any of your own care, such as blood glucose monitoring?

Checking into the Hospital

You'll also want to plan ahead for your admittance to the hospital. Things will go more smoothly if you're prepared for questions and inform people of your diabetes and your care preferences.

Tips for Hospital Admittance

- All patients with diabetes who are admitted to the hospital should have their diabetes clearly identified in the medical record. If you have type 1 diabetes, make sure that the classification shows up in your medical record and remind each new caregiver that your basal insulin may never be omitted.

- Make sure all doctors and nurses and other caregivers are aware that you have diabetes.

- Tell them what medications you are taking for diabetes and any other medications you are taking, including any over-the-counter drugs.

It helps to prepare a legible list of these ahead of time, including how often you take them and in what doses.

- Explain any allergies or other conditions you may have that could affect the actions of medications.

- Speak up about any other medical conditions you may have, including complications of diabetes. High blood pressure may require special treatment before and during surgery. Heart disease medications may require adjustment.

- Tell them about any recent or frequent low blood glucose reactions. Bring your self-monitoring records with you.

- Tell them about your meal plan. Ask to see the hospital's dietitian and explain what type of meal plan you're using, including any special modifications such as less salt, less cholesterol, or less fat.

Blood Glucose Management in the Hospital

Studies have shown that intensive diabetes management is beneficial for people with diabetes who are hospitalized. Your blood glucose control will affect how quickly you recover, how long you are hospitalized, and whether you experience complications during your hospitalization. Your blood glucose needs to be monitored while you are in the hospital, and the results should be available to all members of the health care team. It is a good idea to talk to your provider before any scheduled hospitalization about the plan for achieving your blood glucose targets during your stay.

Insulin

Insulin is the most effective and efficient way to keep blood glucose levels in your target range. Even if you are not on insulin at home, you may need insulin during your hospitalization. You can often go back to oral medications after you get better.

If you are acutely ill, need to be in an intensive care unit, or are recovering from surgery, you should receive insulin intravenously. That way, the nursing staff can react very quickly to blood glucose levels that are too high or low and make adjustments in your dose.

Once you are beginning to recover or your illness becomes better, you can often take insulin injections and achieve the same results. You should receive routine doses of both basal and bolus insulin and corrective doses if your blood glucose level goes out of range. If you see that a component of treatment is missing, ask your physician.

> **Meals in the Hospital**
>
> Your meal plan will be adjusted to give you adequate nutrition for healing. The type of illness or surgery you have will also influence what you are able to eat. If you are unable to eat solid foods, you will be given adequate nutrition intravenously.

If you are used to managing your diabetes at home, you may prefer to give your own injections and do your own blood glucose checks. Ask your provider if that is possible in your hospital and have them write an order so that the rest of the staff will know.

Surgery

If you are facing surgery, it's perfectly normal to feel apprehensive. When you have diabetes, there is even more to think about. People with diabetes can recover about as quickly as anyone, but blood glucose levels can fluctuate around the time of an operation and high blood glucose levels can complicate your recovery and prolong your hospital stay.

Regardless of the cause of your hospital stay, it's essential that your diabetes be closely managed the entire time you are there. By taking an active role and by doing everything you can, you can help yourself recover on schedule.

The first question you will probably ask yourself is whether the surgery is necessary (unless it is an emergency situation). You'll want talk to your provider about the risks and alternatives of surgery as well as how to manage your diabetes during your hospital stay.

Pre-Surgery Questions

- Are there alternatives? What are the consequences of not having the surgery? If you are still in doubt, get a second opinion.

- What are the risks involved and the likelihood of the risks arising? Feel free to ask all of the questions you may have. Even minor surgeries have some degree of risk. You have the right to have that described to you in advance.

- If you want an explanation of tests or other procedures to expect, ask. Unanswered questions can produce anxiety.

- Who will manage your diabetes before, during, and after surgery? Will you be under the care of your diabetes care provider, an endocrinologist, or a hospital physician who specializes in diabetes?

- What is the protocol for managing glucose levels before, during, and after surgery?

Write down your questions prior to meeting with your health care provider, so you remember to ask all of them.

You will receive an intravenous insulin drip prior to and during surgery to keep your blood glucose on target. Ask your diabetes provider to work with your surgeon as much as possible. Certain medications need to be stopped before surgery, some as long as a week ahead of time. Make sure you discuss all of the medications you are taking with your surgeon.

Surgery 101

- The surgeon will meet with you at least once before your operation to explain the surgery and what to expect afterward. It's a good idea to have a list of questions ready.

- The anesthesiologist, who administers the anesthesia to keep you pain free and manages your insulin drip during surgery, will also

→ Lower A1C before Surgery

If your surgery is elective, try to bring your A1C levels as close to normal as possible before you are hospitalized. This will help you withstand the stress of the surgery and may help reduce the chances of infection and speed healing after the operation.

visit you to tell you what to expect and, sometimes, to offer alternatives.

- The nurses caring for you will also be able to answer questions or address concerns you may have.

- After the operation, don't hesitate to ask for medication for pain or nausea. Short-term use of these medications does not affect blood glucose levels.

- You may want a second opinion when a provider recommends surgery. Some insurance companies require second opinions. See chapter 17 for more about second opinions.

Home Health Care and Nursing Homes

Many people today are turning to home health care for a variety of reasons, especially because hospitals prefer to keep hospital stays as short as possible. Home health care services include nursing care and physical, respiratory, occupational, or speech therapy; chemotherapy; nutritional guidance; personal care such as bathing or dressing; and homemaker care.

Home health care can include health professionals who help you when you are bedridden with a long illness or housebound for a short period. They may provide blood testing or send a nurse into your home to administer medicines and other treatments. Home health care workers include professionals, trained aides who help professionals, and volunteers.

Coverage for Home Health Care

- Check with your health insurance plan or your company's benefits officer to see if home health care benefits are covered.

- Don't hesitate to ask the agency you are considering hiring how much they charge for each service, and ask your insurance carrier what services will be covered.

- If Medicare covers you, you may have some limited benefits. Usually, Medicare home health care benefits are restricted to the homebound and bedridden.

- The Department of Veterans Affairs, the military, and worker's compensation may also be other sources of help for home health care.

If full-time care is needed, an extended-care, assisted-living, or nursing home is often the best option. It is important that you visit prospective sites. It is also a good idea to talk to friends, family, neighbors, or coworkers who have family members in these types of facilities.

Resources for Finding Assisted-Living Facilities

- Private or public case management social workers, including those with whom you may be in contact during a hospital stay

- Your local office on aging

- The county or state department of health

- Your primary care provider

- Your religious leader or pastoral counselor

- Local organizations or law firms for the retired or elderly

Assisted living facilities and nursing homes can be very expensive. There are four possible sources of payment: private insurance, Medicare, Medicaid, and self-pay or private pay. Different facilities ask for different types of payments. It is important that you understand what you get for the required fees. The admissions coordinator should provide details of regular monthly charges and exactly what they do—and do not—include. Ask if there is something specific you should know about that is not covered. Ask about how they routinely care for diabetes and how they handle acute situations related to high or low blood glucose episodes.

As an alternative to nursing homes, many people are turning to assisted-living communities or foster care homes. Many of these facilities are suitable for people who do not require full-time nursing care but who might enjoy the benefit of nursing staff and neighbors close at hand.

Check to see what nursing or other services are provided before you choose an assisted-living community. There is a wide array of living situations, from communities that function much like individual apartments, to individual units that provide nursing services, to full-time nursing centers. Check to see whether any of these facilities might meet your needs.

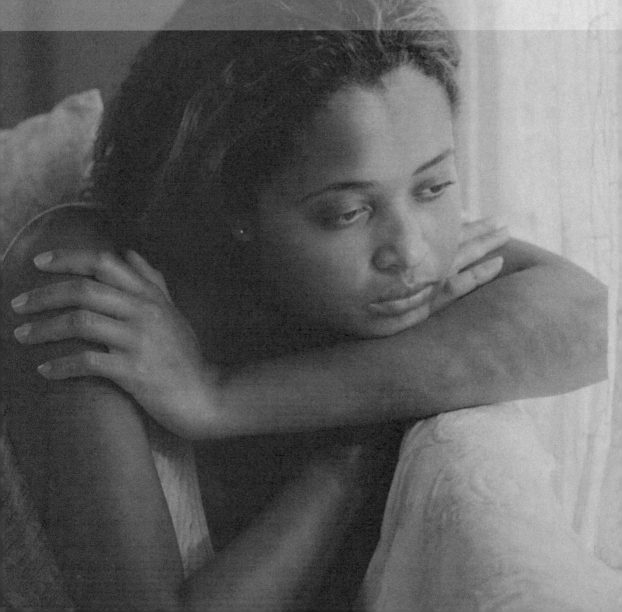

CHAPTER 19

Coping with Diabetes

Everyone has stress and anger in their lives. Yet, managing a chronic condition such as diabetes can add extra frustration and unrest.

When you were first diagnosed with diabetes, you probably had many different feelings. Maybe you tried to shrug diabetes off. Maybe you felt imperfect or that your body had failed you. Perhaps you felt angry and wanted to find something or someone to blame. Maybe you felt sad, blue, or out of sorts.

If you've been living with diabetes for a while, you may have accepted your condition, but you may still feel stress and sadness. Diabetes can cause feelings of depression, isolation, anger, frustration, fear, and guilt.

Finding ways to deal with stress and negative emotions is called coping. It's not the flashiest concept in the world, but it's probably one you'll use on a daily basis as you move forward with your diabetes. It's a fabulous skill that you can continually hone and modify.

Everyone needs a variety of coping skills to use in different situations. There are three important factors in coping: having enough information, feeling in control, and having the support of others.

This chapter will discuss some common feelings and concerns people with diabetes face, as well as strategies for managing these emotions and situations.

Getting in Touch with Your Diabetes

- What part of living with diabetes is the most difficult or unsatisfactory for you?

- How do you feel about this situation?

- How would this situation have to change for you to feel better about it?

- Are you willing to act to improve this situation for yourself?

- What steps could you take to bring yourself closer to where you want to be?

- Can you pick out one thing that you can do to improve things for yourself?

Your Feelings and Concerns

The emotions you experience as you deal with diabetes are generally negative ones. But these negative feelings may actually be useful. For example, denial can be part of nature's way of letting the news of diabetes sink in gradually. Even anger can be an ally in dealing with diabetes if you are able to channel your anger into energy that helps keep you motivated.

The key to dealing with your emotions is to understand your feelings and not try to suppress or deny them. Learning to understand how you are feeling and how your feelings influence your actions is the first step in dealing with your emotions.

Denial

Denial is not necessarily a bad thing. It can help you adjust to living with diabetes. By putting your emotions on hold, you can better deal with the shock of absorbing all of the new information. By pretending you don't have diabetes or that diabetes is not that big of a deal, you can avoid feeling overly stressed out, angry, or depressed as you learn about diabetes and begin to care for yourself.

Eventually, however, denial is no longer helpful or protective. In fact, it can be just the opposite. People who continue to deny the seriousness of diabetes are less likely to take positive steps to manage their blood glucose levels and ultimately to prevent diabetes complications.

Signs of Denial

- Your first reaction to the news that you have diabetes was to try not to think about it or wish it away.

- You tell yourself you'll deal with your diabetes later.

- You convince yourself that the diabetes care providers don't know what they are talking about.

If you feel overwhelmed, talk to your spouse, your close friends, or your diabetes care provider or educator. It may help to take one step at a time. Don't try to change everything all at once. Pick one area that is meaningful for you and start there. Remember that every step in the right direction is a big step.

You may want to consider joining a support group, joining a chat room or message board on the Internet, or seeking counseling. It can be reassuring to know that you have many of the same concerns as others, and they may be able to offer you ideas about ways to cope with diabetes.

Anger

You are likely to experience feelings of anger and frustration in managing your diabetes. You may feel very angry when you are first diagnosed or you may feel quite frustrated after living with diabetes for a while. Your emotions are common reactions to dealing with a difficult condition. It is normal to feel angry over something you feel you can't control. Trying to manage blood glucose levels is often frustrating.

Common Feelings of Anger

- You may feel that life is treating you unfairly.

- You may feel frustrated when all of your hard work doesn't seem to be paying off.

- You may find that feelings of anger coexist with feelings of denial, depression, or anxiety.

- You may find yourself feeling angry whenever you think of having diabetes or when confronted with some of the problems it brings.

- You may find that you lose your temper more quickly in situations that have nothing to do with diabetes. It's as if you are using all of your strength and coping skills to deal with diabetes. There's not much left to deal with life's other stresses and strains.

A good way to deal with anger and other bad feelings is to recognize the feelings, realize that they are common, and find ways to channel your energy.

Tips for Managing Anger

- Start to keep track of your angry episodes and the events that trigger your anger.

- If possible, keep notes or a journal.

- After a few days or even weeks, sit down and review your observations. Try to figure out if there is any sort of pattern.

- See if there are any particular situations or people that make you angry. Does your anger typically occur after sitting in a traffic jam? Does it occur when people start to ask you about your diabetes?

Sometimes just identifying the triggers may not be enough. You may also need to avoid those situations that make you angry. If you find yourself getting hot under the collar every time your spouse asks you about your blood glucose, don't wait until things build up to an angry outburst. In a calm moment, explain that it bothers you. Let your spouse know how he or she can be helpful.

You can let anger eat away at you and make you miserable, or you can think of it as unharnessed energy. Use that energy to do something positive. Your anger may be telling you that you are due for a change in your life.

Educate yourself about diabetes. Learn ways to handle anger without taking it out on others or yourself. For example, go for a walk, count to ten, or walk away from the situation. Many people find that seeing a professional counselor can be helpful initially and as they live with diabetes.

> **Coming to Terms with Diabetes**
>
> You may discover that you have angry feelings because you haven't completely come to terms with your diabetes. If this is the case, think about joining a support group, talking with other people, or seeking the help of a professional counselor.

Stress

Stress is a double-edged sword for people with diabetes, as with many chronic diseases. Stress may contribute to the symptoms of the disease, and living with diabetes can trigger stress.

Stress and Diabetes

Stress doesn't directly cause diabetes. However, for people already headed in that direction, it can push them along a little faster. You may have heard stories of people whose diabetes began after a stressful experience, such as a severe illness or a car accident.

In type 1 diabetes, the immune system mistakenly destroys the insulin-producing cells of the pancreas. This process usually takes many months, perhaps even years, before enough cells are destroyed to lead to diabetes.

A person on the way to developing type 1 diabetes makes less and less insulin. A stressful experience increases the need for insulin. So, the insulin demands brought on by a stressful experience could overwhelm the body's ability to produce insulin.

In type 2 diabetes, the body loses its ability to respond to insulin. As this happens, the pancreas makes less and less insulin. Adding stress-produced hormones, which create more resistance to insulin, could bring on the first symptoms of diabetes.

Stress can have an effect on your blood glucose levels, too. Your body prepares for stress by sending out hormones. High or fluctuating blood glucose and ketone levels may result. If stress is short lived and repetitive, levels of blood glucose and ketones may "bounce" considerably. Some people actually experience a low blood glucose level with an acute stressor.

Depression

Everybody—regardless of whether they have diabetes—goes through periods of feeling down, when they have low energy and don't care to be involved in things going on around them. Depression is serious when these feelings go on for long periods or when they interfere with your quality of life or your ability to care for your diabetes.

The causes, symptoms, prevention, and treatment of depression and other mental health disorders are discussed in detail in chapter 14. If you suspect that you may be experiencing depression, seek help right away. Talk to your health care provider or ask to be referred to a mental health specialist.

Anxiety

Everyone feels nervous or anxious from time to time, especially in a stressful situation. This is normal and, often, even helpful. But if you find that you feel nervous or anxious in situations that are not stressful to most people or if your anxiety is so intense and long lasting that it interferes with day-to-day living, you may have a more serious problem called an anxiety disorder. See more about anxiety disorders in chapter 14.

Alcohol Abuse

If you have diabetes and your blood glucose levels are on target, it is generally safe to drink alcohol occasionally. However, you may have an alcohol abuse problem if you drink too much or have trouble controlling how much alcohol you drink.

Alcohol abuse is even more dangerous for people with diabetes. Many diabetes complications—including nerve damage, eye problems, high blood pressure, kidney disease, and heart disease—can worsen with excessive alcohol use. Long-term alcohol abuse can interfere with how you take care of your diabetes.

Ending alcohol abuse can be very difficult, but it is crucial for many reasons, including your diabetes care. If you have a problem with alcohol, or think you might have a problem, there is help available to you. Talk to your provider, or call your local chapter of Alcoholics Anonymous (AA). Your health care team can help you find the treatment you need to begin the path to recovery.

> **Alcoholism and the Liver**
>
> Alcohol abuse is especially hard on the liver, where your body stores glucose. If your liver is damaged by alcohol, your blood glucose levels may become erratic, and you are more likely to have hypoglycemia.

Take Control

Taking control of your feelings is one of the best—although not always easiest—things that you can do for yourself. This can mean different things for different people. One person may find it helpful to be more assertive with family members. Another person may find relief in practicing yoga or progressive muscle relaxation. In this section, you'll find tips for taking control of your feelings in positive ways.

Handling Stress

Your level of stress depends on you and your environment. Each of us defines what situations we see as stressful and how we respond to the stress.

Both positive and negative situations can be stressful. Change almost always is. How stressful we perceive it to be depends on how good or harmful we find it to be and what else is going on in our lives. Something can feel stressful one day and not the next.

How Do You Act When Stressed?

• Do you anger easily and take your feelings out on others?

• Do you cry easily or become depressed or withdrawn?

Is Your Strategy Working?

To determine whether a strategy is effective, ask yourself: "Did it work? Did I feel better both immediately and later? Is this an effective strategy to use in the future?"

- Do you feel emptiness or apathy?

- Do you reject help from those close to you or want extra attention from them?

- Do you come down too hard on yourself?

Each person deals with stress in his or her own way. We usually behave in ways that are familiar to us. Some of these strategies work; others leave us feeling tense, tired, angry, or sick. Some strategies, such as smoking, drinking too much, and drug abuse, cause other problems. Other techniques and ways of dealing with stress can help us feel more in control, relaxed, and less tense after a stressful event.

Tips for Managing Stress

- Find someone to talk to and who will listen when something is bothering you.

- Join a support group. Your diabetes educator may be able to recommend a group in your area.

- Form a discussion or networking group on any topic or activity that interests you.

- Take up a new hobby or sport, learn a musical instrument, or join a dance class.

- Get moving—join a health club, sign up for an aerobics class, or just take a walk every day.

- Engage in volunteer work.

- Sign up for a class that interests you.

- Think of something you can do that relaxes you and do it—read a book, take a bubble bath, get a massage, or watch a movie.

- Spend time with friends or alone, whichever will replenish you more.

- Pray or meditate. Some church groups offer support for people with diabetes.

- Do a relaxation exercise.

- Take a vacation or even a night away.

- Get a babysitter to give you some extra time alone or with your spouse.

Recognize that everyone has choices in life and that you make your own choices. Pace yourself. Make it a point to identify and anticipate stresses, and create ways to deal with them ahead of time. You may not be able to control traffic jams, an angry boss, or a crying baby, but you do have some control over the way you react to these situations.

Progressive muscle relaxation is a technique that can help relieve stress. The sequence of inhaling, exhaling, and relaxing specific muscles can "take you away" from your current situation. Try it the next time you feel tense.

Progressive Muscle Relaxation

- Close your eyes and breathe slowly and deeply.

- Start with the muscles in your face, working your way down to your feet and toes.

- Inhale. Raise your eyebrows. Tense them. Hold for a count of 3. Relax your eyebrows. Exhale.

- Inhale. Open your mouth and eyes wide. Then close your mouth and eyes tightly. Squeeze. Hold for a count of 3. Relax your eyes and mouth. Exhale.

- Inhale. Bite down on your teeth. Hold for a count of 3. Relax your jaw. Exhale.

- Inhale. Pull your shoulders up. Hold for a count of 3. Relax your shoulders. Exhale.

- Inhale. Tense all the muscles in your arms. Hold for a count of 3. Relax your arms. Exhale.

- Inhale. Tense all the muscles in your chest and abdomen. Hold for a count of 3. Relax your chest and abdomen. Exhale.

- Inhale. Tense all the muscles in your legs. Hold for a count of 3. Relax your legs. Exhale.

- Inhale. Tense all the muscles in your feet. Curl your toes. Hold for a count of 3. Relax your feet. Exhale.

- Inhale. Exhale any tension that may be lingering in your body. Breathe in energy. Take several more deep, slow breaths. Enjoy feeling relaxed.

- Gradually open your eyes.

Boosting Your Self-Esteem

It is much easier to meet life's challenges with a healthy dose of self-esteem. You do better in your work, studies, and personal relationships. And you are more likely to go after what you want out of life when you feel good about yourself.

Unfortunately, diabetes can gnaw away at your sense of self-worth. Some people with diabetes blame themselves for having the illness or its complications. Sometimes, people think less of themselves because they feel different. This can happen whether you are a child, a teenager, or an adult. Some people even wonder if they are being punished when they get diabetes.

Many of our feelings of self-worth stem from the messages we were given as children (both positive and negative) and the messages we give ourselves as adults. One way to boost your feelings of self-worth is to give yourself affirming and positive messages. Recognize your good qualities and give yourself a break, even if no one else does.

Tips for Boosting Self-Esteem

- When you are feeling good about yourself, write down a list of all your strengths and positive qualities. Include things you are especially good at doing.

- When someone compliments you, add it to the list.

- If you have trouble coming up with things to put on the list, ask those around you who like and love you. Often your friends and family are quicker to recognize your strengths than you might be.

- On days when you are feeling down, take out the list and remind yourself of what a great person you are.

How you feel about yourself can affect how you care for your diabetes. Do you believe you deserve to spend the time, effort, and money it takes to care for your diabetes? How do you show yourself respect? If you do it by making choices, others will respect your needs, too. If you need to check your blood glucose right now, do it. Don't be worried about asking others to wait for you while you check.

Be Assertive

One of the ways you can take charge of your diabetes is to learn to be assertive. Most conflicts do not arise out of differences of opinion but out of gaps in communication.

If you are unable to assert yourself, you might find it difficult to talk about your diet or how much time you need to take care of your diabetes. You may be reluctant to have your needs interfere with those of the people around you.

Assertive communication means that both your needs and the needs of the other person are equally important and respected. Assertive statements often begin with "I". For example, "I find it helpful when you don't keep chips in the house." This statement is more effective than blaming or aggressive statements ("You always try to undermine everything I do") or reacting passively and being inwardly resentful.

Tips for Being Assertive

- *Learn to say no.* A simple "no, thank you" communicates to yourself and to others that "I respect myself enough to act in my own best self-interest, and I respect you enough to know that you will understand."

- *Maintain courtesy.* Courtesy is the cornerstone of effective and assertive communication. It relays the assumption that you will treat your needs and those of others equally and that neither will suffer at the other's expense.

- *Be direct.* Direct communication while maintaining courtesy is as important as saying "no" at the appropriate time.

- *Meet your own needs.* Hypoglycemia is an example of an urgent situation in which you must be assertive. Don't put off treatment because you are afraid of offending someone with whom you are interacting.

- *Be firm.* It is important to be firm with both yourself and others. Make a plan about how you will handle certain situations. If pressured, explain your decision directly to others.

- *Maintain self-respect.* If you respect yourself, it will be easier to be assertive.

Making Good Choices

Diabetes is largely a self-managed illness. Unlike more acute illnesses, you provide almost all of your own care.

It is up to you. You are free to decide how much or how little you do to care for your diabetes. Because you benefit from the results of your choices, you have the absolute right to make these decisions.

Many things in our lives are not of our own choosing. Diabetes is not something most people would choose to have. Although you cannot change having diabetes, you do make choices about how you live with it and your attitude toward it. No matter how constrained you may feel, you can often make different choices.

Freedom brings responsibility as well. In fact, freedom and responsibility are two sides of the same coin. Because the choices you make affect your outcomes, you have a great deal of responsibility for your own health and quality of life. It can be overwhelming. There are things that you can do to help you accept this much responsibility.

Tips for Making Good Choices

- Learn all that you can about diabetes. The more you know, the more you are able to weigh the positives and negatives of the choices you have to make.

- Ask your provider for a referral to a diabetes education program in your area.

- Work with your diabetes care provider to develop a plan to manage your diabetes that matches your goals and abilities. Be honest about what you can and cannot do. Remember, you are the one who has diabetes and lives with it each day. You are the expert on yourself and your life.

- Be honest with yourself. It may be tempting to shift the decisions to your health care team or blame the people around you for your outcomes. But when we do not accept responsibility, we become victims of our situation.

Power comes from accepting responsibility for our choices and our lives. Taking responsibility for managing your diabetes gives you power and control over your diabetes and your life.

If you are struggling with this level of responsibility, there are some questions that you can ask yourself to try to understand more about why you feel this way.

Questions of Power and Responsibility

- What stands in the way of accepting responsibility for my diabetes?

- What negative consequences come from feeling forced to behave in certain ways?

- What benefits come from feeling controlled by diabetes?

- What negative consequences come from accepting responsibility for diabetes care?

- What benefits come from accepting responsibility for diabetes care?

- What is one thing can you do this week to take charge of your diabetes care?

Ask for Help When You Need It

Trying to meet the never-ending demands of life with diabetes can make anyone feel frustrated. It's easy to feel cheated when you've met your end of the bargain by doing all that you can, but your blood glucose levels don't reflect your efforts. Wide swings in blood glucose levels can also cause your emotions to change.

If you suspect that this is happening, consider doing some investigative testing. If your mood swings are related to blood glucose fluctuations, talk to your health care team about other ways to manage your diabetes.

Tell the people close to you who want to support you about how you feel. If you need more help dealing with mood swings, ask for a referral to a psychologist or other mental health counselor. You don't have to be alone with diabetes. There is help and support available; you only have to ask for it.

Family Life and Children with Diabetes

I t may be easier to eat what you want and to exercise when you want if you live alone, but friends and family still enter into the picture. You need their support and understanding, and they need yours. If you live with others, you need to take their needs into account as well as your own.

People who are most successful at managing their diabetes have the cooperation and support of their family and friends. It helps when you don't feel alone in meeting the challenge of learning to live with diabetes.

Family Issues

Maybe at first it seems as though you should be able to handle things on your own. After all, your family can't hold your hand and watch you do everything. It is still up to you to manage your diabetes, right? Yes. But having diabetes is bound to affect your family.

Scheduling, family meals, and exercise plans can become sources of conflict when someone has diabetes. Diabetes affects the whole family.

Here, you'll find strategies for approaching the most frequent sources of tension in families.

Scheduling

Life can be demanding. Finding out you have diabetes may upset the delicate balance of your juggling act. You can't tend to your 2-year-old when you're in the middle of giving yourself an insulin shot. Your partner may begin to resent having you check your blood glucose and take insulin just as you're getting dinner on the table. Sex can lose some spontaneity if you have to eat a snack just when the mood is striking.

One way to enlist your family's support is to look at your schedule and routines. Probably the best way to approach this is to enlist their support right away.

Tips for Family Scheduling

- Hold a family meeting and explain how important it is to coordinate insulin doses, physical activity, and meals.

- Ask for suggestions as to how your needs can fit into the family routine.

- Perhaps other family members can do a little more, or it may mean enlisting some outside help.

You may already feel stretched to the limit. Planning meals, checking your blood glucose, and physical activity all take time. Don't be afraid to acknowledge that you can't do it all and that something is going to have to give.

Tip for Scheduling

It's often helpful to write down your usual activities or sit down with your day calendar and try to figure out how to best fit it all in.

Family Meals

Scheduling might not be the only change. Maybe you decide to eat or cook differently. Again, open communication will help. Explain that you are not going on a diet and you are not going to force your family into meager eating conditions. The eating recommendations for people with diabetes are basically guidelines for healthy eating.

The key is getting your family's input. No one likes to be forced into doing something they don't like to do. Your family can also help with your eating plan. For many people, this is the most difficult adjustment to make after being diagnosed with diabetes.

You may want to change some of the foods you eat and when you eat them. It will help you tremendously if the members of your family are willing to accommodate your new plan.

Common Meal Conflicts

- If you're trying to lose weight, you may need to eat smaller portions of certain foods or to avoid some high-calorie foods that your family enjoys. If sticking with your meal plan gnaws at your willpower, ask your family not to eat these foods in front of you, to have them less often, or to not always keep them in the house.

- Your family may object to eating different food and may resent eating on a schedule.

- Always remember that eating well for diabetes is not really a special diet, it just means eating sensibly. Whether you have diabetes or not, eating large amounts of sugar, fats, and salt isn't good for your health.

Physical Activity

Physical activity is also an important part of diabetes management, and your family can participate. Working out benefits everyone, not just those with diabetes. The more you can get your family involved in exercise, the easier it will be for everyone.

Tips for Getting Active with Your Family

- Ask your family to join in! They can walk or jog with you. If not, tell them how they can encourage your efforts.

- Plan family activities that involve some form of physical activity—walking the dog, a nature walk, or a bicycle trip to the corner store.

- An evening stroll or bicycle ride might enhance the quality of life for all family members.

- In addition, helping your children stay fit and at a healthy weight lowers their risk for developing diabetes.

Feelings and Concerns

Let your family know that you might have mood changes. Recognize that your family members will also have feelings about your illness. Learn to talk about your feelings, and try to establish open channels of communication.

Common Feelings and Concerns

- Sometimes you'll be cranky because of diabetes, and sometimes you will feel cranky because of life's demands.

- Your family may express their concern for you by frequently asking about your diabetes or trying to pretend it doesn't exist.

- They may also express their concern by reminding you to take care of your diabetes. It may feel like nagging or that they are becoming the "diabetes police."

- If any of these become a problem, let your family know how they can express their concern in a way that feels supportive to you.

Learn to work with your family members to talk about how you and they are feeling and what to do about it. Maybe you just need a snack or maybe you need to go for a walk. Or maybe your spouse or children need a break. Recognize when there is a problem, and talk about solutions.

Educate Your Family

Sometimes problems arise among family members when they don't really understand the disease. If your teenager is grumpy because he has to wait for you to take an insulin shot before you drive him to the mall, it may be because he doesn't understand how important it is. If your spouse is waving potato chips under your nose when you are trying to cut back, she may not understand the importance of your goal to eat healthily.

Many people think that treating diabetes is as simple as taking insulin a few times a day. Keep in mind that you have the right to ask for the support you need. As a first step, each family member needs to understand what diabetes is, how it is managed, and how to handle emergencies.

Tips for Educating Your Family

- Books, magazines, pamphlets, libraries, support groups, online message boards, and medical professionals can all be of assistance.

- Take a family member with you to some of your health care appointments. By keeping a running list of questions or issues with which they may be concerned, your family can get answers to their questions firsthand.

- Many diabetes education programs encourage family members to attend. The more information they have, the more they can help you and learn to integrate your diabetes management plan into the daily family routines.

Finally, your family should know what to do in an emergency. Make sure they understand the signs of hypoglycemia. Often people with diabetes having a low blood glucose episode will deny that there is a problem or refuse treatment, even though they may be in danger. Make sure your family members can recognize the signs of hypoglycemia and know how to deal with it.

Depending on your family, you can expect different responses to your diabetes and different levels of enthusiasm for helping you work toward your food and exercise goals. Some may join in wholeheartedly, looking at this as a team effort. Other families or family members may resent making changes when they aren't the one who is sick. You need to find the approach that works best for you. In some situations, you may be better off if you go it alone.

Don't Forget Your Partner

If you have diabetes, you know that it can take an emotional toll. But you're not the only one who may feel the stress. Your family members, especially your partner, are likely to share the burden.

The stress on your partner can work two ways. If you shut out your partner completely, he or she may feel isolated and helpless. He or she may feel a need to "rescue" you and resent being left by the wayside. However, if you shift too much of the burden to your partner, he or she may resent having to spend too much effort trying to help you and feel that you should be doing more to help yourself. Many spouses dislike being put in the position of parent or nursemaid.

Common Partner Concerns

• Your mate may worry when the decisions you make about caring for yourself seem wrong.

• He or she may fear the consequences of what will happen, either in an emergency situation or down the road, if you neglect your health.

• Maybe you feel that your spouse is nagging too much.

• Maybe your spouse feels that you are deliberately undermining his or her efforts to support you.

However you are feeling, it is important for both of you to realize that nobody is perfect. Often many of these feelings are due to love, concern, stress, or fear. It is important to acknowledge that these feelings—and probably many other conflicting emotions—do exist.

You may need help learning to communicate. Admitting this is a sign of strength, not a weakness. Confide in your friends. Speak with your spiritual counselor. Consider seeking the help of professional counselors who are trained in coping strategies for people with chronic disease. Your health care provid-

➡ Talk to Your Partner

Try to honestly share your feelings when neither of you is feeling pressured or stressed out. By sharing your feelings and communicating openly, you and your partner may be drawn closer together rather than driven apart.

er may be able to help you find the skilled professional with whom you need to talk.

And finally, don't forget to lighten up. Humor can help you get through stressful times. Laughter helps lighten the load.

Finding Other Sources of Support

Support is important, so if your family isn't able to be supportive or you live alone, you may need to look elsewhere for an extra boost. The American Diabetes Association, counseling, group therapy, and even joining a health club can help you find support outside your family.

American Diabetes Association

One place to start is the American Diabetes Association (ADA). ADA can tell you about support and educational groups that you can attend. By participating in these groups, you can meet other people with diabetes and health care professionals. Whether you are seeking more information or want to talk to people who share your experiences, a support group may be just the thing. You may be able to find a diabetes care partner, and you can support each other.

In addition to education and support groups, ADA can mail you a packet of information on request. They can also answer any questions you may have about diabetes or some of the practical issues in managing diabetes: health care, health insurance, and referrals. They also have books, magazines, and other publications that may help.

Message Boards and Blogs

The Internet is often the first place people turn for information—and support. Message boards can help people with diabetes share feelings, concerns, and strategies. With a message board, you can post an anonymous message and receive comments and advice from other readers.

The ADA hosts several message boards where people with diabetes can discuss specific topics, such as type 1 or type 2 diabetes, parenting a child with diabetes, recent diagnoses, and diabetes technology and equipment.

It can also help to read blogs by other people with diabetes—or even launch your own blog. A blog is an online journal where a person makes regular, often daily, postings about their feelings and activities.

Make sure to read material on the Internet with a critical eye. People may post information that is inaccurate or may not be appropriate for your personal needs. Review Internet-based advice that you find on message boards, blogs, and chat rooms with your health care team before you try it.

Health Clubs

You might also consider joining a health club. Although this is a source you may not have considered, developing a diabetes management program really means developing healthy living habits. People who actively participate in the local health club or fitness center may share similar goals, whether they have diabetes or not. The club may even offer a personal trainer, who can be a tremendous help to you. You might also meet other people with diabetes.

Counseling

Sometimes, despite the help of support groups, and even with a supportive family, you might need extra help. Coping with diabetes and all of the feelings that go along with it is not an easy process.

There are bound to be times when you will need extra support. Your friends and family may not have all the skills you need. Also, new issues may arise during the course of your life or the course of your disease.

Whatever your situation, you may want to consider some form of individual or group counseling for those times when you need extra help. It might help to sort out any difficulties with a professional who can be an objective source of support. A professional therapist can help you examine your problems. Depending on your individual needs, you may want individual, marriage, or family therapy.

You might seem a little put off by the idea of seeing a therapist. Maybe it conjures up negative images, or maybe you think seeing a therapist indicates that there is something wrong with your mental state. Nothing could be further from the truth. Counseling is a healthy way of helping people deal with some of life's difficult problems.

What to Expect from a Therapist

- Counseling involves an ongoing conversation between you and your therapist.

- Your therapist will help you explore your thoughts and feelings and examine how you interact with others and the decisions you make.

- Your therapist may encourage you to tell your story, starting from the beginning. This may help you find a new perspective on the problems in your life and discover the patterns in your actions.

- He or she may also offer suggestions that may help you see the situation from another viewpoint and may help you find new ways of coping.

One of the most important aspects is to find a therapist you trust. You need to feel comfortable with your therapist and feel that he or she is helpful. It often means finding the right personality match. Someone who works well with one person may not necessarily be compatible with someone else. So don't be too discouraged if the first therapist you see doesn't fit your needs. You may need to talk to several before you find one who feels right.

Living with diabetes means adjusting to the complex interplay among family relations, personality, emotions, lifestyle habits, and diabetes management. Therapy will help you learn to take the initiative and necessary action to take charge of your diabetes as well as the conflicting emotions that go along with it.

Group Therapy
While some people benefit from one-on-one encounters with a therapist, others gain more from weekly group therapy sessions. Many people find the combination of approaches to be a double benefit. These groups can foster mutual support, encourage camaraderie, and help combat the depression and isolation that often goes along with a diagnosis of diabetes. Sometimes talking things out with other people helps you find fresh solutions.

What to Expect in Group Therapy

- There are many types of settings and formats for group therapy.

- Some meet in hospitals, clinics, community agencies, and even in therapists' private offices.

- Group therapy should include a trained therapist, a careful selection of group members, and a social structure that includes rules for behavior.

- All therapy groups share the principle that talking about feelings, ideas, and experiences in a safe, respectful atmosphere increases self-esteem, deepens self-understanding, and helps a person get along better with others.

- The group setting gives each member a chance to see how others react to his or her feelings about diabetes and observe how he or she incorporates diabetes into family, work, and play.

Advantages of Group Therapy for People with Diabetes

- It can help you learn that you are not alone.
- You can discuss feelings, worries, and concerns that you may never have dreamed of discussing anywhere else.
- You may discover new approaches to old problems.
- It can help you explore who you are and who you are not.
- It may reduce stress, which in turn may lead to better health.

Children with Diabetes

Any kind of change can upset the family dynamic. How you treat your children and how they interact with each other can be influenced by many factors. Having a child diagnosed with diabetes is a big change that is likely to affect the entire family in ways you never thought possible.

At a time when you, your child, and other children are probably fearful about what the future holds, you will likely be confronted with feelings of anger, resentment, and jealousy upon hearing of a diagnosis of diabetes. While you are trying to gather information and help your child manage his or her diabetes, it is difficult to keep all of the family relationships running smoothly at the same time.

If you have a child with diabetes, your top priority will be to help your child manage the disease while trying to live as normal a life as possible. You will also want to help the rest of the family make a smooth transition into accepting the changes that are inevitable.

Your Child's Health

The first step in helping your child manage his or her diabetes is to learn all you can. Other chapters in this book and Internet resources are a good starting point (see the Resources section at the end of this book for ideas).

Health Care Providers

Some of the first people you'll probably talk with are your child's care provider and diabetes educator. In general, you will need to know how to check your child's blood glucose, how to give insulin if needed, how to use a meal plan, and how to be physically active.

You will also want to know the extent to which your child can begin to take responsibility for his or her own care. If your child is only 2 years old, it is unrealistic to expect her to give herself insulin or check for blood glucose, but if your child is 10, she may very well be capable of checking her own blood glucose. Children mature at different rates. Some may be ready to give their own injections at age 7, but others may not be able to do it until age 11 or older.

In doing your research and helping your child develop a treatment plan, don't forget that every child is different. What works for one child may not work for your child. You already know a lot about your child and what will work best for your family.

Your health care provider should take into consideration your child's age when designing a blood glucose management plan. For example, less stringent goals may be appropriate for younger children.

> ➔ **Health Care Appointments**
>
> Try to schedule appointments that are long enough so that all your questions and concerns can be addressed.

Type 1 Diabetes in Children

Type 1 is the most common form of diabetes in children. Children with diabetes are not just "small adults," and your health care provider should have specific recommendations based on your child's health and age. The American Diabetes Association also publishes books on raising children with diabetes. However, here are a few things to keep in mind.

Children with type 1 diabetes are at risk for complications such as eye, heart, kidney, and other diseases. Therefore, your health care provider should recommend screening for complications based on your child's age and family history.

Common Tests for Children with Type 1 Diabetes

- Test for kidney problems, such as annual screening for microalbuminuria in children aged 10 and older (and who have had diabetes for at least 5 years).

- Test for high cholesterol, including fasting lipid profile in children aged 10 or older. Children with a family history of high cholesterol or cardiovascular disease may be screened earlier.

- Dilated eye exam in children aged 10 and older (and who have had diabetes for 3–5 years).

- Celiac disease screening soon after diagnosis.

- Thyroid disease screening at diagnosis.

- Blood pressure assessment.

Blood Glucose Goals for Type 1 Diabetes by Age-Group

Age	Before Meals (mg/dl)	Bedtime/Overnight (mg/dl)	A1C
Toddlers and younger than 6	100–180	110–200	<8.5%
School age (6–12)	90–180	100–180	<8%
Adolescents and young adults (13–19)	90–130	90–150	<7.5%*

A lower A1C (<7%) is reasonable if it can be achieved without excessive hypoglycemia.

Type 2 Diabetes in Children

Type 2 diabetes is still relatively rare in children. However, it is becoming more common in minority populations. Children with type 2 diabetes should aim to keep blood glucose levels as close to normal as possible, which may be achieved with food and exercise programs or medication. At diagnosis, children with type 2 diabetes may already show signs of complications, so ask your health care provider about appropriate tests and treatments.

Common Tests at Diagnosis for Children with Type 2 Diabetes

- Blood pressure assessment.
- Test for high cholesterol, such as fasting lipid profile.
- Test for kidney problems with microalbuminuria assessment.
- Dilated eye exam.

Children with type 2 diabetes may be at risk for polycystic ovary disease or problems related to obesity, such as sleep disorders, foot problems, and psychosocial concerns. Ask your health care provider if these problems may be affecting your child.

After you meet with your child's diabetes care provider, you will also want to meet with a diabetes educator. A diabetes educator can help you learn to coordinate your child's overall diabetes management plan. This includes balancing your child's meals with his medication or insulin schedule and physical activities.

You will also want to meet with a dietitian and work out an eating plan. Make sure to take into consideration your child's likes and dislikes, how your family usually eats, any cultural or religious influences, how to include treats, and how to handle special events.

Tips for Meal Planning

- You will help your child and your family if you all eat the same foods.

- Don't prepare one dish for the rest of the family and a special meal for your child with diabetes.

- Make sure to involve your child in the meal planning, and ask him what foods he would like to include in his eating plan.

Also talk to your child's teachers and school officials or day care providers about any special needs your child has. (For more on diabetes at school, see the next chapter.) Once you and your child figure out the daily routine and work out ways to deal with special events and circumstances, you will both feel better about living with diabetes.

Parents' Attitudes and Feelings

When you first find out that your child has diabetes, you may be overwhelmed with feelings of shock, disbelief, sadness, anger, or even guilt. It can seem so unfair. You may experience self-doubt as you wonder whether you can give your child the care he or she needs. With all the stresses in your life and all the demands on your time and energy, it may seem that you just won't be able to handle it all.

It can be overwhelming, especially at first. As you learn more about diabetes, you will also learn how to help your child live like any other child. It may take a little work as you figure out how to balance your child's meals with insulin injections and physical activities. You may find that your child takes it all in stride and that the hardest part may be coming to terms with your own feelings.

Don't forget that your child is looking to you for guidance. Your attitude will have a direct impact on how your child sees himself and how he or she comes to terms with this new lifestyle. If you take your child's diabetes in stride, it will be easier for your child to accept it. If you react with anxiety, apprehension, and fear, so will your child.

When you are anxious and concerned about your child, it is tempting to do everything for your child. But even very young children need to have some say in their diabetes care plan.

ADA's Family Link

The American Diabetes Association sponsors a program called Family Link, which allows parents to connect with other parents of children with diabetes. It also sponsors events in local communities. This can be a valuable resource for parents of children with diabetes.

Tips for Encouraging Your Child's Responsibility

• Let your child assume some of the responsibilities of managing diabetes, such as helping to plan meals or snacks.

- Gradually increase the amount of responsibility your child has. But at the same time, make sure your child is able to take on this responsibility.

- Treat shots and blood glucose checks as givens, with no exceptions. You aren't really doing your child a favor if you let diabetes care slide.

> **Be Straightforward**
>
> Deal with diabetes in a matter-of-fact way. Don't downplay your child's fears or concerns, but address them in a straightforward fashion.

- The best way to establish diabetes care habits is for them to become a way of life. As soon as your child sees that these are nonnegotiable, he or she will be more likely to cooperate.

Taking Care of the Rest of the Family

If you have more than one child, the time you spend taking care of diabetes is bound to cause some tension in the family. Siblings may feel jealous of the child with diabetes because of all the attention that he is getting. On the other hand, siblings may give your child with diabetes too much attention, and your child may feel like his siblings are on his case. He may feel that everyone is breathing down his neck.

The best way to deal with diabetes in the family is to treat it openly. Explain to the other children and other family members what is happening, and ask them to be patient as you work things out. Even young children can understand simple information.

In general, you will want to treat your child's diabetes matter-of-factly. Once your child and her siblings come to accept diabetes as a part of your family routine, feelings of anger, jealousy, and fear usually begin to subside.

However, if you continue to experience family turmoil, you might want to consider family counseling. Talk to your child's provider and diabetes educator for help finding a family counselor.

> **Make Siblings Feel Special**
>
> Try to schedule special times with your other children who may feel left out, or ask if they want a job in the overall care of your child with diabetes. A sibling could help record blood glucose readings, for example.

> ### Giving Toddlers a Choice
>
> If your child takes insulin, maybe he or she can choose the injection spot or the finger to poke. This is a good way for your child to get used to having a say in his or her care. It will help him or her to develop a sense of responsibility, so you can gradually let your child assume more and more of the responsibilities of diabetes care as he or she grows older.

Your Child's Changing Role

Just how much you can expect your child to handle with respect to his diabetes care will change as he matures and will depend on his personality. If your child is an infant or toddler when diagnosed, you will be completely responsible for your child's care. But you can and should still keep him involved. You will have to see that your child gets his shots at the right time, and you will have to check his blood glucose and evaluate the results, but you can give your child a voice.

If your child is in preschool, you are still responsible for making sure your child has healthy foods, checks blood glucose whenever necessary, and takes the right type and dose of insulin at the right time. But there is nothing wrong with letting your child begin to take over some of these tasks, with supervision. Insulin pens may make it easier for your child to help with injections.

With your health care team, discuss the developmental stages of your child and when your child can assume some of his or her self-care. As your child matures, he can take on more and more of the tasks. As your child matures during this period, it is essential that she learn to take responsibility for her own care and decisions, because she will often be with friends or at school and out of your watchful vision.

> ### Insulin Pumps
>
> You may want to consider an insulin pump. This can give your child much greater flexibility and independence but is also a big responsibility.

Adolescence is bound to provide the greatest challenges to both you and your child with diabetes. Diabetes is often more difficult to manage due to hormone changes. Children are coming of age and want more freedom. There will be times when your teen resents you and blames you for all the ups and downs of diabetes. This is a normal part of becoming independent and would happen whether or not diabetes was a factor.

Teenage Diabetes Rebellions

- Your teenager may try to rebel by neglecting diabetes care.

- Your child may try to deny the presence of diabetes in an effort to fit in and appear just like everyone else.

- It can be hard to take insulin, count carbohydrates, and check glucose readings at school or when he or she is out with friends.

- It may help to remind your teenager that the best way to fit in and keep diabetes from interfering with life is to keep blood glucose levels on target. A bout of severe hypoglycemia or diabetic ketoacidosis will surely make your child feel different.

It is not uncommon for children and teenagers to feel depressed. Eating disorders, especially among girls, are common. One type of eating disorder among teens with diabetes involves skipping insulin. This allows a person to eat and not gain weight. If you start to suspect that your child is depressed or developing any sort of coping problem, eating disorder, or behavioral problem, seek the help of a professional counselor immediately (see chapter 10 for more on eating disorders).

→ Tip for Adolescents

You might suggest that your child visit a diabetes educator alone. This gives your child a chance to ask questions and establish a relationship that can be helpful in the future as well. When your child is treated like an adult, he or she may act more like an adult. It is critical that your child understands that it is up to her to take charge of her care.

> ### → Diabetes Camp
>
> The ADA sponsors camps for children with diabetes. At camp, kids can make new friends, discover they're not alone with diabetes, and share strategies for managing diabetes. Visit www.diabetes.org or call 1-800-DIABETES for additional information about camps.

Handling Emergencies

Whether your child is a toddler or a teen, it is important that you, your child, and those close to him be aware of the signs that could signal an emergency. Severe hypoglycemia (low blood glucose) and hyperglycemia (high blood glucose) are both emergency situations. Hypoglycemia can lead to unconsciousness and coma. Hyperglycemia can lead to diabetic ketoacidosis (DKA), a life-threatening situation.

To prevent either situation, learn to recognize the warning signs, check your child's blood glucose right away, and treat promptly. Talk to your child's provider in advance about what to do if your child's blood glucose levels fall too low or rise too high. Make sure your child wears an ID at all times that identifies her as having diabetes.

Hypoglycemia
Recommended blood glucose levels are different for children and adults, because of children's high risk and vulnerability to hypoglycemia, relatively low risk of complications before puberty, and developmental and psychological issues.

The blood glucose levels at which hypoglycemia is treated are also often higher than the standard recommendations for adults. Any time your child's blood glucose level falls below the value you have established, he or she may have hypoglycemia. See chapter 8 for more about hypoglycemia, including common signs and treatments.

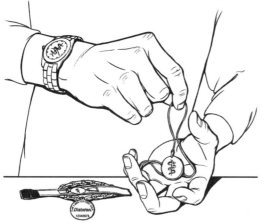

Types of medical identification.

Hyperglycemia and DKA

High blood glucose levels due to insufficient insulin can lead to DKA. This is a life-threatening condition that requires immediate action. Read more in chapter 8 about symptoms of hypergylcemia and DKA and how to check urine for ketones.

➔ Helpful Websites for Parents and Kids

American Diabetes Association
www.diabetes.org/living-with-diabetes/parents-and-kids/

Children with Diabetes Online Community
www.childrenwithdiabetes.com

Work, School, and Travel

Learning to manage your diabetes at work, at school, or during travel will take some extra effort and time. In these situations, you're likely to run into people who don't know about diabetes or encounter circumstances that aren't within your control.

A common theme for managing your diabetes in all of these situations is to be organized and prepared for potential challenges. You may have to take extra time to educate and communicate with people who are unfamiliar with diabetes and its management. This chapter provides tips for talking about diabetes with bosses, colleagues, teachers, and airport security. You'll also find out about your rights in the workplace and schools.

Diabetes in the Workplace

There's really no end to the types of work people with diabetes can do. Today—thanks to the Americans with Disabilities Act and the Rehabilitation Act—there are more and more opportunities for people with diabetes. These two laws guarantee your rights in private employment, local government, and federal government employment.

Diabetes affects each person differently, and each person should be evaluated based on what he or she can do. As long as you are qualified, you can go after almost any job you desire.

You may have an easier time managing your diabetes if you have a regular work schedule. But if your job entails working the late shift or traveling all over the globe, diabetes doesn't have to keep you from pursuing it. Most people can make the necessary adjustments with help from their health care team.

If your employer or prospective employer questions your ability to do your job, explain to them how you are able to manage your diabetes. Emphasize that you are in charge of your diabetes and the discipline you use in taking care of your diabetes is the discipline and determination you will bring to the workplace.

Night Shift

When you work the night shift you may feel out of sync with the rest of the world. While everyone else is eating breakfast, you're ready for your bedtime snack. Adjusting to conventional hours on your days off can also be a challenge. Nevertheless, with careful planning and monitoring, you can learn to make adjustments so that your new routine works for you.

Insulin Adjustments for Night Shift

- If you plan to sleep through the day, you may need to adjust your insulin dose to prevent hypoglycemia while you sleep.

- It may be easier to use a more intensive approach to manage your diabetes. For example, you could take an injection of long-acting insulin at the same time every day and rapid- or short-acting insulin before your meals.

- An insulin pump may also work well. Your health care team can help you make changes.

- If you prefer to stay up until noon and sleep through the afternoon and early evening, your normal morning insulin dose may work just fine. But you may have to make adjustments in your evening dose.

- If your job calls for some nights on and some nights off, then you will need to check your blood glucose levels more often and fine-tune your insulin dose.

If you have type 2 diabetes and are not taking insulin, you may still have to accommodate your work schedule. If you are taking oral medication, eating at a particular time may make a difference. It may be as simple as making sure you eat a snack before sleeping or changing when you eat and work out.

Erratic Hours

You may not work the night shift, but you may have a job that makes you keep odd hours. Meetings with clients may have you eating later than usual. Your job may require lots of travel. Even in the most conventional job setting, there are probably going to be occasions when you're eating or exercising at different times. Whether it happens all the time or once in a while, you'll need to learn how to make adjustments to accommodate changes in routine.

If you tend to keep a crazy schedule, talk to your health care team about an insulin plan that allows for maximum flexibility. Afterwards, check and record your blood glucose levels and evaluate how well your plan worked.

Physical activity can also be affected by changes in schedule. If you are used to a lunchtime jog, but a noontime lunch meeting keeps you from your normal routine, your blood glucose will probably be higher that afternoon. You can compensate by eating less, or, if you're taking insulin, by injecting a little more insulin than usual. If you take your run later in the day, you may find it necessary to eat a larger snack than usual.

Whenever changes in routine require adjustments, be extra diligent about monitoring to keep your blood glucose on target and to learn how to make future adjustments. Be sure to always keep a snack on hand in case your glucose level goes low.

→ Check More Frequently

Whenever you are getting used to a new routine, more frequent blood glucose monitoring will help you decide how to best adjust your daily routine to keep your blood glucose levels in balance.

→ Late Lunches

If you're going to eat a late lunch, try eating your afternoon snack or part of your carbohydrates at your normal lunchtime, and you'll be able to hold off for a while until you eat your full meal. You may also need to delay giving your insulin until your mealtime. It will take a little trial and error, but you will soon figure out how to make adjustments.

Safety on the Job

It is important to always be aware of your blood glucose levels if you operate heavy equipment, if you are involved in public safety jobs like law enforcement or firefighting, or if you drive an automobile. This is especially important for people who take insulin or oral medications that can cause a low blood glucose reaction. A low blood glucose reaction in these situations can result in injury to yourself and others and can have serious employment consequences.

Guidelines for Diabetes and Driving or Operating Heavy Equipment

- Check your blood glucose level before you leave your house or start work.

- If your blood glucose is low (70 mg/dl or less), treat it. Recheck 15 minutes after your first check to be sure your blood glucose level is rising. Otherwise, it is not safe to drive or operate equipment. If your glucose is not rising, treat again, and wait until your blood glucose level has come back up.

- Always take along a fast-acting source of carbohydrate—glucose gel or tablets, hard candy, juice boxes, or raisins. Keep them in your glove compartment, too, so you will always have something available.

- If you feel even minor symptoms of low blood glucose while driving or operating heavy equipment, stop and check your blood glucose. Driving with a low blood glucose level is dangerous. It is better to be a few minutes late or to take a little longer getting the job done than to risk an accident.

- If you can't check your blood glucose and you feel hypoglycemic, stop what you are doing and treat the symptoms. Don't start driving or working again until the symptoms pass. It's a mistake to think you can hold out until you get to your destination or until you finish up the job.

- Always wear diabetes identification.

Armed Forces and Commercial Pilots and Drivers

Federal law requires an employer to evaluate each person with diabetes as an individual, looking at the job in question and how diabetes affects that person. However, there are a few exceptions: the armed forces and commercial pilots and drivers.

→ **ADA Wins Pilot Battle**

Thanks to ADA's efforts, the Federal Aviation Administration (FAA) overturned a 36-year-old blanket ban that prohibited people who use insulin from flying small, private aircraft.

Exceptions to the Law

• The federal government does not allow people who take insulin to enter the armed forces. However, some people who take insulin have been able to remain in the armed forces when diagnosed with diabetes.

• The federal government does not allow people who use insulin to pilot commercial airplanes.

Commercial Drivers' Licenses
The American Diabetes Association (ADA) has worked for years to overturn the so-called "blanket bans" that sometimes prohibit anyone with diabetes from performing certain jobs or participating in other activities. The federal government used to ban people who take insulin from driving large trucks or buses on interstate routes but has now set up a program for individual evaluation of each potential driver. For example, if you were a truck or bus driver with non-insulin-treated diabetes who later began using insulin, you could lose your job.

Tips for Commercial Drivers

• Thanks to the ADA, in 2003, the U.S. Department of Transportation (DOT) instituted an exemption program to allow some people who use insulin to drive commercial vehicles in interstate commerce.

• Under this system, the DOT evaluates each case on an individual basis.

- Currently, drivers must submit an application and go through a physical examination through the DOT to receive an exemption.

In addition, the federal government allows individual states to provide waivers to intrastate drivers who use insulin. These waivers allow commercial drivers to travel within a given state, but only if the goods or people transported are not coming from or going to another state. Contact your state's motor vehicles department to find out if your state has a waiver program for intrastate drivers who use insulin.

The ADA continues to fight for the right for each person with diabetes to be evaluated individually based on how diabetes affects him or her and to not be excluded because of misinformation and stereotypes about diabetes.

Discrimination at Work

Today there are laws to protect against discrimination in the workplace. But unfortunately, discrimination against people with diabetes still exists.

Sometimes people with diabetes are told outright they won't be hired because of their diabetes. But other times discrimination can be subtler. Did you get passed over for a promotion because of your work performance or because your boss was afraid your diabetes might interfere with the added responsibilities? Did you fail to get that job offer because you weren't qualified, or because you told the employer you have diabetes?

Sometimes it's hard to know. The best thing you can do to guard against discrimination in the workplace is to do the best job you can and understand your rights. You can find more information about employment discrimination at www.diabetes.org.

Disability Laws
In 1990, the Americans with Disabilities Act was signed into law. This law protects qualified individuals with disabilities from discrimination. It covers all private-sector employees who work for companies that employ 15 or more people and people who work for state or local governments.

The Rehabilitation Act of 1973 and the Congressional Accountability Act provide similar coverage for people who work for the executive branch of the federal government, companies that receive federal funding, or the legislative branch of the federal government.

Under these federal laws, employers cannot discriminate against you if you have a disability, are qualified for the job, and can carry out the work with or without reasonable accommodation by the employer.

All of the states have their own anti-discrimination laws and agencies responsible for enforcing them. Some state anti-discrimination laws provide more comprehensive protection than federal laws.

In principle, employers are not allowed to discriminate, but in practice some discrimination still occurs. Some employers are slow to change workplace policies, such as bans on hiring anyone who takes insulin, unless they are challenged in court.

American with Disabilities Act: A federal law that protects qualified individuals with disabilities who work in the private sector or for state and local governments from discrimination.

The Rehabilitation Act of 1973: A federal law that protects people with disabilities who work for the executive branch of the federal government or for companies or contractors that receive federal funding from discrimination.

The Congressional Accountability Act: A federal law that provides the same coverage for employees of the legislative branch of the federal government.

Your Rights

A person with diabetes must show that she or he meets the definition of "disability" under the law (specifically, having an actual disability, having a record of a disability, or being regarded as having a disabil-

➔ Diabetes Is a Disability Under the Law

The Rehabilitation Act, the Americans with Disabilities Act, and the Congressional Accountability Act require employers to give people with disabilities an equal opportunity. It may be difficult to think of diabetes as a "disability," but this legal term is necessary to defend your rights.

→ **Americans with Disabilities Amendments Act of 2008**

This new law further protects people from workplace discrimination. It no longer requires that mitigating measures—such as insulin use—be considered when determining whether you have a disability. It considers your endocrine system as a major life activity that can be impaired— and diabetes is therefore a disability.

ity). One type of disability is a limitation in the functioning of a major bodily system, such as the endocrine system. So, under the law, most people with diabetes have to prove that they have limited endocrine function.

Tips about Your Rights

• Courts are required to do an individual assessment of each person.

• The employee must also establish that he or she is qualified for the job in question. A qualified applicant possesses the skill, experience, education, and other job requirements of the position he or she would do with or without reasonable accommodation.

• Employees must also show they were treated unfairly because of their diabetes.

Before these laws were passed, you may have been asked to list any medical conditions on a job application. The employer could then refuse to hire you based on this information. But if you weren't hired, you might not know whether it was because of your qualifications, a bad recommendation, or because of your diabetes.

Current federal law allows an employer to ask an applicant for medical information only after making a job offer and only if all job applicants are asked to provide this information. Then an employer may withdraw a job offer only if the applicant cannot perform the tasks required for the job, even if the employer makes reasonable accommodations.

An employer still has the option of hiring whomever he or she feels is best able to do the job. However, an employer can run into problems if he or she hires someone less qualified while re-

→ **You Can Be Fired**

It is important to keep in mind that if you can't show that you have a disability, have a record of having a disability, or are regarded as having a disability then it is legal under federal law for an employer to refuse to hire you, fire you, or take other adverse action because you have diabetes.

> ➜ **Asking Medical Questions on the Job**
>
> Once you have started working, an employer can only ask medical questions if they are related to the job and consistent with the needs of the business. For example, if an employee falls asleep on the job, an employer may ask if a medical condition is the cause. However, if an employee doesn't look well but is performing his or her job adequately, an employer may not ask whether there is a medical problem.

fusing someone with better qualifications who happens to have diabetes or any other disability.

Reasonable Accommodation

The laws require that employers try to reasonably accommodate people with disabilities. Reasonable accommodation is defined as modification or adjustment of a job or employment practice in order to make it possible for a qualified person with a disability to be employed.

For people with diabetes, employers may have to allow workers to adjust their work schedule or take breaks to eat or check blood glucose so that they can manage their diabetes while on the job.

People with complications from diabetes might need other accommodations, such as a large-screen computer for those with retinopathy or the ability to sit on the job for those with painful neuropathy. The employer must make these accommodations available unless they create an undue burden because of cost or other factors.

Protecting Your Job with FMLA

Another federal law, the Family and Medical Leave Act (FMLA), can help you—and your family—deal with diabetes in the workplace. This law allows workers to take up to 12 weeks of job-protected unpaid leave during any 12-month period to care for their own serious health condition or to care for family members (spouse, child, or parent) with a serious health condition.

Examples of when you might use FMLA for your diabetes would be for a doctor appointment or sick day because of your neuropathy pain (if your employer doesn't allow these accommodations). Or you could use the FMLA to take your child to the emergency room in the event of severe hyperglycemia.

Tips for FMLA

• FMLA absences may be taken in a single 12-week stretch or in shorter intervals, such as a short period to deal with a diabetes-related illness or emergency or a scheduled doctor's appointment.

• Employers who normally pay health insurance premiums must continue to do so for an employee on FMLA leave.

• FMLA applies to most public employers and to those private companies with 50 or more local employees (within 75 miles of the workplace).

• To be eligible, employees must have been with a covered employer for at least 1 year and have worked 1,250 or more hours during the 12 months immediately preceding the date of commencement of FMLA leave.

• When leave is foreseeable, employees must give 30 days' notice.

Some high-level company executives—those who are in the top 10% salary range—may be ineligible for FMLA leave. FMLA offers leave to care for yourself, your spouse, parents, step- and foster parents, minor children, minor step- and foster children, and adult children who are incapable of self-care. FMLA excludes leave care for unmarried partners, in-laws, siblings, grandchildren, and grandparents.

Fighting Back against Discrimination
If you believe that you have experienced discrimination, either in your job or while seeking employment, the best course of action is first to educate and then negotiate. If necessary, litigate and, last, legislate.

Sometimes, dealing with a discrimination problem is as simple as teaching people about diabetes. Many employers don't understand the needs or capabilities of people with diabetes. Sometimes they don't understand the laws that protect you from discrimination.

By educating employers about your needs, limitations, and strengths and by informing them of your rights and their responsibilities, you can resolve many situations in which you suspect discrimination.

Sometimes education alone may not be enough. You may have to negotiate to secure your rights. Your negotiations may be more effective if you first seek legal advice. Seeking legal advice early will maximize your attorney's ability to help you.

> ### → Suggest a Trial Period
>
> If your employer is unwilling to take the steps to resolve a problem, you might suggest a trial period in which you can show how your solution may benefit all involved. You might also consider soliciting outside help, such as elected officials or the media.

Whether you have outside help or not, negotiating involves listening to the concerns of those in the workplace with an open mind and offering solutions to the perceived problems.

If this doesn't help, you may have no choice but to litigate. The litigation process begins by filing an administrative complaint with the appropriate agency.

Filing a Claim

- If you are discriminated against by a private employer or a local government, you must file a charge with the Equal Employment Opportunity Commission (EEOC) and/or the state agency that handles workplace discrimination issues. The EEOC provides free information booklets. Check the Resources section at the end of this book for more information.

- If you work for or are seeking a job with the executive branch of the federal government, you must file a complaint with your agency's Equal Employment Opportunity Office.

- If you have been discriminated against by the legislative branch of the federal government, your claim under the Congressional Accountability Act must be filed with the Office of Compliance.

Be aware that the time limits for filing discrimination claims are very short. Claims with the executive branch of the federal government must be filed within 45 days of the act of discrimination and those with other employers can be due within 180 days of discriminatory treatment. If the agency doesn't resolve the problem to your satisfaction, you can file a lawsuit in federal or state court claiming discrimination on the basis of disability.

If a suit is decided in your favor, the employer may be forced to pay a cash settlement, reverse the discriminatory decision, and pay penalties. To decide on the best course of action, you will want to consult an attorney.

Sources to Contact in Case of Discrimination

- The American Diabetes Association. Call 1-800-DIABETES and ask for the Association's employment discrimination packet. If you have a specific problem, you may also want to fill out a form so that you can talk to the Association's Legal Advocate. A great deal of information is available on the ADA website (www.diabetes.org).

- The Equal Employment Opportunity Commission or your state's anti-discrimination agency. Most states have a commission charged with investigating discrimination.

- Your union representative. If your job is covered by a union contract, your union may be able to help.

It is up to you to prove that you have been discriminated against because of diabetes. Request a written statement saying why you weren't hired or promoted or were let go. There may be other reasons for the employer's decision, and you and your attorney should be aware of them.

Tips for Proving Discrimination

- If an employer is truly discriminating against you on the basis of your diabetes, he or she may not readily admit to it in writing.

- You may have to gather some information to substantiate your claim, such as the employer's job application form, policy manuals, and any rules or regulations cited by the employer as the reason you were dismissed or not hired.

- Save copies of the job advertisement or listing, the job description, and the job performance evaluation criteria.

- You should also compile a list of potential witnesses, including their work titles and how to contact them. Include some information about their duties at work and how they would know about your situation.

- Finally, make a diary of events in chronological order.

Sometimes legislative or regulatory changes are necessary. The ADA works to change laws and policies that are unfair to people with diabetes; for example, ADA successfully fought the "blanket ban" that kept people who use insulin from driving a commercial vehicle in interstate commerce.

Fighting Discrimination: A Success Story

Jeff Kapche always knew he wanted to be a police officer. Kapche passed all the tests and the background check required to join the department as a police officer.

However, the doctor in the city of San Antonio who gave Kapche his physical examination concluded that Kapche, who has type 1 diabetes, could not do the job because of his diabetes. The doctor disqualified Kapche because driving was an "essential function" of the police job, and San Antonio considered drivers who use insulin to be a safety risk to themselves and others.

Kapche appealed the decision, but after a year he had run out of options for internal appeals. He then turned to the American Diabetes Association for help. The ADA helped secure lawyers who argued that blanket bans that disqualify all people with diabetes from a given position, such as a law enforcement position, are both unlawful and medically unnecessary.

It took more than eight years and two trips to the United States Court of Appeals for the Fifth Circuit, but ultimately Kapche's lawsuit resulted in an important victory for workers with diabetes. The appellate court determined that blanket bans against people with diabetes—and specifically Jeff Kapche—were unjustified. Jeff Kapche's struggle helped many people with diabetes to face discrimination on the job.

Job Hunting

Not everyone discriminates against people with diabetes, so don't let the fear of discrimination in the workplace keep you from seeking or reaching your career goals.

Tips for Job Hunting with Diabetes

- Try not to think of diabetes as a defect. It is a part of your life.

- Be prepared by knowing your rights. Remember that employers are not allowed to ask about your health before deciding whether to hire you. Once the job has been offered, they can ask about medical conditions only as they relate to the job as part of the pre-employment physical examination.

- If you wait to disclose your diabetes until after the job has been offered, take a positive approach. Be sure to point out how diabetes helps you be a conscientious employee.

- During your physical exam, if required, accurately describe your condition and how you care for your diabetes. Don't try to change your diabetes care plan immediately before any physical examination. Changes in routine can affect your glucose levels.

- Your company's doctor is probably not a diabetes specialist, and you may need to educate him or her about how you manage your diabetes. Offer input from your treating diabetes physician to help the examining doctor make an accurate diagnosis.

In time, popular thinking will catch up with what many know already: diabetes doesn't have to keep you from doing what you want to do.

Disclosing Diabetes at Work

Whether you tell your employer or fellow employees about your diabetes is completely up to you. There are reasons to tell and reasons not to. Much depends on your particular job circumstances and the people involved. Here are some of the pluses and minuses.

Advantages of Disclosing Diabetes at Work

- If you take insulin or certain oral agents, you may be prone to low blood glucose reactions. This can make you confused and unable to help yourself. If people know you have diabetes, they can help you in the event of such a reaction.

- If you need your employer to make accommodations because of your diabetes (for example, providing time for you to check your blood glucose level in a job that doesn't allow breaks at will), your employer needs to know about your diabetes and why you need the accommodation.

- If your employer is not on official notice that you have diabetes and you suspect that some adverse action is the result of your diabetes, it may be very difficult to prove that your employer discriminated against you because of your diabetes.

- Being open helps people learn more about diabetes. You can help fight prejudice by showing that people with diabetes are just like everyone else. By not telling, you may be sending the message that you have something to be ashamed of.

- When you are open about your diabetes, you may be surprised to learn how many others have diabetes themselves or in their families. You can help each other.

- When you talk about your diabetes, other people can learn about the symptoms and treatment. As a result, people you know get the help they need if they suspect that they may also have diabetes.

Disadvantages of Disclosing Diabetes at Work

- You may want to maintain your privacy. Just as you wouldn't necessarily talk about how much money you make, you might not want to discuss your diabetes, which is just as personal.

- If you don't tell, you are less likely to lose a job promotion or job offer because of your diabetes. However, diabetes can be difficult to hide if you need to take breaks or leave a meeting to monitor blood glucose or take medications. Although laws protect against discrimination, it is not always easy to prove.

Diabetes at School

Adjusting to diabetes in school can be challenging. This is true whether your child has been living with diabetes and is entering school for the first time or changing schools or is already in school and has been recently diagnosed with diabetes.

You want to make sure your child is given the same opportunities as other children, but you also want to make sure your child is safe at school and that any special needs are met. And you definitely don't want your child to feel like an outcast.

Diabetes Medical Management Plan

The best approach to dealing with diabetes in schools is to communicate openly with the school's administration and teachers and, if your child agrees, with the other children in class. Make sure your child's school staff understands what it means to have diabetes, how your child manages his or her diabetes, and what needs your child has.

Your child's school may already have a policy in effect to deal with the needs of children with chronic illnesses, including diabetes. However, you and your child's health care team will need to develop an individual plan—called a Diabetes Medical Management Plan (DMMP)—to address your child's specific health care needs.

The plan spells out the medical care your child should receive at school, including information about blood glucose monitoring, meals and snacks, insulin, and emergency care, which may include the administration of glucagon.

Some children are capable of self-care, whereas other children will need a great deal of help. All children with diabetes will need help in the event of an emergency.

ADA has developed a sample DMMP, which is available on the Internet for printing or downloading at www.diabetes.org or by calling 1-800-DIABETES and asking for a school discrimination packet. A sample DMMP form is located in the Resources section of this book, on p. 447–453.

Diabetes Medical Management Plan: An individualized plan for your child's health developed by you and your child's health care team. It may also be referred to as a health care plan or physician's orders or another name.

Details of a DMMP

- A child should be able to receive assistance with blood glucose monitoring and insulin or glucagon administration if needed.

- A child can eat whenever and wherever necessary. This includes keeping snacks or glucose tablets close at hand.

- A child can go to the bathroom or water fountain when necessary.

- A child can participate fully in all school activities, including extracurricular activities such as sports or field trips, with diabetes care provided by trained school staff members.

- Option to refrain from exams or physical activity when blood glucose levels are too high or too low.

- A child should be able to eat lunch on schedule, with enough time allotted to finish eating.

- A child can be excused for tardiness in case of a blood glucose problem.

- A child should be allowed to check blood glucose levels in the classroom or wherever he or she happens to be (if the child is capable of this self-management task).

- A child is allowed to be absent, without penalty, for medical appointments and diabetes-related illnesses.

Section 504 Plan and Individualized Education Program

The implementation of a DMMP by the school is called a Section 504 plan if it is developed under the federal Rehabilitation Act or an Individualized Education Program (IEP) if it is developed under the Individuals with Disabilities Education Act. For example, a physician and parents develop a DMMP. The school, with input from parents, develops the 504 or IEP plan. You'll want to ensure that your school has one of these plans in place so that your child's needs are met. A model Section 504 plan is located in the Resources section of this book, on p. 455–463.

Communicate and Educate

Sitting down with your child's teachers, school nurse, school administrators, and other personnel and discussing your child's needs is important. Schools that are reluctant to accommodate a child's diabetes needs may not actually understand diabetes.

It is your responsibility to educate your child's school staff about your child's diabetes so that they understand that the needs of a child with diabetes are not unreasonable. In turn, it is the school's job to make sure your child is medically safe and has the same opportunities as other students.

Tips for Talking with Schools about Diabetes

- If your child is entering a school for the first time, meet several weeks before school starts with the school principal, school nurse, teachers, and other school personnel who will have direct contact with your child.

- If your child is already enrolled in school but has been recently diagnosed with diabetes, meet with school personnel before your child returns to school.

- Before meeting with school personnel, it is important to meet with your child's health care team and work out a DMMP for your child.

In your initial meeting with school personnel, discuss what is in your child's DMMP and how these needs will be met.

It is also important to understand how school policies and protocols might affect the diabetes care your child receives while at school and to educate and work with school personnel to make any needed adjustments. Discuss any concerns you might have and be sure to find out what concerns your child may have. Open communication at this stage is critical to establishing a positive working relationship.

Topics to Discuss in School Meetings

- Provide a brief explanation of diabetes, clarify any misconceptions, and explain the consequences of blood glucose levels that are too high or too low and the appropriate corrective actions.

- Find out whether there is a nurse on duty to assist with routine care and to handle emergencies and, when a nurse isn't available, which adults will be trained to provide care to your child during the school day and at all school-sponsored extracurricular activities.

- Determine what time your child will be eating lunch and whether there is a designated snack time for all children.

- Make sure your child will have immediate access to a snack and a quick-acting form of glucose whenever necessary.

- Also, it is especially important to talk with school personnel, including your child's physical education teacher, about the impact of food, insulin, and physical activity on blood glucose levels and how to prevent and respond to hypoglycemia.

Classroom Blood Glucose Monitoring and Self-Management

People with diabetes must manage their blood glucose levels through the careful balance of food, exercise, and medication. Blood glucose monitoring is an essential component to good health. It is the only way of making sure blood glucose levels are maintained within your child's target range.

Your child's immediate access to diabetes equipment and self-care is important so that symptoms don't get worse and so that she or he doesn't miss valuable classroom instruction or other school activities.

You may want your child to check his or her blood glucose levels and promptly treat wherever he or she is at school or during a school-related activity. However, this depends on your child's age, level of experience and skill, and personal preference.

Good diabetes care depends on self-management. However, because of your child's age, maturity level, or level of experience or skill, he or she may not be able to handle various aspects of diabetes care alone. Trained school personnel will be needed to check blood glucose levels, to administer insulin or medication, or to recognize and treat hypoglycemia (and administer glucagon) or hyperglycemia.

Training of School Personnel

Diabetes care training for school nurses and other school personnel should be developed and implemented by diabetes educators, school nurses or other qualified health care providers, and school administrators. There are three levels of training that school personnel should receive.

Levels of Training Appropriate for School Personnel

1. Some school personnel will need to be trained to perform actual diabetes care tasks, such as blood glucose monitoring, insulin administration, glucagon administration, and recognition and treatment of hypoglycemia or hyperglycemia. They should also receive a general overview of diabetes and explanation of type 1 and type 2 diabetes, education about nutrition and exercise, and an explanation of legal rights and responsibilities of parents and schools. School personnel should be trained to ensure that a trained person is available during the school day and at all school-sponsored events, field trips, before- and after-school activities, and extracurricular activities.

2. Other staff members who have primary responsibility for a student with diabetes need to understand how to recognize when your child needs help, what accommodations are needed, and how to locate a diabetes-trained person who can provide it.

3. All school personnel should receive a brief overview of diabetes and how to get help when needed.

Appropriately trained school personnel will help to ensure a safe school environment for your child and will enable her or him to participate in all school-sponsored events and to achieve optimal academic performance.

Your Child's Rights

Once you have met with school personnel and discussed your child's needs, as set out by his or her DMMP, hopefully the school will accommodate your child. Almost all schools are required by law to provide aids and related services to meet the needs of children with diabetes. Three federal laws may play an important role at school.

Federal Laws Regarding Diabetes at School

- Section 504 of the Rehabilitation Act of 1973 protects individuals with disabilities from discrimination in any federally funded program, including public school systems.

- The Americans with Disabilities Act provides similar protection in all public and private schools, except schools run by religious institutions.

- Both laws have been found to protect children with diabetes.

- The Individuals with Disabilities Education Act (IDEA) guarantees "free appropriate public education including special education and related service programming for all children with disabilities." This law only applies to those children whose diabetes adversely affects their ability to learn. This can occur when your child's blood glucose levels are often very high or low at school, if your child misses a lot of school due to diabetes-related complications, or if your child has another disability that affects learning.

- You can ask your school district to evaluate your child to determine which laws apply.

After you have discussed your child's DMMP with school personnel, the next step is to determine how the school will treat your child. It is important to write down just what steps are going to be taken. That way, everyone—from student to parent to school staff—knows their responsibilities.

The accommodation may be documented in either a 504 plan or in an IEP. The document should specifically state your child's disability, needs, accommodations, and how these accommodations will be delivered.

The plan sets out a blueprint for making sure your child has the same opportunities to participate in all academic and school-sponsored activities as children without disabilities. Typically, an IEP is more specific than a 504 plan with regard to your child's academic needs.

Tips for Working with Schools

- Make sure to think through what things are important to your child's well-being and include those in the plan.

- You are more likely to get greater cooperation from the school officials if you show a willingness to understand their concerns, but maintain a firm position on how your child's needs must be met.

- Try to encourage the attitude that you are all members of the same team.

If you feel that your child's school is not meeting your needs, you have no choice but to take stronger action. You may want to contact an attorney for help in deciding the best course of action. You may consider filing an administrative complaint with the U.S. Department of Education or through the school district or state appeal process. Do not delay in getting legal help. Administrative appeal and other actions need to be started quickly or you lose the ability to pursue them.

In working with school officials to meet your child's needs, it helps to know your rights. You have the right to request that your child be evaluated for services, and if eligible, you have several other rights.

Your Public School Rights

- You can schedule a meeting with school officials. You have a right to bring an advocate, attorney, or experts to this meeting to better explain your child's diabetes management.

- You can develop a plan to accommodate the unique needs of your child. This plan should precisely set out the types of special services your child needs to receive.

- You can withhold signing a plan if it does not meet your child's needs. Be reasonable, but stand firm if your child's needs are not being accommodated.

- You should be notified and review any proposed changes in your child's plan, be included in any conference or meeting held to review the plan, and review and consider changes before they are implemented.

More School Resources from the ADA

The American Diabetes Association has long been involved in working to end discrimination against students with diabetes. To further these efforts, ADA launched the Safe at School campaign to ensure that students with diabetes are safe at school and can fully participate in all school activities. You can find more information about the campaign at ADA's website (www.diabetes.org/safeatschool).

Written materials are also available from the ADA that explain diabetes care in a school setting. One example of an ADA pamphlet is "Children with Diabetes: Information for Schools and Child Care Providers." The ADA's packet on school discrimination can be obtained at www.diabetes.org or by calling 1-800-DIABETES. You can also discuss a specific school or day care problem with an ADA Legal Advocate.

More School Resources

- The National Diabetes Education Program's "Helping the Student with Diabetes Succeed: A Guide for School Personnel" is available from www.ndep.nih.gov/resources/school.htm. The National Institutes of Health, the Centers for Disease Control and Prevention, the U.S. Department of Education, the ADA, and many other diabetes and education organizations developed this comprehensive guide.

- ADA's Diabetes Care Tasks at School Training Modules are available from www.diabetes.org/schooltraining.

Travel and Diabetes

In today's world, almost everyone is on the go. You're bound to have changes in your daily schedule and routine, whether jumping on a plane several times a month or riding the train every now and then. However, your diabetes should not get in the way of your travel. With a little advance planning, you can go anywhere and do almost anything. But there are a few things you should be aware of that will make your diabetes care that much easier.

Air Travel

Traveling through airports and on airplanes is a drag these days. The extra time involved in checking your bags, going through security, and boarding with carry-on luggage can leave anyone exasperated. You'll need to be extra organized with your diabetes supplies and medications to make sure things go smoothly. Here are a few tips.

Tips for Packing

- You will want to take enough supplies and medication for your trip plus extras in case you get delayed, you misplace something along the way, or you decide to stay longer.

- Make sure that all your diabetes supplies are in your carry-on bag. You can't count on your luggage getting to your destination at the same time you do.

- You should also be sure to pack snacks to carry with you and have accessible whenever you may feel your blood glucose going low.

- If you take insulin or other injectable medications, make sure they are in your carry-on bag. The luggage compartments on airplanes are often very cold, and your insulin could freeze. Also, your bag could be left in the hot sun and the insulin could get too warm.

- If you use an insulin pump, take an alternate source of insulin in case your pump stops working while you are away from home. Most pump companies will send another one to your destination by express mail, but you need a way to take insulin in the meantime.

Carry-On Luggage Checklist

Medications
- Insulin or other injectable medications or pens
- Syringes, pen needles, or pump supplies
- Oral diabetes medications
- Glucose tablets or other source of quick-acting carbohydrate
- Snacks, such as dried fruit or crackers
- Antibiotic ointment
- Other prescribed medications
- Glucagon kit
- Anti-nausea and anti-diarrhea medications

Blood Monitoring Equipment
- Test strips
- Lancets
- Blood sampling device and a spare
- Glucose meter
- Hand-washing gel or alcohol wipes
- Spare batteries for glucose meter
- Cotton or tissues

Airport Security

Much has changed in airports and airport security in the past few years. The important thing to keep in mind is that your diabetes equipment and medications are necessary and permitted through security checkpoints.

However, new restrictions on everyone traveling may mean that it takes a little longer to get through security than it did in the past. Being patient and organized when you arrive at security will make things go more smoothly.

New rules implemented by the U.S. Transportation Security Administration (TSA) may affect people who use insulin pumps. If you use an insulin pump, you may be required to undergo more comprehensive screening, including hand and explosives checks of all of your carry-on luggage. Be aware of these new rules, and allow extra time to pass through security.

Security regulations allow anyone to pass through security with 3.4 ounces or less of liquids, aerosols, or gels. These items must be put in one quart-size, sealable bag. However, larger volumes of prescription liquids and other liquids needed by people with disabilities and medical conditions are allowed through airport security. They must be declared to the TSA officer on duty.

Some Allowed Prescription and Other Liquids

- All prescription and over-the-counter medications (liquids, gels, and aerosols), including petroleum jelly, eye drops, and saline solution for medical purposes.

- Liquids, including water, juice, or liquid nutrition, or gels for passengers with a disability or medical condition.

- Life-support and life-sustaining liquids, such as bone marrow, blood products, and transplant organs.

- Items used to augment the body for medical or cosmetic reasons such as mastectomy products, prosthetic breasts, bras or shells containing gels, saline solution, or other liquids.

- Gels or frozen liquids that are needed to cool disability-related or medically related items used to treat disabilities or medical conditions.

The TSA has developed specific advice for travelers with diabetes. You should notify the security agent that you have diabetes and that you are carrying diabetes medication and supplies with you.

TSA-Allowed Diabetes Supplies and Equipment

- Insulin and insulin-loaded dispensing products (vials or box of individual vials, jet injectors, biojectors, epipens, infusers, and preloaded syringes).

- Unlimited number of unused syringes when accompanied by insulin or other injectable medication.

- Lancets, blood glucose meters, blood glucose meter test strips, alcohol swabs, and meter-testing solutions.

- Insulin pump and insulin pump supplies (cleaning agents, batteries, plastic tubing, infusion kit, catheter, and needle), but must be accompanied by insulin.

- Glucagon emergency kit.

- Urine ketone test strips.

> → **Request a Visual Inspection**
> You can always ask to have a visual inspection of your diabetes medication and supplies.

- Unlimited number of used syringes when transported in a disposal container or other similar hard-surface container.

- Sharps disposal containers or similar hard-surface disposal container for storing used syringes and test strips.

- Insulin in any form or dispenser must be clearly identified.

Although not required, it is a good idea to take a letter from your diabetes care provider saying that you have diabetes. This is particularly helpful if you are traveling overseas.

For more information or to report unfair treatment by security personnel, contact the Transportation Security Administration at 1-866-289-9673 or www.tsa.gov.

Meals during Air Travel
Many flights no longer offer food service. Ask at the desk before you board the plane if there will be a meal or snack. You can purchase something at the airport to carry on the plane and eat around your usual mealtime or before you board.

If a meal will be served, you can order a special meal in advance. Most airlines have low-sugar, low-fat, low-salt, and low-cholesterol meals available on request. Most airlines require that you request special meals at least 24–48 hours in advance. However, many people prefer to get the regular meals and choose which food to eat.

Tips for Meals on Airlines

- Mealtimes on the plane can be somewhat unpredictable. So don't inject your premeal insulin until your meal has been served. Bad weather, a bumpy flight, or air traffic can delay service.

- Take along extra snacks in case your meal is delayed, there is no meal service, or there is no time to buy food at the airport.

- You may want to tell your flight attendant that you have diabetes, especially if you are traveling alone. That way, your airline crew will be prepared should any emergency arise. If there is a meal delay, he or she may be more willing to see that you get your meal as soon as possible.

- If you order a diet soda from beverage service, ask for the can or watch the flight attendant pour your drink. This can prevent you from accidentally getting a regular soda that could raise your blood glucose too high.

Also be aware that air travel can be dehydrating, so you'll feel better at the end if you drink lots of fluids. Avoid alcohol because it can only add to dehydration.

Time Zones
Crossing time zones can sometimes be confusing. Should you be eating according to east coast or west coast time? If you are in the air, when should you inject your next dose of insulin?

Tips for Time Zones

- In general, when you lose hours from your day (traveling from west to east), you may need less insulin.

- When adding hours to your day (traveling from east to west), you may need an extra dose of insulin.

- If you are uncertain of how to work your insulin and meals into your travel and business plans, take a copy of your itinerary and work schedule to your diabetes care provider. He or she can suggest some sample routines to try.

- Your health care team can help you adjust your intermediate-acting insulins for travel days. Long-acting and rapid-acting insulins and insulin pumps are usually easier to manage.

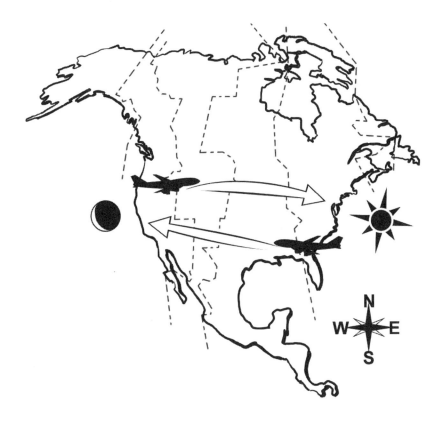

- If you are crossing several time zones or traveling overseas, it will probably take a day or two to get adjusted to the new schedule.

Car, Train, and Bus Travel

If you are traveling by automobile or other types of ground transportation, you often have more flexibility in your schedule, but there are still things to think about. You need to be sure that your insulin is properly stored. Extreme temperatures—either hot or cold—may reduce the potency of your insulin. Even backpacks or cycle bags can get too hot in warm weather.

You don't have to routinely store open insulin bottles in the refrigerator. But putting insulin in glove compartments and trunks and even in a locked car in a parking lot can cause the insulin to overheat. If there is a danger of overheating, keep insulin in an insulated container. The other caution is very cold weather. Insulin left overnight in a car trunk can freeze. Once insulin freezes, it loses all potency and needs to be discarded.

General Tips for Travel

The key to successful traveling, especially when you have diabetes, is careful planning. Think of contingencies that might arise or any particular needs that you might encounter and develop a plan in advance. You may want to ask your health care provider for advice on how to pack and what to bring on your trip.

Tips for Travel

• Wear a medical ID bracelet or necklace that says you have diabetes.

• Keep a prescription for insulin and other medications on hand. This is especially important if your travel plans are subject to frequent changes.

• To be safe, pack twice as much injectable medication and blood glucose monitoring equipment as you think you will need. Pack your supplies in your carry-on luggage, so you'll always have them within reach.

• Don't get separated from your supplies. Get used to carrying a tote bag, fanny pack, or backpack with your injection supplies such as insulin, syringes, meter, lancets, glucose gel or tablets, glucagon kit, and some food.

Tips for Traveling Abroad

• If you are traveling abroad, learn how to say, "I have diabetes" and "Sugar or orange juice, please," in the language of the country you are visiting. If you find the words difficult to say, write the phrase on a piece of paper and show it to the person with whom you're trying to communicate.

• If you are overseas and need medical attention—and you have a choice—think about contacting the nearest American consulate,

American Express, or a local medical school for a list of English-speaking doctors.

- If you find yourself running low on insulin while abroad, remember that insulin sold outside the United States is sometimes a different strength. If you buy insulin that is a different strength (U-40 or U-80), you must also buy new syringes to match the new insulin to avoid errors in dosing.

- If you are going overseas, call the ADA for a list of International Diabetes Federation groups.

Physical Activity during Travel
You've got everything under control. You are exercising regularly and eating well. Then your boss decides to send you out of town at the last minute to meet with some prospective clients. In situations like this and others, how will you manage? Fear not. You may not be able to schedule a 2-hour workout session, but here are a few suggestions to keep your program on track.

Tips for Exercising during Travel

- Pack a pair of comfortable walking shoes and some athletic socks. It is easier to squeeze a brisk walk into a busy schedule than most other activities and can be done in almost any locale.

- If your schedule is jammed with long meetings, try getting up a little earlier and squeeze in a walk after breakfast. On long car trips, stop every 2 hours and take a brisk 10-minute walk.

- If you are attending a conference, wear comfortable shoes. You'll be more likely to walk around the exhibit hall, walk outside to a restaurant, or take a stroll in a nearby park if your feet aren't killing you. You will also be less likely to injure your feet.

- Take along your exercise equipment when packing your bags. If space is tight, take a swimsuit or walking shoes. If you are driving, you might be able to take a racquet and balls, golf clubs, skis, a soccer ball, or even a bicycle.

- Suggest that the whole family participate. Play with your children or grandchildren, organize a game of tag or touch football, or go for a walk. Everyone will benefit from the activity, and it's nice to spend time together.

- Before booking your hotel, ask if it has a health club, swimming pool, or exercise room. Some hotels provide access to a nearby fitness center.

- Check with health clubs in the area you are visiting to see if you can buy a few days of use. If you belong to a national health club chain, see if they have clubs in the city you are visiting.

Eating during Travel

Eating on the road can be more unpredictable than eating at home or as part of your daily routine. To keep things on target, check your blood glucose levels more often than usual, even if you have type 2 diabetes.

Eating different foods and different eating and exercise schedules can affect your blood glucose. Keep snacks on hand in case your blood glucose levels start to drop or you have an insulin reaction. Also, talk to your health care team about adjusting your insulin and meal schedules when crossing time zones.

Book Your Ticket

We're traveling more than ever and farther from home these days. Your job may demand that you travel or you may live on the other side of the country from your family and friends. Managing your diabetes on the road or in the air will probably take adjustment. However, you'll learn tricks and personal strategies the more often you travel. So, if your diabetes has been keeping you from traveling, book a ticket or hop in the car. The world awaits you.

Sample Forms

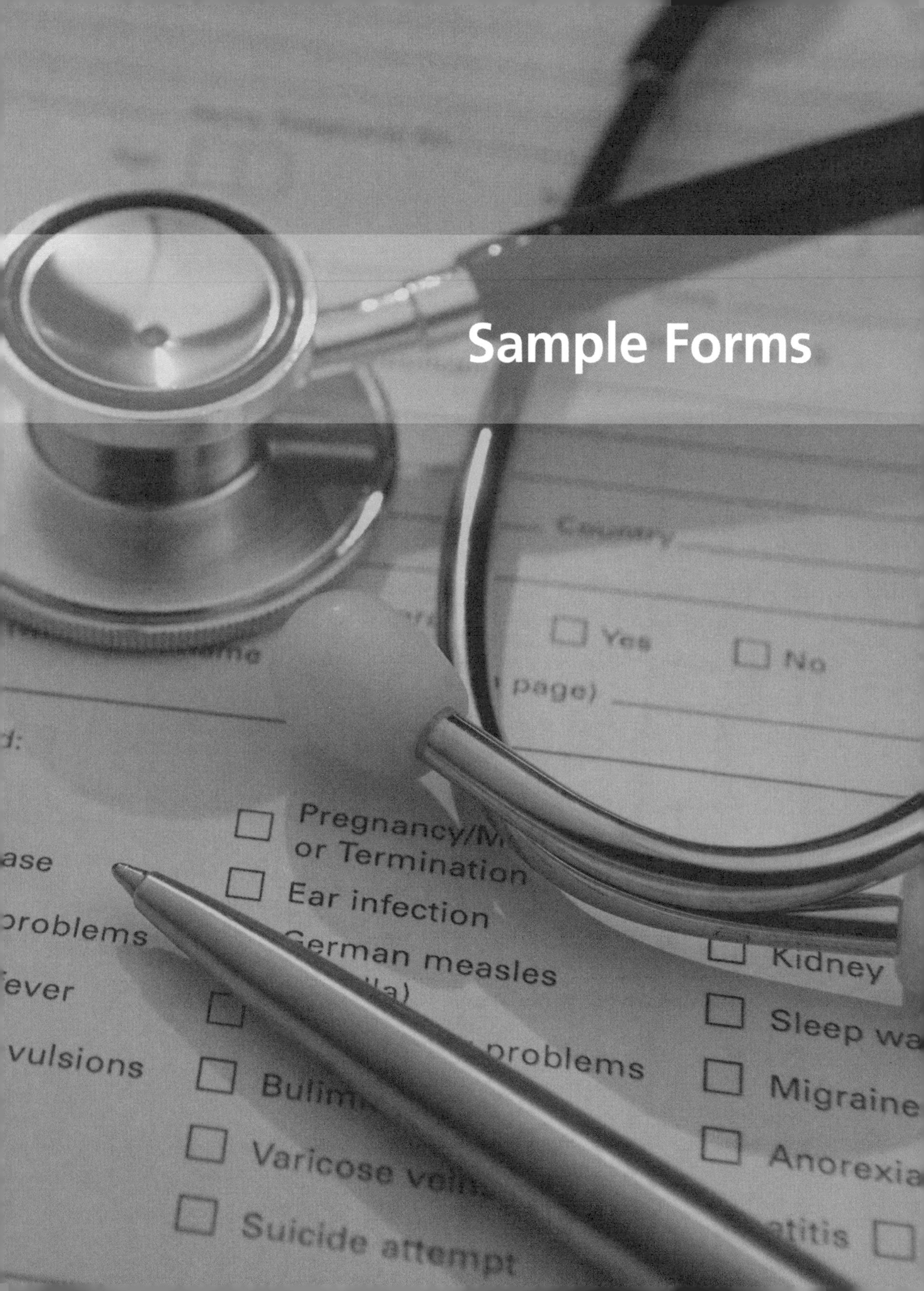

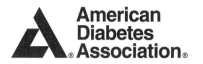 **American Diabetes Association**®

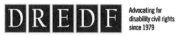 **DREDF** Advocating for disability civil rights since 1979

DISABILITY RIGHTS EDUCATION & DEFENSE FUND

Date of Plan: _____

Diabetes Medical Management Plan

This plan should be completed by the student's personal health care team and parents/guardian. It should be reviewed with relevant school staff and copies should be kept in a place that is easily accessed by the school nurse, trained diabetes personnel, and other authorized personnel.

Effective Dates: _____

Student's Name: _____

Date of Birth: _____ Date of Diabetes Diagnosis: _____

Grade: _____ Homeroom Teacher: _____

Physical Condition: ❑ Diabetes type 1 ❑ Diabetes type 2

Contact Information

Mother/Guardian: _____

Address: _____

_____

Telephone: Home_____ Work _____ Cell _____

Father/Guardian: _____

Address: _____

_____

Telephone: Home _____ Work _____ Cell _____

Student's Doctor/Health Care Provider:

Name: _____

Address: _____

Telephone: _____ Emergency Number: _____

Other Emergency Contacts:

Name: _____

Relationship: _____

Telephone: Home_____ Work _____ Cell _____

Notify parents/guardian or emergency contact in the following situations: _____

_____

_____

Blood Glucose Monitoring

Target range for blood glucose is ❏ 70–150   ❏ 70–180   ❏ Other _____

Usual times to check blood glucose _____

Times to do extra blood glucose checks (check all that apply)

❏ before exercise

❏ after exercise

❏ when student exhibits symptoms of hyperglycemia

❏ when student exhibits symptoms of hypoglycemia

❏ other (explain): _____

Can student perform own blood glucose checks?   ❏ Yes   ❏ No

Exceptions: _____

_____

Type of blood glucose meter student uses:_____

Insulin

Usual Lunchtime Dose

Base dose of Humalog/Novolog /Regular insulin at lunch (circle type of rapid-/short-acting insulin used) is _____ units or does flexible dosing using _____ units/ _____ grams carbohydrate.

Use of other insulin at lunch: (circle type of insulin used): intermediate/NPH/lente _____ units or basal/ Lantus/Ultralente _____ units.

Insulin Correction Doses

Parental authorization should be obtained before administering a correction dose for high blood glucose levels. ❏ Yes ❏ No

_____ units if blood glucose is _____ to _____ mg/dl

_____ units if blood glucose is _____ to _____ mg/dl

_____ units if blood glucose is _____ to _____ mg/dl

_____ units if blood glucose is _____ to _____ mg/dl

_____ units if blood glucose is _____ to _____ mg/dl

Can student give own injections?   ❏ Yes ❏ No

Can student determine correct amount of insulin?   ❏ Yes ❏ No

Can student draw correct dose of insulin?   ❏ Yes ❏ No

Type of blood glucose meter student uses:_____

_____ Parents are authorized to adjust the insulin dosage under the following circumstances:

_____

_____

For Students with Insulin Pumps

Type of pump: _____ Basal rates: _____ 12 am to _____

_____ _____ to _____

_____ _____ to _____

Type of insulin in pump_____

Type of infusion set: _____

Insulin/carbohydrate ratio: _____ Correction factor: _____

Student Pump Abilities/Skills: *Needs Assistance*

Count carbohydrates	❏ Yes	❏ No
Correct bolus amount for carbohydrates consumed	❏ Yes	❏ No
Calculate and administer corrective bolus	❏ Yes	❏ No
Calculate and set basal profiles	❏ Yes	❏ No
Calculate and set temporary basal rate	❏ Yes	❏ No
Disconnect pump	❏ Yes	❏ No
Reconnect pump at infusion set	❏ Yes	❏ No
Prepare reservoir and tubing	❏ Yes	❏ No
Insert infusion set	❏ Yes	❏ No
Troubleshoot alarms and malfunctions	❏ Yes	❏ No

For Students Taking Oral Diabetes Medications

Type of medication: _____ Timing: _____

Other medications: _____ Timing: _____

Meals and Snacks Eaten at School

Is student independent in carbohydrate calculations and management? ❏ Yes   ❏ No

Meal/Snack	Time	Food content/amount
Breakfast	_____	_____
Mid-morning snack	_____	_____
Lunch	_____	_____
Mid-afternoon snack	_____	_____
Dinner	_____	_____

Snack before exercise?   ❏ Yes   ❏ No

Snack after exercise?   ❏ Yes   ❏ No

Other times to give snacks and content/amount: _____

_____

Preferred snack foods:_____

_____

Foods to avoid, if any: _____

Instructions for when food is provided to the class (e.g., as part of a class party or food sampling event):

_____

_____

Exercise and Sports

A fast-acting carbohydrate such as _____ should be available at the site of exercise or sports.

Restrictions on activity, if any: _____ student should not exercise if blood glucose level is below _____ mg/dl or above _____ mg/dl or if moderate to large urine ketones are present.

Hypoglycemia (Low Blood Sugar)

Usual symptoms of hypoglycemia:_____

_____

Treatment of hypoglycemia: _____

_____

Glucagon should be given if the student is unconscious, having a seizure (convulsion), or unable to swallow.

Route _____, Dosage _____, site for glucagon injection: _____arm, _____thigh, _____other. If glucagon is required, administer it promptly. Then, call 911 (or other emergency assistance) and the parents/guardian.

Hyperglycemia (High Blood Sugar)

Usual symptoms of hyperglycemia: _____

_____

Treatment of hyperglycemia: _____

_____

Urine should be checked for ketones when blood glucose levels are above _____ mg/dl.

Treatment for ketones: _____

_____

Supplies to Be Kept at School

_____ Blood glucose meter, blood glucose test strips, batteries for meter

_____ Lancet device, lancets, gloves, etc.

_____ Urine ketone strips

_____ Insulin pump and supplies

_____ Insulin pen, pen needles, insulin cartridges

_____ Fast-acting source of glucose

_____ Carbohydrate containing snack

_____ Glucagon emergency kit

Signatures

This Diabetes Medical Management Plan has been approved by:

_____   _____
Student's Physician/Health Care Provider   Date

_____   _____
Student's Physician/Health Care Provider   Date

I give permission to the school nurse, trained diabetes personnel, and other designated staff members of _____ school to perform and carry out the diabetes care tasks as outlined by _____'s Diabetes Medical Management Plan. I also consent to the release of the information contained in this Diabetes Medical Management Plan to all staff members and other adults who have custodial care of my child and who may need to know this information to maintain my child's health and safety.

Acknowledged and received by:

_____   _____
Student's Parent/Guardian   Date

_____   _____
Student's Parent/Guardian   Date

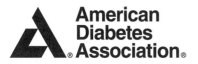 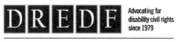

DISABILITY RIGHTS EDUCATION & DEFENSE FUND

Sample Section 504 Plan

The attached sample Section 504 Plan was developed by the American Diabetes Association (ADA) and the Disability Rights Education and Defense Fund, Inc. (DREDF).

Model 504 Plan for a Student with Diabetes

[NOTE: This model 504 Plan lists a broad range of services and accommodations that might be needed by a child with diabetes in school. The plan should be individualized to meet the needs, abilities, and medical condition of each student and should include only those items in the model that are relevant to that student. Some students will need additional services and accommodations that have not been included in this model plan.]

Section 504 Plan for _____

School _____ School Year_____

Student's Name _____

Birth Date _____ Grade _____

Type _____diabetes   Disability_____

Homeroom Teacher _____ Bus Number_____

Objectives/Goals of This Plan

Diabetes can cause blood glucose (sugar) levels to be too high or too low, both of which affect the student's ability to learn as well as seriously endangering the student's health both immediately and in the long term. The goal of this plan is to provide the special education and/or related aids and services needed to maintain blood glucose within this student's target range, and to respond appropriately to levels outside of this range in accordance with the instructions provided by the student's personal health care team.

References

- School accommodations, diabetes care, and other services set out by this Plan will be consistent with the information and protocols contained in the National Diabetes Education Program Helping the Student with Diabetes Succeed: A Guide for School Personnel, June 2003.

Definitions Used In This Plan

1. *Diabetes Medical Management Plan (DMMP):* A plan that describes the diabetes care regimen and identifies the health care needs of a student with diabetes. This plan is developed and approved by the student's personal health care team and family. Schools must do outreach to the parents and child's health care provider if a DMMP is not submitted by the family. [Note: School districts may have other names for the plan. If so, substitute the appropriate terminology throughout.]

2. *Quick Reference Emergency Plan:* A plan that provides school personnel with essential information on how to recognize and treat hypoglycemia and hyperglycemia.

3. *Trained Diabetes Personnel (TDP):* Non-medical school personnel who have been identified by the school nurse, school administrator, and parent who are willing to be trained in basic diabetes knowledge and have received training coordinated by the school nurse in diabetes care, including the performance of blood glucose monitoring, insulin and glucagon administration, recognition and treatment of hypoglycemia and hyperglycemia, and performance of ketone checks, and who will perform these diabetes care tasks in the absence of a school nurse.

1. Provision of Diabetes Care

1.1 _____ At least _____ staff members will receive training to be Trained Diabetes Personnel (TDP), and either a school nurse or TDP will be available at the site where the student is at all times during school hours, during extracurricular activities, and on school-sponsored field trips to provide diabetes care in accordance with this Plan and as directed in the DMMP, including performing or overseeing administration of insulin or other diabetes medications (which, for pump users, includes programming and troubleshooting the student's insulin pump), blood glucose monitoring, ketone checks, and responding to hyperglycemia and hypoglycemia, including administering glucagon.

1.2 _____ Any staff member who is not a TDP and who has primary care for the student at any time during school hours, extracurricular activities, or during field trips shall receive training that will include a general overview of diabetes and typical health care needs of a student with diabetes, recognition of high and low blood glucose levels, and how and when to immediately contact either a school nurse or a TDP.

1.3_____ Any bus driver who transports the student must be informed of symptoms of high or low blood glucose levels and provided with a copy of the student's Quick Reference Emergency Plan and be prepared to act in accordance with that Plan.

2. Trained Diabetes Personnel

The following school staff members will be trained to become TDPs by _____ (date):

_____

_____

_____

3. Student's Level of Self-Care and Location of Supplies and Equipment

3.1 As stated in the attached DMMP:

(a) The student is able to perform the following diabetes care tasks without help or supervision:

_____

_____

_____

and the student will be permitted to provide this self-care at any time and in any location at the school, at field trips, at sites of extracurricular activities, and on school buses.

(b) The student needs assistance or supervision with the following diabetes health care tasks:

_____

_____

_____

(c) The student needs a school nurse or TDP to perform the following diabetes care tasks:

_____

_____

_____

3.2 The student will be permitted to carry the following diabetes supplies and equipment with him/her at all times and in all locations:

_____

_____

3.3 Diabetes supplies and equipment that are not kept on the student and additional supplies and will be kept at:

_____

3.4 Parent is responsible for providing diabetes supplies and food to meet the needs of the student as prescribed in the DMMP.

_____

_____

4. Snacks and Meals

4.1 The school nurse or TDP, if school nurse is not available, will work with the student and his/her parents/guardians to coordinate a meal and snack schedule in accordance with the attached DMMP that will coincide with the schedule of classmates to the closest extent possible. The student shall eat lunch at the same time each day, or earlier if experiencing hypoglycemia. The student shall have enough time to finish lunch. A snack and quick-acting source of glucose must always be immediately available to the student.

4.2 The attached DMMP sets out the regular time(s) for snacks, what constitutes a snack, and when the student should have additional snacks. The student will be permitted to eat a snack no matter where the student is.

4.3 The parent/guardian will supply snacks needed in addition to or instead of any snacks supplied to all students.

4.4 The parent/guardian will provide carbohydrate content information for snacks and meals brought from home.

4.5 The school nurse or TDP will ensure that the student takes snacks and meals at the specified time(s) each day.

4.6 Adjustments to snack and meal times will be permitted in response to changes in schedule upon request of parent/guardian.

5. Exercise and Physical Activity

5.1 The student shall be permitted to participate fully in physical education classes and team sports except as set out in the student's DMMP.

5.2 Physical education instructors and sports coaches must have a copy of the emergency action plan and be able to recognize and assist with the treatment of low blood glucose levels.

5.3 Responsible school staff members will make sure that the student's blood glucose meter, a quick-acting source of glucose, and water are always available at the site of physical education class and team sports practices and games.

6. Water and Bathroom Access

6.1 The student shall be permitted to have immediate access to water by keeping a water bottle in the student's possession and at the student's desk, and by permitting the student to use the drinking fountain without restriction.

6.2 The student shall be permitted to use the bathroom without restriction.

7. Checking Blood Glucose Levels, Insulin and Medication Administration, and Treating High or Low Blood Glucose Levels

7.1 The student's level of self-care is set out in section 3 above, including which tasks the student can do by himself/herself and which must be done with the assistance of, or wholly by, either a school nurse or a TDP.

7.2 Blood glucose monitoring will be done at the times designated in the student's DMMP, whenever the student feels her/his blood glucose level may be high or low, or when symptoms of high or low blood glucose levels are observed.

7.3 Insulin and/or other diabetes medication will be administered at the times and through the means (e.g., syringe, pen, or pump) designated in the student's DMMP for both scheduled doses and doses needed to correct for high blood glucose levels.

7.4 The student shall be provided with privacy for blood glucose monitoring and insulin administration if the student desires.

7.5 The student's usual symptoms of high and low blood glucose levels and how to respond to these levels are set out in the attached DMMP.

7.6 When the student asks for assistance or any staff member believes the student is showing signs of high or low blood glucose levels, the staff member will immediately seek assistance from the school nurse or TDP while making sure an adult stays with the student at all times. Never send a student with actual—or suspected—high or low blood glucose levels anywhere alone.

7.7 Any staff member who finds the student unconscious will immediately contact the school office. The office will immediately do the following in the order listed:

1. **Contact the school nurse or a TDP (if the school nurse is not on site and immediately available) who will confirm the blood glucose level with a monitor and immediately administer glucagon (glucagon should be administered if no monitor is available);**

2. **Call 911 (office staff will do this without waiting for the school nurse or TDP to administer glucagon); and**

3. **Contact the student's parent/guardian and physician at the emergency numbers provided below.**

7.8 School staff including physical education instructors and coaches will provide a safe location for the storage of the student's insulin pump if the student chooses not to wear it during physical activity or any other activity.

8. Field Trips and Extracurricular Activities

8.1 The student will be permitted to participate in all school-sponsored field trips and extracurricular activities (such as sports, clubs, and enrichment programs) without restriction and with all of the accommodations and modifications, including necessary supervision by identified school personnel, set out in this Plan. The student's parent/guardian will not be required to accompany the student on field trips or any other school activity.

8.2 The school nurse or TDP will be available on site at all school-sponsored field trips and extracurricular activities, will provide all usual aspects of diabetes care (including, but not limited to, blood glucose monitoring, responding to hyperglycemia and hypoglycemia, providing snacks and access to water and the bathroom, and administering insulin and glucagon), and will make sure that the student's diabetes supplies travel with the student.

9. Tests and Classroom Work

9.1 If the student is affected by high or low blood glucose levels at the time of regular testing, the student will be permitted to take the test at another time without penalty.

9.2 If the student needs to take breaks to use the water fountain or bathroom, check blood glucose, or to treat hypoglycemia or hyperglycemia during a test or other activity, the student will be given extra time to finish the test or other activity without penalty.

9.3 The student shall be given instruction to help him/her make up any classroom instruction missed due to diabetes care without penalty.

9.4 The student shall not be penalized for absences required for medical appointments and/or for illness. The parent will provide documentation from the treating health care professional if otherwise required by school policy.

10. Communication

10.1 The school nurse, TDP, and other staff will keep the student's diabetes confidential, except to the extent that the student decides to openly communicate about it with others.

10.2 Encouragement is essential. The student will be treated in a way that encourages the student to eat snacks on time, and to progress toward self-care with his/her diabetes management skills.

10.3 The teacher, school nurse, or TDP will provide reasonable notice to parent/guardian when there will be a change in planned activities such as exercise, playground time, field trips, parties, or lunch schedule, so that the lunch, snack plan, and insulin dosage can be adjusted accordingly.

10.4 Each substitute teacher and substitute school nurse will be provided with written instructions regarding the student's diabetes care and a list of all school nurses and TDPs at the school.

11. Emergency Evacuation and Shelter-in-Place

11.1 In the event of emergency evacuation or shelter-in-place situation, the student's 504 Plan and DMMP will remain in full force and effect.

11.2 The school nurse or TDP will provide diabetes care to the student as outlined by this Plan and the student's DMMP, will be responsible for transporting the student's diabetes supplies and equipment, will attempt to establish contact with the student's parents/guardians and provide updates, and will provide and receive information from parents/guardians regarding the student's diabetes care.

13. Parental Notification

13.1 *NOTIFY PARENTS/GUARDIANS IMMEDIATELY IN THE FOLLOWING SITUATIONS:*

- Symptoms of severe low blood sugar such as continuous crying, extreme tiredness, seizure, or loss of consciousness.

- The student's blood glucose test results are below _____, or remain below _____ 15 minutes after consuming juice or glucose tablets.

- Symptoms of severe high blood sugar such as frequent urination, presence of ketones, vomiting, or blood glucose level above _____.

- The student refuses to eat or take insulin injection or bolus.

- Any injury.

- Insulin pump malfunctions cannot be remedied.

- Other: _____

  _____

13.2 Emergency Contact Instructions

Call parent/guardian at numbers listed below. If unable to reach parent/guardian, call the other emergency contacts or student's health care providers listed below.

EMERGENCY CONTACTS:

Parent's/Guardian's Name	Home Phone Number	Work Phone Number	Cell Phone Number
Parent's/Guardian's Name	Home Phone Number	Work Phone Number	Cell Phone Number

Other emergency contacts:

Name	Home Phone Number	Work Phone Number	Cell Phone Number
Name	Home Phone Number	Work Phone Number	Cell Phone Number

_____	_____	_____	_____
Name	Home Phone Number	Work Phone Number	Cell Phone Number

_____	_____	_____	_____
Name	Home Phone Number	Work Phone Number	Cell Phone Number

Student's Health Care Provider(s):

Name: _____ Phone Number _____

This Plan shall be reviewed and amended at the beginning of each school year or more often if necessary.

Approved and received:

_____   _____
Parent/Guardian   Date

Approved and received:

_____   _____
School Administrator and Title   Date

_____   _____
School Nurse   Date

Resources

For the Visually Challenged

American Council of the Blind
2200 Wilson Boulevard, Suite 650
Arlington, VA 22201
Phone: 202-467-5081
Toll-Free Phone: 800-424-8666

Website: www.acb.org

National information clearinghouse and legislative advocate that publishes a monthly magazine in Braille, large print, cassette, and computer disk versions.

American Foundation for the Blind
2 Penn Plaza, Suite 1102
New York, NY 10121
Phone: 212-502-7600
Toll-Free Phone: 800-232-5463
E-mail: afbinfo@afb.net

Website: www.afb.org

Works to establish, develop, and provide services and programs that assist visually challenged people in achieving independence.

American Printing House for the Blind
1839 Frankfort Avenue
P.O. Box 6085
Louisville, KY 40206-0085
Phone: 502-895-2405
Toll-Free Phone: 800-223-1839
E-mail: info@aph.org

Website: www.aph.org

Deals with the publication of literature in all media (Braille, large type, recorded) and manufacture of educational aids. Newsletter provides information on new products.

Lighthouse International
111 E. 59th St
New York, NY 10022
Toll-Free Phone: 800-829-0500

Website: www.lighthouse.org

A national health association dedicated to fighting vision loss through prevention, treatment, and empowerment.

National Federation of the Blind
200 East Wells Street
Baltimore, MD 21230
Phone: 410-659-9314

Website: www.nfb.org

Membership organization providing information, networking, and resources. Some aids and appliances available through national headquarters. A division called the Diabetics Action Network provides resources for people with diabetes.

National Library Service for the Blind and Physically Handicapped (NLS)
Library of Congress
1291 Taylor Street, NW
Washington, DC 20542
Phone: 202-707-5100
Toll-Free Phone: 888-657-7323
E-mail: nls@loc.gov

Website: www.loc.gov/nls

Free library program of Braille and audio materials circulated to eligible borrowers.

Recording for the Blind & Dyslexic (RFB&D)
20 Roszel Road
Princeton, NJ 08540
Toll-Free Phone: 800-221-4792
E-mail: custserv@rfbd.org

Website: www.rfbd.org

Library for members with print disabilities. Provides educational materials in recorded and computerized form.

The Seeing Eye, Inc.
10 Washington Valley Road
Morristown, NJ 07963
Phone: 973-539-4425
E-mail: info@seeingeye.org

Website: www.seeingeye.org

Offers guide-dog training and instruction on working with a guide dog.

For Amputees

American Amputee Foundation
P.O. Box 94227
North Little Rock, AR 72190
Phone: 501-835-9290
E-mail: info@americanamputee.org

Website: www.americanamputee.org

Offers peer counseling for new amputees and their families. Provides information and referral to vendors. Maintains a list of support groups throughout the United States. Publishes a newsletter.

National Amputation Foundation
40 Church Street
Malverne, NY 11565
Phone: 516-887-3600
E-mail: amps76@aol.com

Website: www.nationalamputation.org

Sponsor of Amp-to-Amp program, in which a new amputee is visited by an amputee who has resumed normal life. Provides information and educational materials.

For Finding Long-Term or Home Care

National Association for Home Care and Hospice

228 7th Street, SE
Washington, DC 20003
Phone: 202-547-7424

Website: www.nahc.org

Largest trade association representing home care agencies and hospices. Free information for consumers about how to choose a home care agency.

For Finding General Health and Doctor Information

American Board of Medical Specialties

222 North LaSalle Street, Suite 1500
Chicago, IL 60601
Phone: 312-436-2600

Website: www.abms.org

Record of physicians certified by 24 medical specialty boards. Directories of certified physicians organized by city of medical practice and alphabetically by physician names are available in many libraries and online.

American Medical Association

515 N. State Street
Chicago, IL 60654
Toll-Free Phone: 800-621-8335

Website: www.ama-assn.org

Help in finding a doctor and other resources for patients.

MedicAlert Foundation

2323 Colorado Avenue

Turlock, CA 95382

Toll-Free Phone: 888-633-4298

Website: www.medicalert.org

To order a medical ID bracelet.

For Finding Diabetes Educators and Dietitians

American Association of Diabetes Educators

200 W. Madison Street, Suite 800

Chicago, IL 60606

Toll-Free Phone: 800-338-3633

E-mail: aade@aadenet.org

Website: www.diabeteseducator.org

Referral to local diabetes educators and other patient resources.

American Dietetic Association

120 South Riverside Plaza, Suite 2000

Chicago, IL 60606-6995

Phone: 312-899-0040

Toll-Free Phone: 800-877-1600

Website: www.eatright.org

Nutrition information, guidance, and referral to a registered dietitian.

For Finding Foot Professionals

American Board of Podiatric Surgery

445 Fillmore Street

San Francisco, CA 94117-3404

Phone: 415-553-7800

E-mail: info@abps.org

Website: www.abps.org

Referral to a local board-certified podiatrist.

Pedorthic Footwear Association
2025 M Street, NW, Suite 800
Washington, DC 20036
Phone: 202-367-1145
Toll-Free Phone: 800-673-8447

Website: www.pedorthics.org

Find a local certified pedorthist (a person trained in fitting prescription footwear).

For Finding Mental Health Professionals

American Psychiatric Association
1000 Wilson Boulevard, Suite 1825
Arlington, VA 22209
Phone: 703-907-7300
Toll-Free Phone: 888-357-7924
E-mail: apa@psych.org

Websites: www.psych.org and www.healthyminds.org

Referral to your state psychiatric association for referral to a local psychiatrist. Healthyminds.org provides mental health information.

American Psychological Association
750 First Street, NE
Washington, DC 20002-4242
Phone: 202-336-5500
Toll-Free Phone: 800-374-2721

Website: www.apa.org

Referrals to local psychologists and other patient resources.

National Association of Social Workers (NASW)
750 First Street, NE, Suite 700
Washington, DC 20002-4241
Phone: 202-408-8600

Websites: www.helpstartshere.org and www.socialworkers.org

Help finding a social worker in your area.

American Association for Marriage and Family Therapy
112 S. Alfred Street
Alexandria, VA 22314-3061
Phone: 703-838-9808

Website: www.aamft.org

Professional association of marriage and family therapists. Information on marriage and family therapists in your area.

American Association of Sexuality Educators, Counselors, and Therapists
1444 I Street, NW
Washington, DC 20005
Phone: 202-449-1099
E-mail: aasect@aasect.org

Website: www.aasect.org

Professional association of sexuality educators, counselors, and sex therapists. Information on finding a professional in your area and other patient resources.

For Finding Eye Doctors

American Academy of Ophthalmology
P.O. Box 7424
San Francisco, CA 94120-7424
Phone: 415-561-8500

Website: www.aao.org

General information about ophthalmology as well as help in locating an ophthalmologist.

American Optometric Association
243 N. Lindbergh Boulevard
St. Louis, MO 63141
Toll-Free Phone: 800-365-2219

Website: www.aoa.org

Help in finding an optometrist in your area.

For Heart and Other Organ Information

American Heart Association
7272 Greenville Avenue
Dallas, TX 75231
Toll-Free Phone: 800-242-8721

Website: www.heart.org

Information about cardiovascular disease and stroke for patients and caregivers.

The Neuropathy Association
60 E. 42nd Street, Suite 942
New York, NY 10165
Phone: 212-692-0662
E-mail: info@neuropathy.org

Website: www.neuropathy.org

For information about disorders that affect the peripheral nerves.

National Kidney Foundation
30 E. 33rd Street
New York, NY 10016
Phone: 212-889-2210
Toll-Free Phone: 800-622-9010

Website: www.kidney.org

For donor cards and information about kidney disease and transplants.

United Network for Organ Sharing
P.O. Box 2484
Richmond, VA 23218
Phone: 804-782-4800
Toll-Free Phone: 888-894-6361

Website: www.unos.org

For information about organ transplants and a list of organ transplant centers in the U.S.

American Chronic Pain Association
P.O. Box 850
Rocklin, CA 95677
Toll-Free Phone: 800-533-3231
E-mail: acpa@pacbell.net

Website: www.theacpa.org

To learn more about chronic pain and how to deal with it.

For Travelers

Centers for Disease Control and Prevention
Travelers' Health
1600 Clifton Road
Atlanta, GA 30333
Toll-Free Phone: 800-CDC-INFO
E-mail: cdcinfo@cdc.gov

Website: www.cdc.gov/travel

Provides health information for international travelers.

International Association for Medical Assistance to Travellers
1623 Military Road, #279
Niagara Falls, NY 14304
Phone: 716-754-4883

Website: www.iamat.org

Travel advice and membership directory of doctors in foreign countries who speak English and who received postgraduate training in a developed country.

International Diabetes Federation
Chausée de la Hulpe 166
B-1170 Brussels, Belgium
Phone: +32-2-5385511
E-mail: info@idf.org

Website: www.idf.org

An umbrella organization of over 200 diabetes associations throughout the world dedicated to preventing and curing diabetes.

For Physical Activity

American College of Sports Medicine
P.O. Box 1440
Indianapolis, IN 46206-1440
Phone: 317-637-9200

Website: www.acsm.org

For information about health and fitness.

Diabetes Exercise and Sports Association
310 West Liberty, Suite 604
Louisville, KY 40202
Phone: 502-581-0207
Toll-Free Phone: 800-898-4322

Website: www.diabetes-exercise.org

For people with diabetes and for health care professionals interested in exercise and fitness at all levels.

President's Council on Fitness, Sports, and Nutrition
1101 Wootton Parkway, Suite 560
Rockville, MD 20852
Phone: 240-276-9567

Websites: www.fitness.gov and www.presidentschallenge.org

For information about physical activity, exercise, fitness, and nutrition.

For Schools and Students

Disability Rights Education and Defense Fund
3075 Adeline St., Ste. 210
Berkeley, CA 94703
Phone: 510-644-2555
Toll-Free Phone: 800-348-4232
E-mail: info@dredf.org

Website: www.dredf.org

Law and policy center dedicated to protecting and advancing the civil rights of people with disabilities.

National Dissemination Center for Children with Disabilities (NICHCY)
1825 Connecticut Ave, NW, Suite 700
Washington, DC 20009
Phone: 202-884-8200
Toll-Free Phone: 800-695-0285
E-mail: nichcy@aed.org

Website: www.nichcy.org

Provides information on disabilities in children, laws relating to children with disabilities, and effective educational practices.

National Diabetes Education Program (NDEP)
1 Diabetes Way
Bethesda, MD 20814-9692
Toll-Free Phone: 888-693-6337

Website: www.ndep.nih.gov

NDEP is a federal partnership of the National Institutes of Health, the Centers for Disease Control and Prevention, and more than 200 public and private organizations. The NDEP school guide can be found at www.ndep.nih.gov/ media/Youth_NDEPSchoolGuide.pdf.

United States Department of Education
400 Maryland Avenue, SW
Washington, DC 20202

Office for Civil Rights
Phone: 202-453-6100
Toll-Free Phone: 800-421-3481
E-mail: ocr@ed.gov

Website: www.ed.gov/ocr

Contact the Office for Civil Rights to report any educational discrimination, request information on civil rights compliance programs, and get information on procedures for filing discrimination complaints.

Office of Special Education and Rehabilitative Services
Phone: 202-245-7468

Website: www.ed.gov/osers

The Office of Special Education and Rehabilitative Services' mission is to improve results and outcomes for people with disabilities of all ages. It pro-

vides support to parents and individuals, school districts, and states in three areas: special education, vocational rehabilitation, and research.

For People Over 50

American Association of Retired Persons (AARP)
601 E Street, NW
Washington, DC 20049
Toll-Free Phone: 888-687-2277
E-mail: member@aarp.org

Website: www.aarp.org

Largest membership organization in the nation, offering services from prescription drug to insurance and other discounts.

National Council on the Aging
1901 L Street, NW, 4th Floor
Washington, DC 20036
Phone: 202-479-1200

Website: www.ncoa.org

Advocacy group concerned with developing and implementing high standards of care and high quality of life for the elderly. Referral to local agencies concerned with the elderly.

For Equal Employment Information

American Bar Association
Commission on Mental and Physical Disability Law
740 15th Street, N.W.
Washington, DC 20005
Phone: 202-662-1570
Toll-Free Phone: 800-285-2221
E-mail: cmpdl@abanet.org

Website: www.abanet.org/disability

Provides information and technical assistance on all aspects of disability law.

Disability Rights Education and Defense Fund, Inc.
3075 Adeline St., Ste. 210
Berkeley, CA 94703
Phone: 510-644-2555
Toll-Free Phone: 800-348-4232

Website: www.dredf.org

Provides technical assistance and information to employers and individuals with disabilities on disability rights legislation and policies.

Equal Employment Opportunity Commission (EEOC)
131 M Street, NE
Washington, DC 20507
Phone: 202-663-4900
Toll-Free Phone: 800-669-4000
E-mail: info@eeoc.gov

Website: www.eeoc.gov

The EEOC is responsible for enforcing federal laws that make it illegal to discriminate against a job applicant or an employee because of the person's race, color, religion, sex (including pregnancy), national origin, age (40 or older), disability, or genetic information. It is also illegal to discriminate against a person because the person complained about discrimination, filed a charge of discrimination, or participated in an employment discrimination investigation or lawsuit.

For Health Insurance Information

AARP Health
P.O. Box 1017
Mongomeryville, PA 18936
Customer Service: 800-444-6544
Service Line: 800-523-5800
Claims Line: 800-523-5880

Website: www.aarphealthcare.com

The AARP provides comprehensive health care and insurance information. AARP also administers health insurance plans, including individual, group, student, Medicare supplemental, and short-term health insurance.

Medicare Hotline
Centers for Medicare and Medicaid Services
7500 Security Boulevard
Baltimore, MD 21244-1850
Toll-Free Phone: 800-MEDICARE

Website: www.medicare.gov

For information and various publications about Medicare.

Social Security Administration
Social Security Administration
Office of Public Inquiries
Windsor Park Building
6401 Security Boulevard
Baltimore, MD 21235
Toll-Free Phone: 800-772-1213

Website: www.ssa.gov

For information about Social Security.

The Robert Wood Johnson Foundation
P.O. Box 2316
Route 1 and College Road East
Princeton, NJ 08543
Toll-Free Phone: 877-843-7953

Website: www.rwjf.org

An independent philanthropy dedicated to improving the health of Americans. The website has publications and research on health insurance coverage.

For More Information on Diabetes

American Diabetes Association (National Office)
1701 North Beauregard Street
Alexandria, VA 22311
Toll-Free Phone: 800-DIABETES (800-342-2383)
Website: www.diabetes.org

ADA's website has a wealth of information on diabetes, living with diabetes, and community events. Call ADA's hotline to receive free pamphlets or subscribe to the monthly magazine Diabetes Forecast. Visit ADA's online bookstore for the latest books on diabetes.

National Institute of Diabetes and Digestive and Kidney Diseases (NIDDK)

Office of Communications and Public Liaison
NIDDK, NIH
Building 31, Room 9A06
31 Center Drive, MSC 2560
Bethesda, MD 20892-2560
Phone: 301-496-3583

Website: www.niddk.nih.gov

The NIDDK is an Institute of the National Institutes of Health. The website contains information for patients on diabetes care and research.

Diabetes Monitor

Website: www.diabetesmonitor.com

This in-depth website features information on medications and research and has a mentor section.

Index

pioglitazone, 174, 176
pituitary glands, 310
placenta, 46
plasma, 70, 73
plasma glucose test, 15
pneumococcal vaccine, 259
pneumonia, 96, 256
pneumonia vaccine, 324
podiatrist, 157, 160, 335–336, 357
point of service (POS), 352–353
poison, 29
polio, 29
polycystic ovarian syndrome
(PCOS), 46, 276–277, 403
polydextrose, 125
polyunsaturated fats, 126
portion control, 146–147
portions, 141
postpartum thyroiditis, 300
poultry, 125, 139–140
pramlintide acetate, 177, 222
prediabetes, 20
preeclampsia, 48, 299
preexisting condition, 345, 348–
349. *See also* Health Insurance
Portability and Accountability
Act (HIPAA) of 1996
Pre-Existing Conditions Plan
(PCIP), 349
preferred provider organization
(PPO), 352–353
pregnancy. *See also* gestational
diabetes
alcohol, 132
angiotensin-converting enzyme
(ACE) inhibitors, 291
artificial sweeteners, 124, 132
baby's risk for type 1 diabetes,
289
baby's risk for type 2 diabetes,
289–290
after birth, 300
birth control, 284, 311
blood glucose and, 284
blood glucose monitoring, 63
caffiene, 132
contractions, 166
diabetes complications, 291
diabetic ketoacidosis (DKA), 97
exercise, 166
eye exam schedule, 334
fear of, 281
gestational diabetes, 45–53, 295

health care providers, 292
health insurance, 350–351
hypoglycemia unawareness, 89,
296
infections, 255
insulin during, 295
insulin pumps, 208
intensive diabetes management
(IDM), 112, 118
meal planning and, 131–132
morning sickness, 297
multiple daily injections, 217
obesity, 131
physical activity, 165, 298
self-monitoring blood glucose
(SMBG), 58
statins, 291
tests, 298
tight control, 292
type 2 diabetes, 295
vitamins and minerals, 128
weight goals, 297
women's health, 288–303
premenstrual syndrome (PMS), 272
premixed (biphasic) insulin,
185–186, 188, 219
prenatal vitamins, 128
preparation, 85
pre-pregnancy exam, 290–291
prescription drug plans, 359
prescription drugs, 178, 436, 440.
See also medications
primary care physician, 338
private insurance, 351–356
progesterone, 273, 275, 277–278,
285
progestin implant, 285
progressive muscle relaxation, 383
proliferative retinopathy, 160, 239,
242
prostate cancer, 309
prostate exam, 324
prosthesis, 261, 309
protamine, 185
proteins, 27, 36, 123, 125
proteinuria, 244
pseudoephedrine, 102
psychiatrists, 333
psychologists, 333
psychotherapy, 266, 309
pulse, 323
purchasing resources, 81–83
Pyriminil, 29

R
race, 28, 38–39, 47
raloxifene, 271
random plasma glucose test, 18–19,
26, 36
rapid-acting insulin analogs, 184–
185, 187, 216, 218–222, 412
rashes, 260
rat poison, 29
receptors, 36
record keeping, 103, 274–275. *See
also* logbook
rectal exam, 324
red meat, 139
reduced foods, 136
registered dietitian (RD), 49, 122,
292, 294, 328–332
registered nurse (RN), 328
regular insulin (Humulin R, Novolin R), 185, 187–188, 191,
198, 221–222
Rehabilitation Act of 1973, 411,
417, 427, 431
relaxation exercises, 252
repaglinide, 85, 173, 176
reproductive system, 273
research, 109–111, 228–229, 272
resources
alcoholism, 381
assisted-living facilities, 370
blood glucose monitoring tools,
67
children, 409
Children's Health Insurance
Program (CHIP), 351
discrimination, 416, 421–422
financial, 119
glycemic index (GI), 134
health care reform, 345
health insurance, 347, 350
home health care, 370
Medicare, 350, 358–359
Medigap, 359
nutritional, 331
parents, 409
prescription drug plans, 360
preventive care health insurance,
352
school, 433
respiratory distress, 48, 172, 300
restaurants, 140–141
resting heart rate, 154
retail pharmacy, 178

Other Titles from the American Diabetes Association

American Diabetes Association Month of Meals Diabetes Meal Planner
by American Diabetes Association

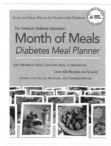

The bestselling Month of Meals™ series is all here—newly updated and collected into one complete, authoritative volume! Forget about the hassle of planning meals and spending hours making menus fit your diabetes management. With this invaluable guide, you'll have millions of daily menu combinations at your fingertips. Simply pick a menu for each meal, prepare your recipes, and enjoy a full day of delicious meals tailored specifically to you. It's as easy as that!

Order no. 4679-01; Price $22.95

Stress-Free Diabetes
by Joseph P. Napora, PhD, LCSW-C

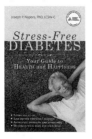

Did you know that stress can be unhealthy and dangerous, particularly for people with diabetes? Don't give stress power over your health. Reduce your stress and take charge of your life! Learn how to use these helpful stress busters to improve your diabetes care and yourself: problem solving, become emotionally smart, recognize and reframe unhealthy beliefs, use humor to stay positive, live mindfully, and practice meditation.

Order no. 4890-01; Price $16.95

50 Things You Need to Know about Diabetes: Expert Tips for Taking Control
by Kathleen Stanley, CDE, CN, RD, LD, MSEd, BC-ADM

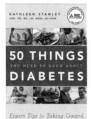

Cut through the confusion, jargon, and conflicting information about diabetes care and get the simple advice you need about eating right, exercising, and staying healthy. Learn how to interpret A1C and eAG numbers, keep your love life happy, and avoid depression and burnout. Make your life easier—and a lot healthier!

Order no. 4884-01; Price $17.95

Diabetes Meal Planning Made Easy, 4th Edition
by Hope S. Warshaw, MMSc, RD, CDE, BC-ADM

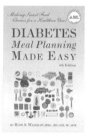

This new edition of the meal-planning bestseller uncovers the secrets to healthy eating with diabetes—from the basics of what to eat to the practical skills of shopping, planning nutritious meals, and even eating healthy restaurant meals. You don't have to change your life to eat healthy, but you might be surprised to learn how eating healthy can change your life!
Order no. 4706-04; Price $16.95

15-Minute Diabetic Meals
by Nancy S. Hughes

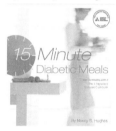

What can you cook in 15 minutes? It's time to find out! With over 200 time-saving recipes, *15-Minute Diabetic Meals* shows you how to cut corners by using convenience items and making smart choices at the grocery store to make healthy meals in a snap. You'll be amazed at what you can prepare in absolutely no time.
Order no. 4676-01; Price $18.95

The Heart-Smart Diabetes Kitchen:
Fresh, Fast, and Flavorful Recipes Made with Canola Oil
by the American Diabetes Association and CanolaInfo

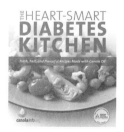

Bring the taste of fresh, natural ingredients and wholesome meals to your table. Featuring over 150 recipes made with canola oil, this cookbook allows you to serve dishes that are low in saturated fat and cholesterol but high in flavor in no time. It's just what the doctor, and your inner chef, ordered.
Order no. 4677-01; Price $18.95

To order these and other great American Diabetes Association titles, call **1-800-232-6733** or visit **http://shopdiabetes.org**.
American Diabetes Association titles are also available in bookstores nationwide.